THE
CHEST

ATLAS *of* TUMOR RADIOLOGY v. 3

PHILIP J. HODES, M.D., *Editor-in-Chief*

Sponsored by

THE AMERICAN COLLEGE OF RADIOLOGY

—with the cooperation of:

AMERICAN CANCER SOCIETY
AMERICAN ROENTGEN RAY SOCIETY
CANCER CONTROL PROGRAM, USPHS
EASTMAN KODAK COMPANY
JAMES PICKER FOUNDATION
RADIOLOGICAL SOCIETY OF NORTH AMERICA

THE
CHEST

by

ROY R. GREENING, M.D.

*Department of Radiology, Swedish Hospital Medical Center,
and Clinical Professor of Radiology, University of Washington,
School of Medicine, Seattle, Wash.*

and

J. HAYNES HESLEP, M.D.

Spohn Hospital, Corpus Christi, Tex.

YEAR BOOK MEDICAL PUBLISHERS · INC.

35 EAST WACKER DRIVE, CHICAGO

Editor's Preface

In 1960, the Committee on Radiology of the National Research Council began to consider the preparation of a tumor atlas for radiology similar in concept to the Armed Forces Institute of Pathology's "Atlas of Tumor Pathology." So successfully had the latter filled a need in pathology that it seemed reasonable to establish a similar resource for radiology. Therefore a subcommittee of the Committee on Radiology was appointed to study the concept and make recommendations.

That original committee, made up of Dr. Russell H. Morgan (Chairman), Dr. Marshall H. Brucer and Dr. Eugene P. Pendergrass, reported that a need did indeed exist and recommended that something be done about it. That report was unanimously accepted by the parent committee.

Soon thereafter, there occurred a normal change of the membership of the Committee on Radiology of the Council. This was followed by a change of the "Atlas" subcommittee, which now included Dr. E. Richard King (Chairman), Dr. Leo G. Rigler and Dr. Barton R. Young. To this new subcommittee was assigned the task of finding how the "Atlas" was to be published. Numerous avenues were explored; none seemed wholly satisfactory.

With the passing of time, it became increasingly apparent that the American College of Radiology had to be brought into the picture. It had prime teaching responsibilities; it had a Commission on Education; it seemed the logical responsible agent to launch the "Atlas." Confident of the merits of this approach, the entire Committee on Radiology of the Council became involved in focusing the attention of the American College of Radiology upon the matter.* In 1964, as the result of their persuasiveness, the Board of Chancellors of the American College of Radiology named an ad hoc committee to explore and define the scholarly scope of the "Atlas" and the probable costs. In 1965, the ad hoc committee recommended that the College

---

* At that time, the Committee on Radiology included, in addition to the subcommittee, Drs. John A. Campbell, James B. Dealy, Jr., Melvin M. Figley, Hymer L. Friedell, Howard B. Latourette, Alexander Margulis, Ernest A. Mendelsohn, Charles M. Nice, Jr., and Edward W. Webster.

sponsor and publish the "Atlas." Accordingly, an Editorial Advisory Committee was chosen to work within the Commission on Education with authority to select an Editor-in-Chief. At the same time, the College provided funds for starting the project and began representations for grants-in-aid without which the "Atlas" would never be published.

No history of the "Atlas of Tumor Radiology" would be complete without specific recording of the generous response of the several radiological societies, as well as the private and Federal granting institutions whose names appear on the title page and below among our acknowledgments. It was their tangible evidence of confidence in the project that provided everyone with enthusiasm and eagerness to achieve our goal.

The "Atlas of Tumor Radiology" includes all major organ systems. It is intended to be a systematic body of pictorial and written information dealing with the roentgen manifestations of tumors. No attempt has been made to provide an atlas equivalent of a medical encyclopedia. Nevertheless the "Atlas" is designed to serve as an important reference source and teaching file for all physicians, not radiologists alone.

The thirteen volumes of the "Atlas" are: *The Hemopoietic and Lymphatic Systems,* by Gerald D. Dodd and Sidney Wallace; *The Bones and Joints,* by Gwilym S. Lodwick (published); *The Chest,* by Roy R. Greening and J. Haynes Heslep (published); *The Gastrointestinal Tract,* by George N. Stein and Arthur K. Finkelstein; *The Kidney,* by John A. Evans and Morton A. Bosniak (published); *The Lower Urinary Tract, Adrenals and Retroperitoneum,* by Morton A. Bosniak, Stanley S. Siegelman and John A. Evans; *The Breast,* by David M. Witten (published); *The Head and Neck,* by Gilbert H. Fletcher and Bao-Shan Jing (published); *The Brain and Eye,* by Ernest W. Wood, Juan M. Taveras and Michael S. Tenner; *The Female Reproductive System,* by G. Melvin Stevens (published); *The Endocrines,* by Howard L. Steinbach and Hideyo Minagi (published); *The Accessory Digestive Organs,* by Robert E. Wise and Augustine P. O'Keeffe; and *The Spine,* by Bernard S. Epstein.

Some overlapping of material in several volumes is inevitable, for example, tumors of the female generative system, tumors of the endocrine glands and tumors of the urinary tract. This is considered to be an asset. It assures the specialist completeness in the volume or volumes that concern him and provides added breadth and depth of knowledge for those interested in the entire series.

The broad scope of the "Atlas of Tumor Radiology" has precluded its preparation by a single or even several authors. To maintain uniformity of format, rather rigid criteria were established early. These included manner of presentation, size of illustrations, as well as style of headings, sub-headings and legends. The authors were encouraged to keep the text at a minimum, freeing as much space as possible for large illustrations and meaningful legends. The "Atlas" is to be just that, an "atlas," not a series of "texts." The authors were urged, also, to keep the bibliography brief.

The selection of suitable authors for the "Atlas" was extremely difficult, and to a degree invidious. For the final choice, the Editor-in-Chief accepts full responsibility. It is but fair to record, however, that his Editorial Advisory Committee accepted his recommendations. The format of the "Atlas," too, was the choice of the Editor-in-Chief, again with the concurrence of his advisory group. Should the "Atlas of Tumor Radiology" fall short of its goals, the fault will lie with the Editor-in-Chief alone; his Editorial Advisory Committee was selfless in its dedication to the purposes of the "Atlas," rendering invaluable advice and guidance whenever asked to do so.

As medical knowledge expands, medical concepts change. In medicine, the written word considered true today may not be so tomorrow. The text of the "Atlas," considered true today, therefore may not be true tomorrow. What may not change, what may ever remain true, may be the illustrations of the "Atlas of Tumor Radiology." Their legends may change as our conceptual levels advance. But the validity of the roentgen findings there recorded should endure. Thus, if the fidelity with which the roentgenograms have been reproduced is of superior order, the illustrations in the "Atlas" should long serve as sources for reference no matter what revisions of the text become necessary with advancing medical knowledge.

ACKNOWLEDGMENTS

The American College of Radiology, its Commission on Education, the Editorial Advisory Committee, the authors and the Editor-in-Chief wish to acknowledge their grateful appreciation:

1. For the grants-in-aid so willingly and repeatedly provided by The American Cancer Society, The American Roentgen Ray Society, The Cancer Control Program, National Center for Chronic Disease Control (USPHS Grant No. 59481), The James Picker Foundation, and the Radiological Society of North America.

2. For the superb glossy print reproductions provided by the Radiography Markets Division, Eastman Kodak Company. Special mention must be

made of the sustained interest of Mr. George R. Struck, its Assistant Vice-President and General Manager. We applaud particularly Mr. William S. Cornwell, Technical Associate and Editor Emeritus of Kodak's *Medical Radiography and Photography*, as well as his associates, Mr. Charles C. Heckman and Mr. David Edwards and others in the Photo Service Division whose expertise provided the "Atlas" with its incomparable photographic reproductions.

3. To Year Book Medical Publishers, for their personal involvement with and judicious guidance in the many problems of publication. There were occasions when the publisher questioned the quality of certain illustrations. Almost always the judgment of the authors and the Editor-in-Chief prevailed because of the importance of the original roentgenograms and the singular fidelity of their reproduction.

4. To the Associate Editors, particularly Mrs. Anabel I. Janssen, whose talents lightened the burden of the Editor-in-Chief and helped establish the style of presentation of the material.

5. To the Staff of the American College of Radiology, especially Messrs. William C. Stronach, Otha Linton, Keith Gundlach and William Melton, for continued conceptual and administrative efforts of unusual competence.

This volume is the result of the collaboration of a superb clinical scholar and a young associate of rare inquisitiveness. By demanding constantly of Dr. Greening the "reasons why," Dr. Heslep honed his teacher's powers of observation to a level that enabled him to enunciate verbally that which experience had rendered intuitive and routine. It had become commonplace for a glance to suffice for Dr. Greening to deal easily with roentgen problems (an experience not uncommon among peers). It was commonplace too for him to explain easily the reasons for coming consistently to the correct diagnosis. What bothered the student (Dr. Heslep) was an insatiable curiosity about the less common, the roentgen nuances that suggested pathophysiologic process "A" rather than process "B" to Dr. Greening. This constant demand for explanation of "reasons why" was a challenge rarely left unanswered. Eventually it became the catalyst that enriched both student and teacher and made possible this volume of the "Atlas of Tumor Radiology."

Those interested in chest tumors will find here material that is easily grasped and upon which to build. The authors have made no attempt to illustrate the innumerable faces of chest tumors. Their concern instead has been to present basic radiologic pathophysiologic principles, enriched by carefully chosen illustrative material, each example to serve as a hallmark and keystone in decision making.

The "Atlas of Tumor Radiology" is being published at a time when massive scientific effort is taking place at an unprecedented rate and on an unprecedented scale. We hope that our final product will provide an authoritative summary of our current knowledge of the roentgen manifestations of tumors.

PHILIP J. HODES
Editor-in-Chief

Emeritus Professor of Radiology,
Thomas Jefferson University, Philadelphia, Pa.
Professor of Radiology, University of Miami School of Medicine,
Miami, Florida

Editorial Advisory Committee

HARRY L. BERMAN   VINCENT P. COLLINS   E. RICHARD KING
LEO G. RIGLER   PHILIP RUBIN

Authors' Preface

IN the present state of our knowledge, the successful treatment of tumors of the chest is still dependent on early diagnosis. In spite of new procedures, the main method of detection remains the roentgen study of the chest. To acquire the greatest skill in evaluation of the chest radiograph one not only must have an intimate knowledge of the normal anatomy of the chest but must learn how anatomic interrelationships will project a three-dimensional image on a one-dimensional plane. The effects of various projections and additional procedures to enhance the delineation of a suspected abnormality must be learned. As a help, we present in Part 1 some basic principles for obtaining the most useful radiographic information.

Illustrations have been selected to demonstrate major relationships between normal structures and pathologic changes. Whereas the entire chest is usually demonstrated, accompanying enlargements of the abnormal area are also presented to enhance minor differences in the character of shadows which may allow definitive, specific diagnoses. Many shadows, obviously, can represent a variety of diseases. For the most part, no differential diagnosis is offered, but emphasis is placed on characteristics which suggest the most likely conclusion. For example, it is not thought to be of value to list the more than 150 possibilities of diagnosis in patients with diffuse nodular pulmonary lesions. Pertinent clinical history many times leads to proper interpretation, and wherein this applies, it is so indicated.

For some diseases, more than one illustration is presented to indicate some of the variations possible with the disease process. A rather large series of lymphomas and carcinoma of the lungs is provided because of the innumerable variations of these neoplasms. In spite of the wide spectrum of shadows, there is still a basic similarity in presentation and development which suggests the proper diagnosis and which we hope to emphasize. In general, when multiple examples are given, very obvious lesions are presented initially and succeeded by more and more subtle, hard-to-detect abnormalities. This again is especially true for the large group of lymphomas and squamous cell lesions.

A few examples of special procedures are given in lesions in which they are believed to be most helpful, either for diagnosis or for the management of the patient.

We wish to express our grateful appreciation to the many people who supplied us with illustrative material. We are especially indebted to the Editor-in-Chief, Dr. Philip J. Hodes, for his tolerance, understanding and most helpful advice during a rather trying period that finally made this volume possible.

Though the selection of material was made with the thought of finding the best and most graphically useful radiographs, such was not always possible. Grateful and humble respect, indeed awe, are accorded Mr. William Cornwell for the magnificently prepared photographs of the material selected. The publisher has faithfully reproduced these illustrations in an outstanding manner.

ROY R. GREENING
J. HAYNES HESLEP

PART 1

General Radiologic Considerations, 1

PART 2

Bronchogenic Carcinoma, 9

PART 3

Lymphomas, 151

PART 4

Mediastinal Tumors, 211

PART 5

Parenchymal Tumors, 345

PART 6

Tumors of the Pleura and Chest Wall, 411

PART 7

Metastatic Tumors, 443

Index, 499

PART 1

General Radiographic Considerations

General Radiographic Considerations

THE MOST COMMONLY UTILIZED RADIOGRAPHIC EXAMINATION is that of the chest. Yet in spite of constant use, it probably remains the most difficult of all radiographic studies to interpret accurately. For the physician who would become skilled in the evaluation of this clinical aid, not only is a broad medical background a necessity, but a thorough knowledge of technical variations is imperative to produce a suitable and informative radiograph in any given situation. In addition, much must be learned about the methods of production and the significance of a variety of adjunctive radiographic studies.

It has been well shown that a mass in the chest as large as 10 cm may not be detected on excellent survey radiographs if such a mass lies in areas of pleural reflections or diaphragmatic curves or is adjacent to the cardiac or major vascular shadows. Masses of similar size in the main pulmonary parenchyma can be overlooked completely if there are small amounts of respiratory motion. Cardiac and vascular motions also contribute to tissue blurring. Ideally for static radiographs one would hope to obtain images of extreme sharpness, similar reproducible densities throughout, with no motion, in exactly the same phase of the cardiac cycle and amount of respiratory effort. If possible, the elimination of the bony thorax and an ability to see through or around the heart and major vessels would allow one to visualize all areas of the lung, pleura and mediastinum. Unfortunately at this time all of these criteria cannot be met in any single examination.

Phototimers or, better, ionization chambers are being used to obtain chest radiographs of similar reproducible density; however, almost exactly similar patient positioning is essential to achieving identical results. Great variations in the patient's age, size, nutritive status and pulmonary aeration, either voluntary or involuntary, affect reproducible densities with this apparatus, making it not quite as helpful as was originally hoped. To obtain comparable respiratory efforts, attempts at making radiographs at the peak of inspiration by placing a heat-sensing device below the nostrils and using the altered temperature at the precise moment of changing respiration to trigger the x-ray exposure have been helpful. This is of great value in infants and children but somewhat less useful in co-operative adults.

A standard 72 in. radiation source–film distance has been used for many years and still seems to be an adequate general compromise. In certain circumstances one may wish to increase the distance to eliminate all distortion or to increase distortion and magnify the chest image by decreasing the focal spot–patient distance and increasing the patient–film distance. In the latter situation, the smallest focal spot is necessary to obtain sharp images. For routine standard chest radiographs, focal spot size of the x-ray tube is not critical because of the relatively long distance between tube, object and film.

Shadows of the chest are best demonstrated by taking advantage of scattered radiation from the patient's tissues. However, beyond certain thicknesses scatter becomes a disadvantage and a stationary or movable grid must be interposed, thus introducing another set of variables. Such aids do make visual perception of shadows in the hard-to-see areas more difficult, generally requiring more studied analysis of the results. Numerous methods to amplify suspected abnormalities have been developed for use if only simple standard equipment is available. These include the varying of chemical processing and the blocking of light from one of the intensifying screens in an entire cassette or in one-half of a cassette. Films of differing sensitivity or single emulsion films may be useful especially when limited radiographic apparatus is available.

Each physician interested in studying diseases of the chest should develop methods adaptable to his particular available apparatus.

Variations in cardiac size from systole to diastole may be as great as 1–1.5 cm in a normal person. Similarly, variations in sizes of veins and arteries may vary from 3–5 mm in the region of larger vessels and progressively less as one proceeds peripherally. During ordinary radiography such changes go undetected, as multiple cardiac pulsations will occur during a single radiographic exposure. These motions all contribute to image unsharpness. In special situations, exposures using times from 1 to several milliseconds can be used. We may hope that one day all routine chest radiography will be made in such ultrashort times. The addition of a triggering device from the R-wave of the electrocardiograph, if made at the millisecond level, will allow one to make radiographs in exactly reproducible phases of the cardiac cycle. The result is a radiograph of strikingly different appearance and would seem to be more diagnostic.

With the detection of a suspected abnormality, it often is necessary to carry out added radiographic procedures to come to the most likely conclusion. Investigations utilizing 250 kv, 1–2 million volt or cobalt therapy machines for radiography to eliminate multiple examinations have been of help in some instances. Radiographs produced in this manner result in almost complete obliteration of the bony thoracic cage and accentuate air-containing and blood-filled tissues in a single radiograph (Fig. 58). Unfortunately, the physical characteristics of the radiation emitted at these high-energy ranges alter intensifying screen characteristics as well as the characteristics of radiographic film. Special lead intensifying screens are of some help, as is industrial film. The mechanical problems involving timing devices, controlled rate of shutter operations and relatively low instantaneous radiation outputs leave these methods for future development.

For survey purposes single posteroanterior radiographs of 35, 70 and 100 mm, 14×17 in. paper, or standard film radiographs are all used. It once was thought that an ideal initial examination for any patient with a chest complaint must include fluoroscopy plus exposures on inspiration and expiration, lateral projection and overexposed radiographs. If an abnormality was detected, added studies including oblique, lordotic, stereoscopic, magnification and body-section radiographs were resorted to.

The simplest, most valuable procedure to supplement the initial survey radiograph is careful fluoroscopic study of the chest. In this examination one must observe diaphragmatic and rib cage motion. The two sides of the chest and entire diaphragm on each side must be compared. Any local changes in diaphragmatic motion or segmental alterations must be recorded. Coughing or sniffing may exaggerate small changes.

The fanning movements of the vessels in the lung, their changing relationships with one another and the cardiac margins as well as changes in the size of the trachea and major bronchi during respiration and coughing must be observed. Variations in ventilation manifested by density changes in the fluoroscopic image reflect altered air movement. These may be in segments, lobes or an entire lung. Localized lobar or segmental alterations in ventilation may be enhanced by deep, slow inspiration and expiration much as is utilized for auscultation of the chest. The addition of a final forced expiration may accentuate minor ventilatory changes. During such maneuvers, like areas of the lung must be compared which normally appear similar. Unfortunately, the technical improvement of constant brightness controls in the new x-ray machines makes chest fluoroscopy to detect small ventilatory changes difficult. The use of fluorodensitometry to record these changes in ventilation by graphic methods gives one an objective means of evaluating such findings, eliminates the constant brightness control problem and does not require a skilled fluoroscopist. Recording the fluoroscopic images on video tape or by motion pictures allows consultation and study of respiratory movements at leisure; these recordings also provide an excellent teaching modality. Inspiration and expiration exposures on the same or separate radiographs are useful for measuring diaphragmatic and rib cage motion as well as for recording the movements of the vessels in the lung and are of help in recording altered ventilation. Causes for variations may not always be found, but if a current study differs from a previous one, this change may be quite significant and makes continued observation imperative.

Familiarity with normal vascular outlines in the hilar regions in postero-anterior, oblique and lateral radiographs is essential. In studying each series of radiographs, one must be able to identify and follow the course of the vessels starting from their origin (Figs. 6, 12, 25 and 26). If these structures cannot be identified clearly, an abnormality is present. It is then imperative that further studies be made, and these must be extensive enough to find the cause of the vascular alteration. Such changes may reflect local tumors (primary or secondary) or may indicate vascular disease or inflammatory processes, recent or old. Localized decrease of vascular size in the central area of the lung may be an early indication of the presence of a neoplasm. This may be in the hilar regions or nearby pulmonary parenchyma. Rarely are peripheral lesions associated with hilar vascular changes. Local vascular alterations, however, are frequently present adjacent to peripheral neoplasms.

In lateral projections similar vascular identification must be made. Normal relationships between vessels, trachea and the tracheal bifurcations must be so well learned that recognition of their variations becomes reflex. Throughout this volume, emphasis is placed on the detection of tumors in the lateral radiograph.

Body-section radiography (tomography) has become an integral part of most questionable chest examinations. For this, an understanding of the characteristics of one's body-section device is a necessity. Standard test objects to evaluate and periodically monitor such units are available and should be used. A variety of movements available in the same or different units gives considerable latitude in accentuating or obscuring various structures. With experience one learns the best motion and thickness of slice needed to portray the abnormality optimally. This may vary with the nature of the abnormality. Lesions containing tiny calcifications may best be shown in thin sections, while vague ill-defined lesions may be portrayed best by zonography.

Bronchography is of prime importance in the differential diagnosis of chest disease. Contrast agents containing iodine or barium may be used. Some day, it is hoped, nebulization or dusting may permit bronchography without disturbing pulmonary function.

The roentgen changes produced by tumors include apparent bronchial amputation, abnormal stretching of major or smaller bronchi, asymmetrical narrowing of a bronchus, "thumb printing" within an opacified bronchus and, perhaps least reliably, "rat-tail" narrowing. Occasionally a polypoid tumor itself is outlined. Whatever the abnormality, the roentgen study should be complete even though the definitive diagnosis must await biopsy.

The understanding of the abnormalities depicted on radiographs of the chest is dependent on a knowledge of the anatomic patterns of the broncho-pulmonary segments. This is important not only to discovery of early disease but to an understanding of the progress or regression of disease processes. The Jackson-Huber classification is most commonly used.[6]

In special instances all of one's skills may still fail to detect the cause for persistent pulmonary symptoms. If all studies apparently show no abnormality, occasionally random body-section radiographs made in antero-posterior and lateral projections, and rarely in oblique positions, to bring smaller bronchi into parallel focus, may be revealing. This study has repeatedly unveiled small metastatic pulmonary foci in patients in whom amputation or radical operative procedures have been planned optimistically as curative measures. Finally, if the results of all modalities, including bronchoscopy and cellular washings, prove normal, one may have to resort to re-examinations in three to six months (Figs. 15, 26 and 36). On occasion, we have ultimately found small lesions by the latter methods as long as one year after exhausting all resources initially but retaining a constant suspicion of the presence of a neoplasm.

Pulmonary arteriography and venography as well as bronchial arteriography should be in the armamentarium of the physician skilled in roentgenography of the chest, even though their value has been disappointing in the detection and evaluation of early lesions. These procedures have more value in study of the extent of known neoplastic lesions.

Several examples of developing neoplasms are presented (Figs. 15, 36, 44 and 46). In some instances the lesion was initially undetected, in others the primary interpretation was incorrect, while in some instances patients refused recommended treatment. On a few occasions we have followed patients refusing treatment with known primary pulmonary cancer for as long as 10 years. Slow progression has occurred; but in at least one instance, death 10 years after the initial diagnosis was not from the neoplasm but from a vascular disorder. Rigler recorded retrospective studies in patients whose lesions long remained unrecognized, some from 7–10 years. Despite the relative slow growth of some pulmonary tumors, it remains of paramount importance to recognize abnormalities as early as is possible, at which time every known diagnostic modality must be used for definitive diagnosis.

BIBLIOGRAPHY

1. Abrams, H. L.: *Angiography* (Boston: Little, Brown & Company, 1971).
2. Campbell, J. A.: The diaphragm in roentgenology of the chest, Radiol. Clin. North America 1:395, 1963.
3. Deutschberger, O.: *Fluoroscopy in Diagnostic Radiology* (Philadelphia: W. B. Saunders Company, 1963).
4. Di Rienzo, S.: *Radiologic Exploration of the Bronchus* (Springfield, Ill.: Charles C Thomas, Publisher, 1949).
5. Fraser, R. G., and Pare, J. A. P.: *Diagnosis of Diseases of the Chest* (Philadelphia: W. B. Saunders Company, 1970).
6. Jackson, C. L., and Huber, J. F.: Correlated anatomy of the bronchial tree and lungs with a system of nomenclature, Dis. Chest 9:319, 1943.
7. Krause, G. R., and Lubert, M.: Anatomy of bronchopulmonary segments: Clinical applications, Radiology 56:333, 1951.
8. Liebow, A. A.: Pathology of carcinoma of the lung as related to the roentgen shadow, Am. J. Roentgenol. 74:383, 1955.
9. Lillington, G. A., and Jamplis, R. W.: *A Diagnostic Approach to Chest Diseases* (Baltimore: Williams & Wilkins Company, 1965).
10. Mayer, E., and Maier, H. C.: *Pulmonary Carcinoma* (New York: New York University Press, 1956).
11. Meschan, I.: *An Atlas of Normal Radiographic Anatomy* (Philadelphia: W. B. Saunders Company, 1951).
12. Nelson, W. W., *et al.*: Barium sulfate and bismuth subcarbonate suspensions as bronchographic contrast media, Radiology 72:829, 1959.
13. Rigler, L. G.: The roentgen signs of carcinoma of the lung, Am. J. Roentgenol. 74:415, 1955.
14. Rigler, L. G., and Hertzman, E. R.: Planigraphy in the diagnosis of the pulmonary nodule, Radiology 65:692, 1955.
15. Schinz, H. R., *et al.* (ed.): *Roentgen Diagnostics* (1st Am. ed., trans. by J. T. Case) (New York: Grune & Stratton, Inc., 1953).
16. Shanks, S. C., and Kerley, P. (eds.): *A Textbook of X-ray Diagnosis* (3rd ed.; Philadelphia: W. B. Saunders Company, 1962), Vol. II.
17. Simon, G.: *Principles of Chest X-ray Diagnosis* (New York: Appleton-Century-Crofts, Inc., 1971).

PART 2

Bronchogenic Carcinoma

General Characteristics

THE TERMINOLOGY regarding carcinoma of the lung is confusing. If one regards a bronchogenic tumor as a neoplasm arising from mucosa one would have to include squamous cell carcinoma, oat cell carcinoma, giant cell carcinoma, undifferentiated carcinoma, adenocarcinoma, as well as tumors arising from mucous glands such as carcinoid, adenocystic carcinoma and mucoepidermoid carcinoma. Respiratory bronchial epithelium also may give rise to a bronchiolar carcinoma. Microscopically, there is variation in the criteria used by pathologists in the diagnostic naming of many of these tumors. Some prefer only one diagnostic term, "carcinoma of the lung," since multiple sections of any lung neoplasm show a pleomorphic structure involving all of the epithelial elements in the area of origin. In spite of conflicting pathologic opinions, certain radiographic patterns seem to be more common in certain types of tumors. Thus, although considered by some to be an artificial grouping, we have grouped our cases according to the nature of the cellular components.

The incidence of carcinoma of the lung seems to be increasing in both men and women, with a greater increase in women at present. The peak incidence is between the ages of 40 and 65, but lesions have been discovered in children below the age of 10. Since these tumors can mimic almost any type of pulmonary lesion, including aneurysms of the veins, arteries or heart, a high index of suspicion must be maintained by anyone reviewing chest radiographs, especially of middle-aged people, but always remembering that these neoplasms can occur at almost any age.

Sixty to 75% of carcinomas of the lung involve a main bronchus; they may also arise in the periphery of the lung. Characteristically, growth extends through the bronchial wall but tends to spare the cartilages for some time. Growth along the bronchial walls produces thickening which can be seen microscopically but may not be sufficient to be portrayed in a roentgenogram until its total thickness is at least 3 mm. These tumors begin as firm, warty roughening of the mucosa which narrows the lumen. Bronchi widen and narrow with inspiration and expiration; therefore if strategically located these tumors may cause abnormal segmental, lobular, lobar or even entire lung ventilation early. Unfortunately most patients are not examined during this relatively silent period, which may last for years. Since our routine method of radiographic study does not include altered physiologic function, incorporation of such studies would seem a useful method in early cancer detection. One of us has had an opportunity to study all chests by means of radiographs on inspiration and expiration and lateral projections as well as fluoroscopy for a number of years. In this time, only a handful of patients with hyperaeration was discovered. In one of these, with a lobular area of hyperaeration, distant metastatic disease was already present at the time of discovery of a small primary endobronchial lesion. Conversely, a series of patients who refused treatment had been followed and demonstrated slowly progressive pulmonary neoplasms for up to 12 years. Several of these people died of other causes and with little pulmonary disability. Technical improvements in equipment with routine use of fluorodensitometry may one day provide a useful tool for the early detection of pulmonary neoplasms with abnormal ventilation alone.

Lung cancer can produce almost any type of shadow seen in a chest roentgenogram depending on the location and adjacent tissues involved. Whereas early lesions involve mainly bronchial walls, they frequently may appear as pulmonary nodules. When they do, certain features point to their malignant nature. Size is only important in that the larger nodule is more apt to be malignant. With small nodules, shape is extremely important (Figs. 8, 15, 34 and 35); a nodule with irregular branching pseudopods extending into adjacent lung is most certainly a malignant lesion. With this shape, the presence of calcium in or adjacent to the nodule in no way precludes its malignant nature. To define these contours, body-section radiography is imperative.

Bronchography (Figs. 41–43) is of great help in diagnosis in patients with abnormal shadows and indeterminate results of tomography or bronchoscopy. On occasion, bronchial washings or sputum cytology may be positive and the source remain unknown. Bronchography may allow a definitive diagnosis and location. In some instances it may furnish a map for biopsy.

Although any tumor may become necrotic as it increases in size, the squamous cell lesions tend to slough their surface cells earlier, thus being likely to cavitate as relatively small tumors (Fig. 14). It is not unusual to find thick-walled cavities in small peripheral tumors, either primary or secondary. Cavities may not be delineated as often as they occur because of our tendency to perform body-section radiography with the patient supine. One will discover many more cavities if such studies are done with the patient in both supine and erect positions. The typical appearance of these cavities is of a thick, shaggy, irregularly walled lesion (Figs. 9–11); however, on occasion, thin-walled, emphysematous-appearing cavities will be found with squamous cell neoplasms (Fig. 16). Fluid levels (Fig. 10) may or may not be present and may appear and disappear from time to time with no change of symptoms. One must not be misled by the presence of acid-fast organisms in such a patient, as both diseases can coexist (Figs. 46–48).

No extensive discussion regarding the etiology of lung cancer is intended; however, the well-known association between such tumors and certain occupations should be mentioned, notably that among the cobalt miners in Schneeberg, Germany. Ore mined by these people contains uranium, arsenic and cobalt. Radon from uranium ore is a proved carcinogenic agent. The role of arsenic and cobalt in the production of lung cancer is uncertain. Chromium, asbestos and coal tar products are established as etiologic agents. The association with scars in the lung seems to be very important even though the distribution of lung carcinoma may be the same for patients who have had tuberculosis and those who have not, as suggested by Snider and Placik[19] in their analysis of 124 patients. There does seem to be a relationship between pulmonary scars and carcinoma whether the scars are from tuberculosis, infarction, trauma or other causes (Figs. 46–48). Any so-called local reactivation of old granulomatous processes should be regarded with suspicion as to the development of adjacent neoplasia. The question of whether or not systemic tuberculosis may predispose to pulmonary cancer has not been answered.

Thoracic inlet tumors with the superior pulmonary sulcus syndrome usually are produced by well-differentiated squamous cell tumors which invade the chest wall by direct extension (Figs. 5 and 7). Primary bronchial cleft tumors, primary bone tumors, in rib or vertebra, as well as sympathetic nerve tumors may produce the same syndrome, consisting of shoulder pain, weakness of the arm with or without edema and rib and/or vertebral bony destruction plus a mass at the thoracic inlet. Horner's syndrome is present 90% of the time.

Adenocarcinomas usually arise in the periphery of the lung; they are uncommon and difficult to diagnose. A few examples are presented. The incidence in men and women is equal.

Alveolar cell carcinoma may mimic a variety of pulmonary disease processes, appearing as solitary pulmonary nodules, miliary types of lesions as well as bronchopneumonic patches in one or both lungs or as pneumonic areas in lobular, lobar or entire lung segments. When found as a solitary nodule the margins are ill-defined and spiculated much like squamous cell lesions. A high index of suspicion of the presence of such lesions is the most important aid to early diagnosis.

A large number of predominant squamous cell tumors is presented to emphasize their enormous variation in pattern. Large, easy to see, classic types are shown first, followed by subtle, difficult to detect lesions. Gradual development of squamous cell lesions is emphasized because there seems to be a long clinically silent period in most patients, during which time the tumors are slowly progressive and for the most part may be successfully treated at this stage.

In the chest, angiography has been used with varying degrees of success, depending on the nature of the abnormality. Of prime helpfulness in the recognition of suspected vascular abnormalities, the procedure has been used far more often in the presence of mediastinal abnormalities than for lesions apparently arising in the lung or pleura. There will be occasions, however, when even parenchymal or pleural lesions may require angiography, particularly in suspected sequestrations of the lungs. Angiograms have been included in several illustrations in this volume of the Atlas which amply document the role and value of angiography. In the main, however, we have concerned ourselves only with noninvasive radiologic procedures of routine applicability. For similar reasons, we have omitted the role of the various isotope scanning procedures, ultrasound and thermography.

BIBLIOGRAPHY

1. Abrams, H. L.: *Angiography* (Boston: Little, Brown & Company, 1971).
2. Boyden, E. A.: The distribution of bronchi in gross anomalies of the right upper lobe, particularly lobes subdivided by the azygos vein and those containing pre-epiarterial bronchi, Radiology 58:797, 1952.
3. Davis, E. W., *et al.*: The solitary pulmonary nodule, J. Thoracic Surg. 32:728, 1956.
4. Demy, N. G., and Adler, H.: Asbestosis and malignancy, Am. J. Roentgenol. 100:597, 1967.
5. Di Rienzo, S.: *Radiologic Exploration of the Bronchus* (Springfield, Ill.: Charles C Thomas, Publisher, 1949).
6. Fleischner, F. G.: Mediastinal lymphadenopathy in bronchial carcinoma, Radiology 58:48, 1952.
7. Garland, L. H.: A three step method for diagnosis of solitary pulmonary nodules, Canad. M. A. J. 83:1079, 1960.
8. Greenspan, R. H.: Pulmonary angiography in lesions of the chest, Radiol. Clin. North America 1:315, 1963.
9. Hinshaw, H. C.: *Diseases of the Chest* (3rd ed.; Philadelphia: W. B. Saunders Company, 1956).
10. Mayer, E., and Maier, H. C.: *Pulmonary Carcinoma* (New York: New York University Press, 1956).
11. Michelson, E., and Salik, J. O.: The vascular pattern of the lung as seen on routine and tomographic studies, Radiology 73:511, 1959.
12. Miller, R. F., *et al.*: Bronchogenic cysts, Am. J. Roentgenol. 70:771, 1953.
13. Molnar, W., and Riebel, F. R.: Bronchography: An aid in the diagnosis of peripheral pulmonary carcinoma, Radiol. Clin. North America 1:303, 1963.

14. Nelson, W. W., *et al.*: Barium sulfate and bismuth subcarbonate suspensions as bronchographic contrast media, Radiology 72:829, 1959.
15. Rigler, L. G.: The roentgen signs of carcinoma of the lung, Am. J. Roentgenol. 74:415, 1955.
16. Rigler, L. G., and Hertzman, E. R.: Planigraphy in the diagnosis of the pulmonary nodule, Radiology 65:692, 1955.
17. Shanks, S. C., and Kerley, P. (eds.): *A Textbook of X-ray Diagnosis* (3rd ed.; Philadelphia: W. B. Saunders Company, 1962), Vol. II.
18. Simon, G.: *Principles of Chest X-ray Diagnosis* (New York: Appleton-Century-Crofts, Inc., 1971).
19. Snider, G. L., and Placik, B.: Relationship between pulmonary tuberculosis and bronchogenic carcinoma: Topographic study, Am. Rev. Resp. Dis. 99:229, 1969.
20. Steinberg, I., and Finby, N.: Great vessel involvement in lung cancer: Angiocardiographic report on 250 consecutive proved cases, Am. J. Roentgenol. 71:807, 1959.

Figure 1.—Squamous cell carcinoma of the right upper lobe.

A, posteroanterior radiograph: Showing a large, slightly lobulated, solid-appearing mass occupying a major portion of the right upper lobe (**a**). There is some depression and narrowing of the right main stem bronchus (**b**). No calcification is evident within the mass, but there is slight compression of some adjacent lung with minor displacement of a few surrounding parenchymal vessels (**c**).

B, close-up view of the lesion in **A**.

C, lateral radiograph: Revealing the spherical nature and lobulated margins of the mass. The apparent fluid level (**arrow**) is an artifact. In general, the larger a solitary pulmonary nodule is, the more likely it is to be a malignant process.

A 70-year-old man had had cough for a long period and, recently, blood-streaked sputum. A right pneumonectomy was performed. The pathologic examination revealed a huge squamous cell carcinoma with some local mediastinal extension. Necrosis was present in the central area of the mass. In spite of apparent adequate removal of the local tumor, the patient died of distant metastases about one year after excision.

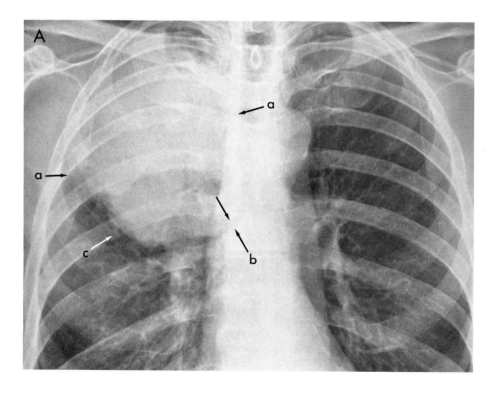

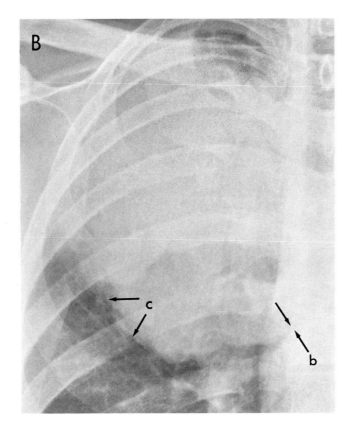

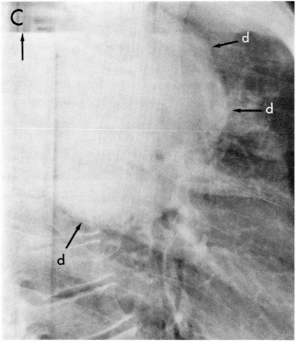

Figure 1 · Squamous Cell Carcinoma: Right Upper Lobe / 17

Figure 2.—Squamous cell carcinoma of the right apex.

  A, posteroanterior radiograph: Showing a sharply demarcated round mass (**arrows**) in the apical portion of the right upper lobe. There is faint suggestion of bone destruction in the right third rib (**a**). The trachea is deviated slightly to the left (**b**) and the lower air column obscured.

  B, lateral exposure: Revealing the smooth edges and spherical shape of the tumor (**arrows**). The tracheal airway is completely obscured by the mass, which is denser than the cardiac shadow.

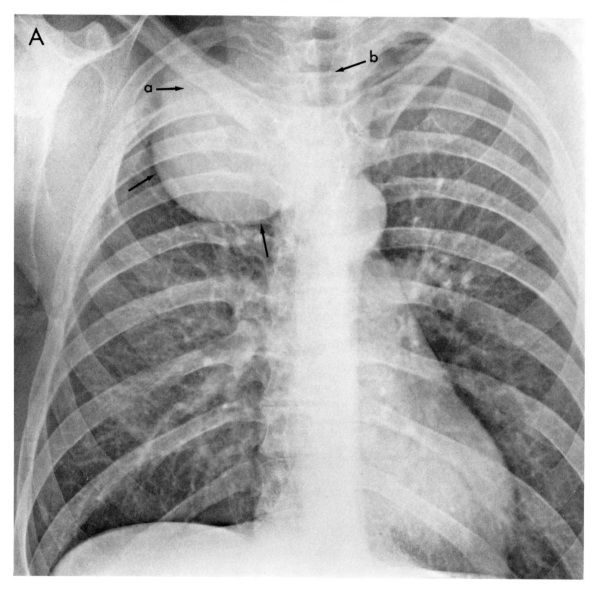

A 50-year-old man who was a heavy smoker complained of a painful right shoulder. No real evidence of Horner's syndrome was present; the painful shoulder and rib destruction suggested a sulcus tumor. Thoracotomy revealed the large mass fixed to and invading the posterior portions of the right third rib. Pathologic diagnosis was squamous cell carcinoma.

Figure 2, courtesy of Dr. H. S. Neal, Media, Pa.

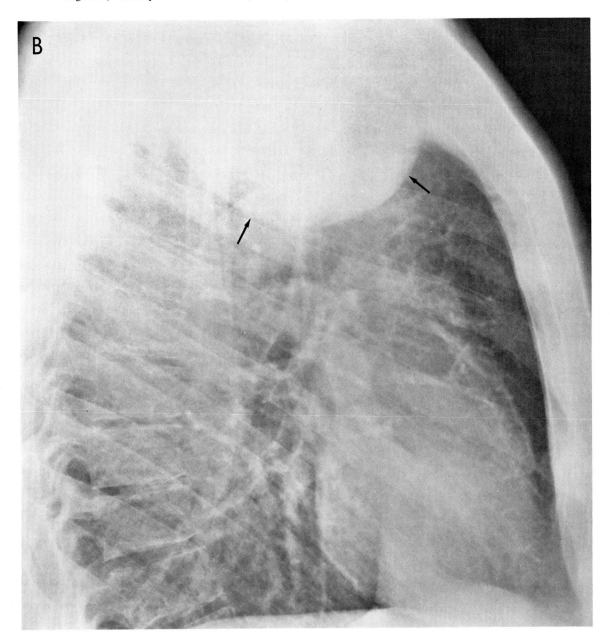

Figure 2 · Squamous Cell Carcinoma: Right Apex / 19

Figure 3.—Squamous cell carcinoma of the left apex.

A, posteroanterior radiograph: Delineating a large lobulated mass occupying the major portion of the apical posterior portion of the left upper lobe. The second intercostal space (**a**) is widened, and there is minimal irregularity along the inferior margin of the second rib (**b**).

B, lateral view: Revealing evidence of lobulation (**arrows**).

C, left subclavian venogram: Demonstrating invasion by the mass (**arrow**) and some reversal of flow into adjacent neck veins (**c**).

A 62-year-old woman had had severe left shoulder pain for several months. Biopsy study of the mass revealed a squamous cell cancer.

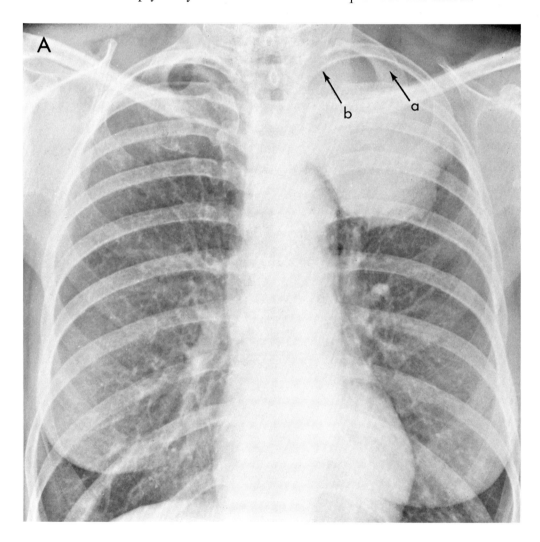

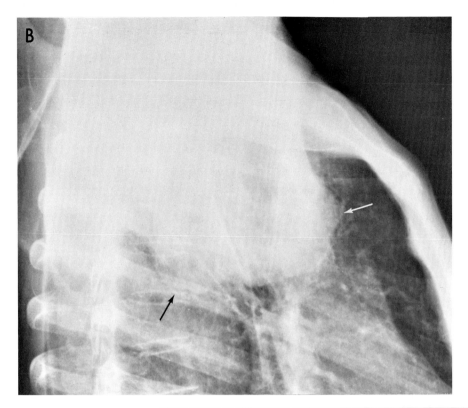

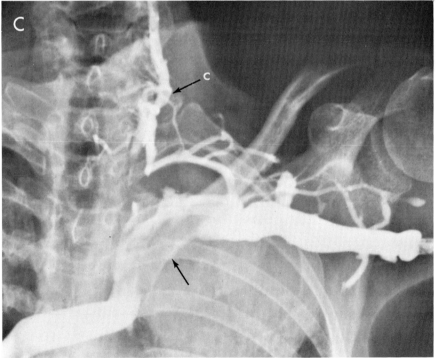

Figure 3 · Squamous Cell Carcinoma: Left Apex / 21

Figure 4.—Squamous cell carcinoma of the right upper lobe.

A, posteroanterior radiograph: Showing a large mass that occupies the major portion of the right upper lung field. There is considerable apical pleural thickening, and the mass blends into the mediastinum in the region of the ascending aorta.

B, lateral view: Defining the general limits of the tumor (**arrows**).

C, right subclavian venogram: Indicating invasion of the innominate vein distally (**a**) and almost complete obstruction proximally (**b**).

A 54-year-old man with a chronic cough finally consulted his physician because of symptoms of a superior vena caval obstruction. Scalene node biopsy revealed squamous cell carcinoma. Radiation therapy afforded some palliation.

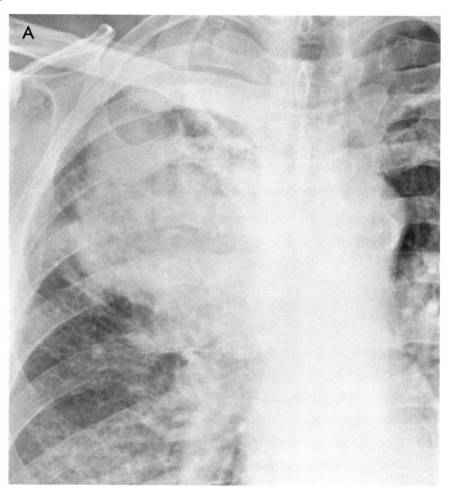

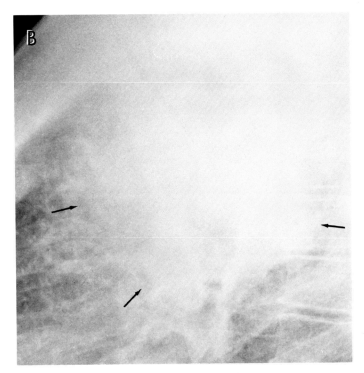

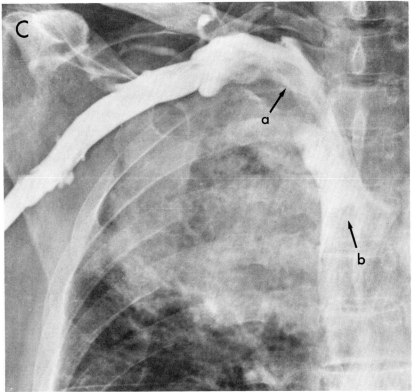

Figure 4 · Squamous Cell Carcinoma: Right Upper Lobe / 23

Figure 5.—Squamous cell carcinoma of the right upper lobe with metastases.

A, posteroanterior radiograph: Revealing a smooth-edged ovoid mass in the right upper lobe (**arrow**) with extensions to the right apex apparently involving the pleura (better seen in the magnified view in **C**). The trachea and main stem bronchus are obviously patent.

B, magnified view of lesion in **A**: Revealing extension of the tumor into the subapical pleura (**arrows**).

C, lateral exposure: Demonstrating the tumor's position in the superior mediastinum (**arrows**) somewhat behind the trachea (**a**), extending along it and blurring its air shadow (**b**). Note the slightly enlarged node (**c**).

A 54-year-old man who had smoked two packages of cigarets a day for many years saw his physician because of a rather heavy feeling in the right side of his chest. Thoracotomy revealed a large mass in the right upper lobe with extension to the paratracheal and hilar nodes. Pathologic study revealed squamous cell carcinoma.

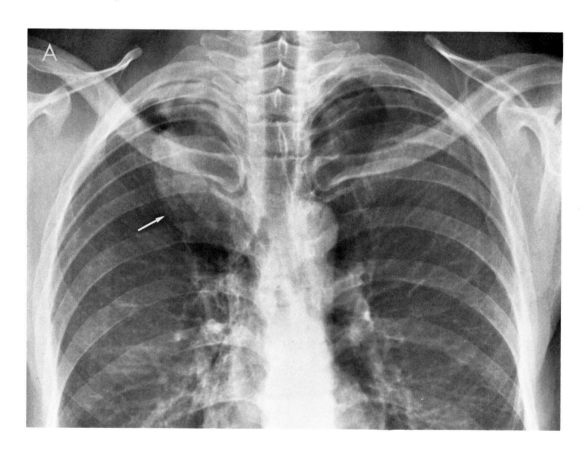

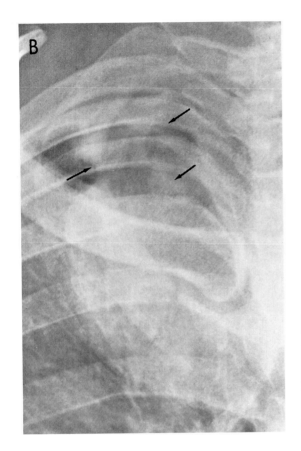

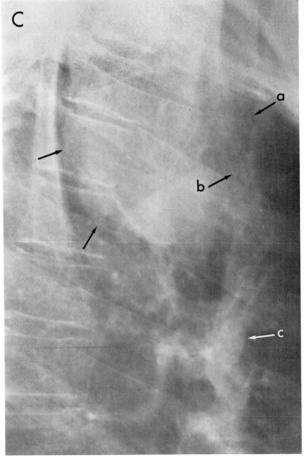

Figure 5 · Squamous Cell Carcinoma: Right Upper Lobe / 25

Figure 6.—Squamous cell carcinoma with hilar and paratracheal nodal metastases.

A, posteroanterior radiograph: Revealing hilar and paratracheal masses with sharply demarcated margins (**arrows**). The vascular structures in the right hilar area are obscured. Some distortion of the bronchus intermedius is present (**a**).

B, lateral projection: Showing the soft tissue mass in the superior mediastinum (**arrows**) slightly superimposed on the air shadow of the trachea (**b**). The sharply outlined hilar nodal mass is clearly evident (**c**).

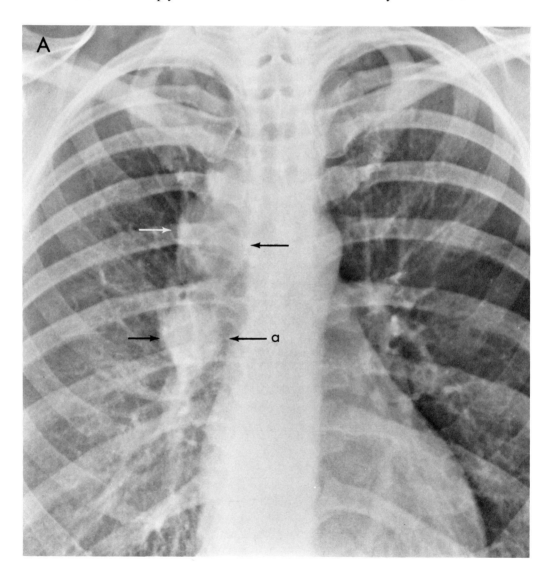

A 48-year-old man had a recent history of blood-streaked sputum. He had been a heavy smoker for more than 20 years. Recently the character of his cough had changed. The general physical examination yielded essentially normal results. At right pneumonectomy some of the mass had to be peeled away from the superior vena cava. Pathologic examination revealed a primary squamous cell carcinoma in the right upper lobe with mediastinal extension into paratracheal and hilar nodal groups.

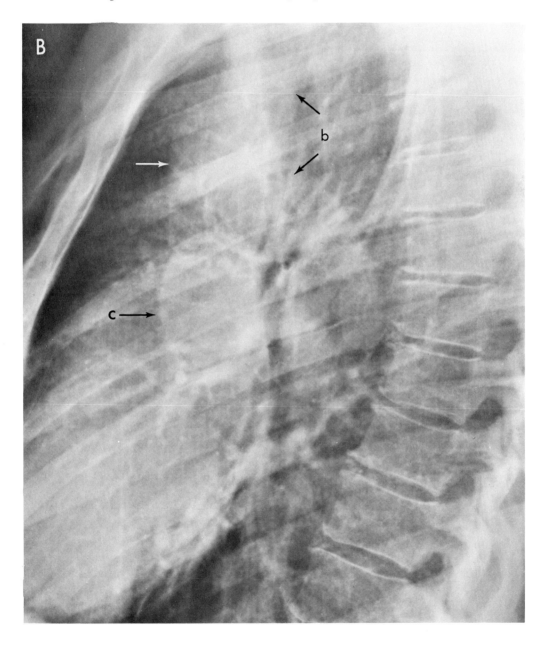

Figure 6 · Squamous Cell Carcinoma with Metastases / 27

Figure 7.—Squamous cell carcinoma with rib destruction.

Posteroanterior exposure: Revealing the left second rib destroyed (**a**) by a soft tissue mass in the left apex (**arrows**). This mass lies within the chest and differs sharply from extrapulmonary masses that invade the ribs (seen Fig. 180).

A 65-year-old man had had a painful left shoulder and neck for about four months. He denied having any cough or productive sputum but had smoked two packages of cigarets for many years. Needle biopsy revealed typical squamous cell carcinoma. Radiation therapy provided symptomatic relief for about one year.

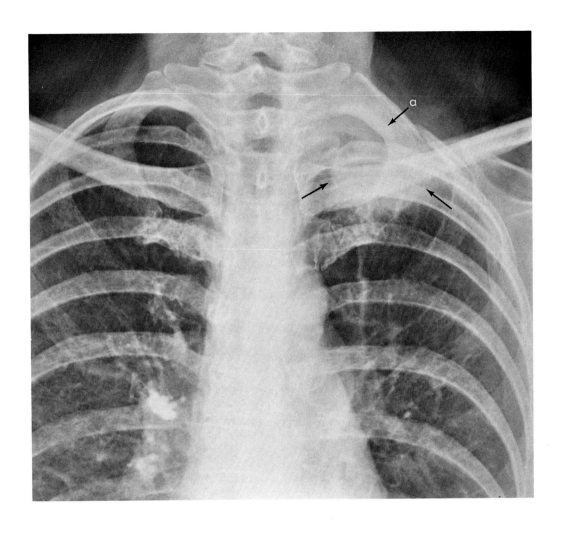

Figure 7 · Squamous Cell Carcinoma Involving a Rib / 29

Figure 8.—Squamous cell carcinoma of the left lower lobe.

A, posteroanterior radiograph: Revealing a rather ill-defined soft tissue mass in the left lower lobe (**arrows**). Its margins are somewhat difficult to delineate in conventional radiographs because they fade into the surrounding parenchyma.

B, lateral body-section radiograph through the central portion of the mass: Demonstrating the margins of an ovoid mass (**arrows**) with several pseudopods (**a**) extending into the pulmonary parenchyma of the left lower

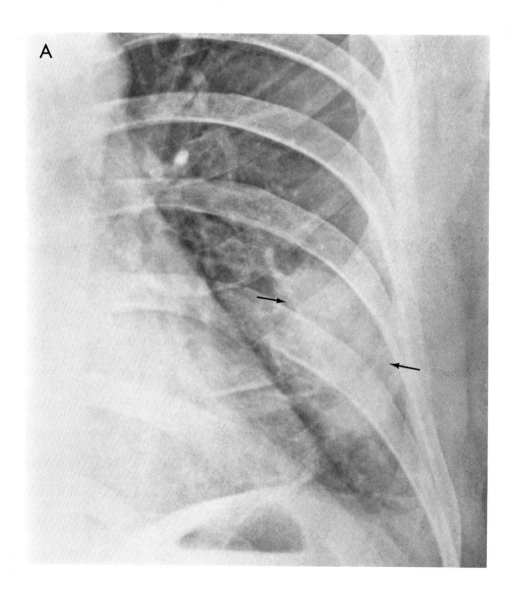

lobe. Part of this mass adjoins the oblique fissure (**b**). No hilar or mediastinal nodal changes were evident.

A 50-year-old man with cough and blood-streaked sputum had had some recent fever and sweating. Results of the general physical examination and routine laboratory studies were within normal limits. Pneumonectomy revealed a lesion well confined to the left lower lobe and abutting on the oblique fissure. The lesion proved to be a squamous cell carcinoma without hilar extension or vascular invasion.

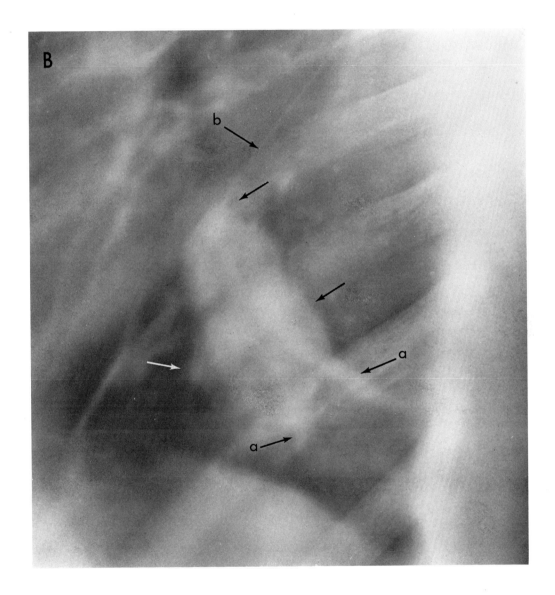

Figure 8 · Squamous Cell Carcinoma: Left Lower Lobe / 31

Figure 9.—Squamous cell carcinoma of the right middle lobe.

A, posteroanterior radiograph: Revealing an ovoid dense lesion (**arrows**) in the region of the right middle lobe. The adjoining blood vessels seem normal, as do the remaining portions of the chest.

B, magnification of the lesion in **A**: Delineating the shaggy irregular border.

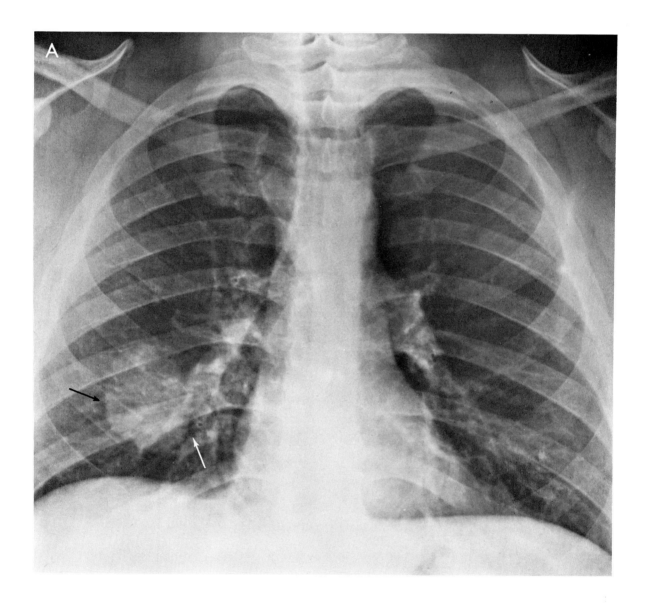

C, posteroanterior body-section study: Revealing a notched upper border (**a**) of the lesion. There is no evidence of an associated blood vessel to explain the notching. The notching is a coincidental finding that some believe to be highly characteristic of malignant lung disease.

A 37-year-old man, a food-handler weighing 230 lb., required a chest x-ray study to satisfy the city health authorities. The mass was discovered at this time. Thoracotomy revealed a solid mass in the right middle lobe with no mediastinal invasion. Pathologic diagnosis was squamous cell carcinoma.

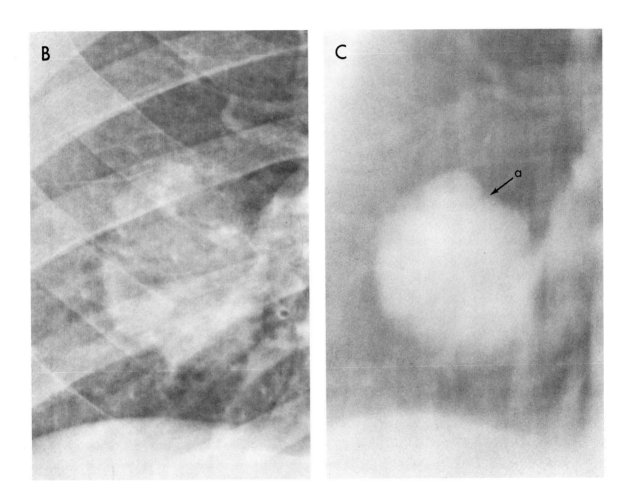

Figure 9 · Squamous Cell Carcinoma: Right Middle Lobe / 33

Figure 10.—Cavitary squamous cell carcinoma.

A, posteroanterior close-up examination: Revealing a large mass (**arrows**) in the right upper lobe and an air–fluid level (**a**) which occupies the posterior portion of the right upper lobe. The inner margins are nodular and shaggy (**b**). There is some parenchymal reaction adjacent to the lower margin of the lesion (**x**).

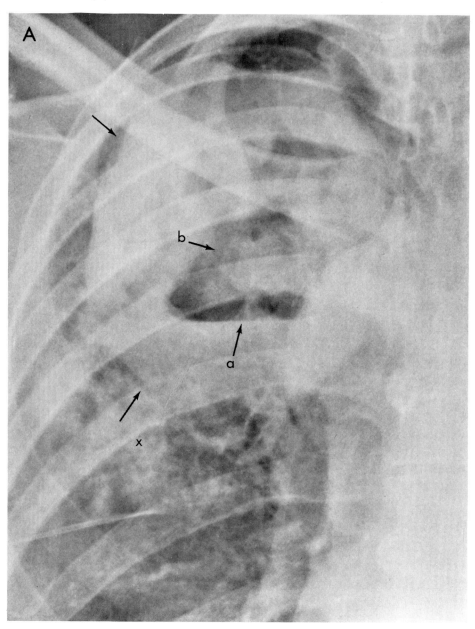

B, posteroanterior body-section radiograph of the area in **A**: Accentuating the nodular and shaggy inner margin of the cavity (**b**). Note the thickness of the wall of the cavity (**y**) as well as its lobulated outer margin (**c**).

A 64-year-old woman who was a heavy smoker complained of chills, fever and cough productive of purulent sputum. Pneumonectomy was performed. Pathologic study revealed a large cavitating squamous cell carcinoma with an infected necrotic center.

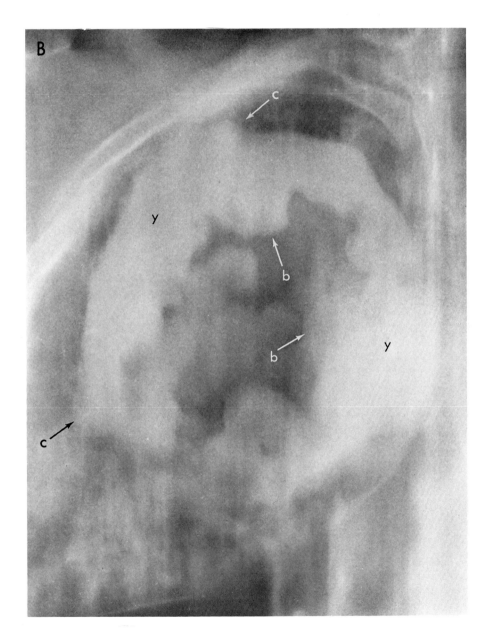

Figure 10 · Squamous Cell Carcinoma: Cavitation / 35

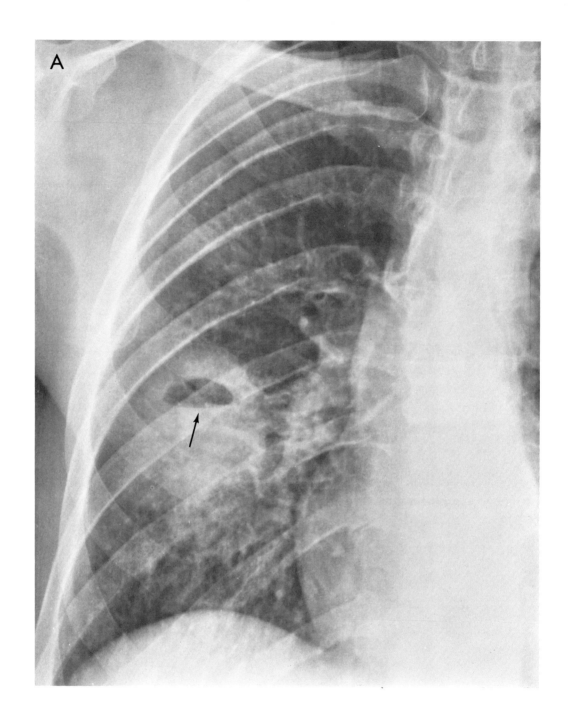

Figure 11.—Cavitary squamous cell carcinoma.

A, posteroanterior radiograph: Revealing a large ill-defined mass in the right middle lung field with an air–fluid level (**arrow**).

B, anteroposterior supine tomogram: Demonstrating the irregular and nodular inner wall of a thick-walled cavity (**arrows**) with an ill-defined spiculated outer margin (**a**). In the supine study, the fluid is dependent, allowing one to obtain a true outline of the wall of the mass.

A 60-year-old woman had had fever and hemophysis for about three weeks. Right lower lobectomy was performed. Pathologic study revealed a cavitating squamous cell carcinoma.

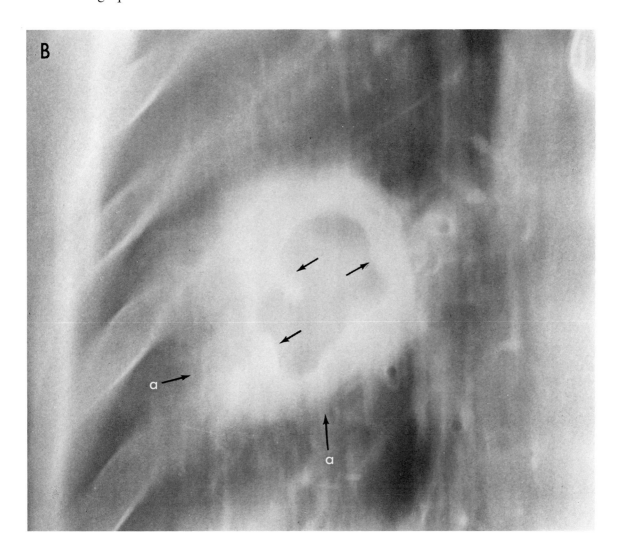

Figure 11 · Squamous Cell Carcinoma: Cavitation / 37

Figure 12.—Squamous cell carcinoma of the right upper lobe with multiple cavities.

A, posteroanterior exposure: Revealing a large multilobulated mass (**arrows**) with at least one thin-walled cavitating lesion in the right upper lobe. The lesion could represent either a cavity with multiple pockets or several separate cavities. A portion of the mass fades into the surrounding parenchyma (**a**). The tracheal airway is narrowed (**b**), and there is loss of the outline of the superior vascular margins in the right hilar region (**y**).

B, close-up view of lesion in **A.**

C, lateral exposure: Showing the lesion to occupy the posterior portions of the right upper lobe (**arrows**). Distortion of adjacent hilar vessels and narrowing of the trachea are clearly visible at **b**.

A 50-year-old man complained of chills, fever and rusty sputum. Right pneumonectomy revealed extension of the lesion to the mediastinal, paratracheal and hilar lymph nodes. In spite of the narrowed trachea, the tumor could be peeled from the wall. Microscopic study revealed a large squamous cell carcinoma containing a thin-walled multiloculated abscess.

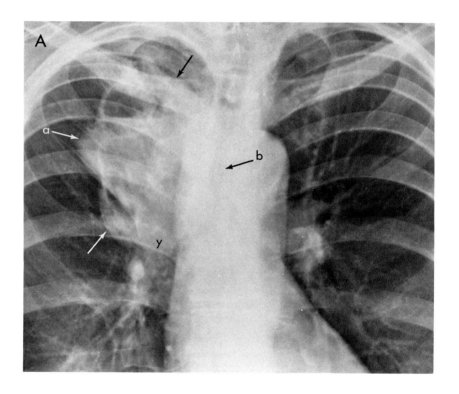

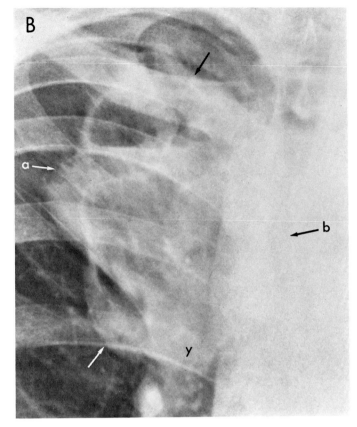

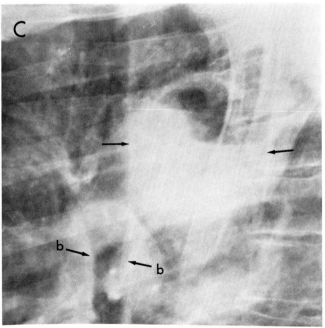

Figure 12 · Squamous Cell Carcinoma with Abscess / 39

Figure 13.—Cavitating squamous cell carcinoma.

A, posteroanterior close-up view: Showing a large, ragged, cystlike, moderately thick walled cavity. A well-defined solid inferior shadow (**arrow**) is present adjacent to the right hilus.

B, supine body-section study through the cavitating lesion: Revealing the nodular thick-walled nature of the cavity. Radiating striae (**a**) are rather suggestive of malignant disease. The inferior solid mass (**arrow**) is seen with its sharp-edged lateral margins. Note that the medial edge (**x**) is ill defined and consonant with malignant disease.

C, posteroanterior view 10 days after **A**: Revealing considerable collapse of the cavity. Thickness of its walls is unchanged, and it retains its ragged appearance. There is no change in the inferior mass (**arrow**).

A 55-year-old man was hospitalized complaining of fever for 2 days, right-sided chest pain, shortness of breath and a cough productive of yellowish brown sputum. For the preceding 3 months he had noted increasing fatigue, anorexia, nonproductive cough and a 15 lb. weight loss. He had smoked two packages of cigarets daily for 20 years. About 6 weeks after the initial examination a thoracotomy was performed and both masses were removed. Squamous cell cancer was present in each area.

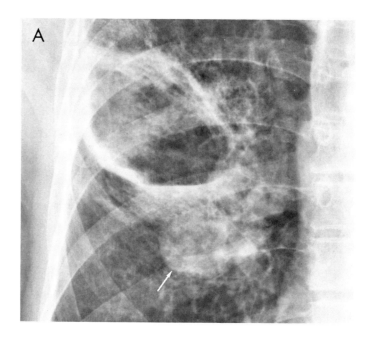

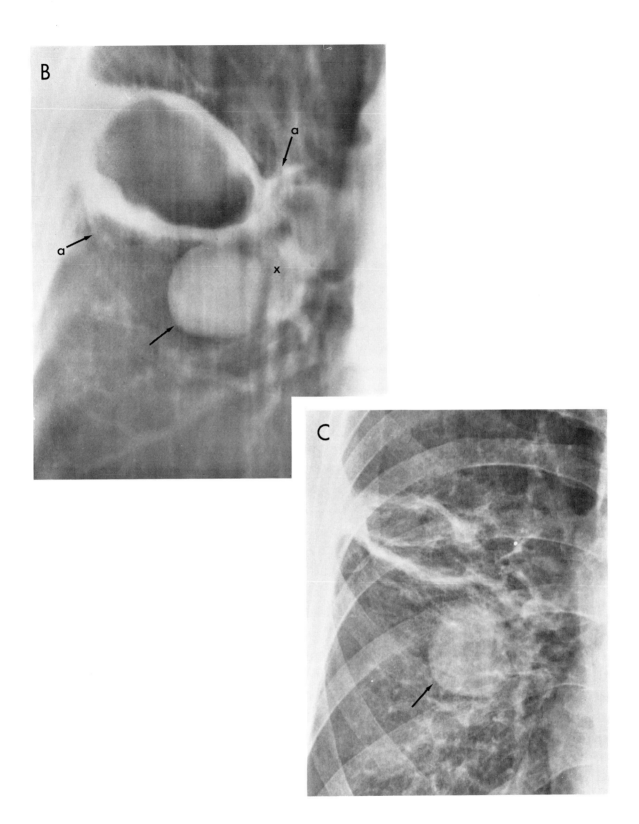

Figure 13 · Squamous Cell Carcinoma: Cavitation / 41

Figure 14.—Developing squamous cell carcinoma.

   A, posteroanterior exposure: Revealing a small density (**arrow**) considered to be an old scar.

   B, close-up view of lesion in **A**: Showing it not to be as linear as one might expect an old healed scar to be. It has a certain bulbous masslike quality of suspicious nature.

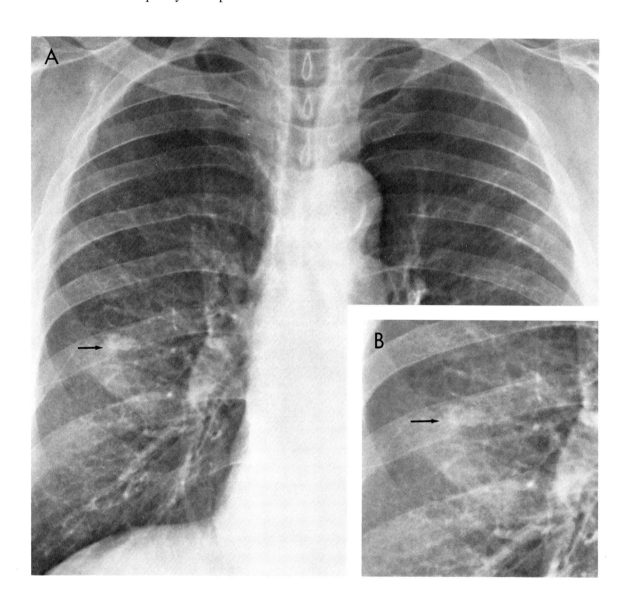

C, three years later, magnification of a portion of a posteroanterior radiograph: Disclosing a nodular mass (**arrow**) with irregular margins; the original lesion seen in **A** has gotten larger.

D, body-section study: Revealing a small cavity (**a**). The pseudopods (**b**) extending into adjacent lung suggest cancer.

A 54-year-old man was asymptomatic for over three years after the firs examination. A subsequent right middle and lower lobectomy revealed nodule essentially confined to the right middle lobe. The pathologic diagnos was squamous cell carcinoma. One hilar node contained metastatic tumor.

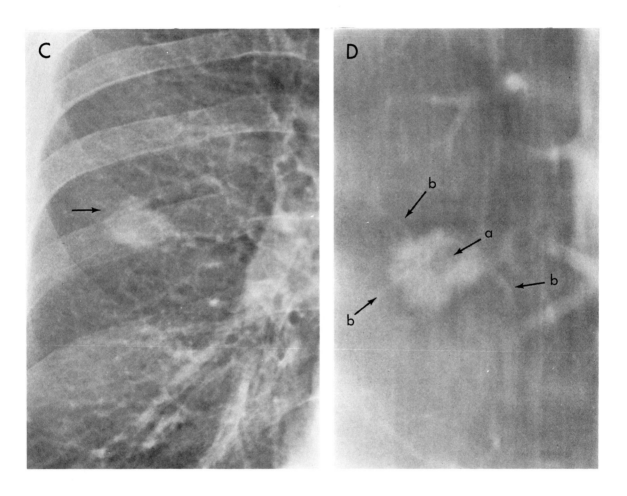

Figure 14 · Developing Squamous Cell Carcinoma / 43

Figure 15.—Squamous cell carcinoma with a small cavity.

A, posteroanterior radiograph: Revealing an ill-defined mass in the right first anterior interspace (**arrow**). The radiologists had difficulty convincing the patient's physician of the presence of a mass, and even after agreeing that something was present, the physician thought it was probably an inflammatory process and refused further study at this time.

B, close-up of lesion in **A**.

C, posteroanterior projection, two months later: Again revealing the rather ill-defined lesion in the right upper lobe (**arrow**).

D, one month after **C**: Demonstrating the abnormal right upper lobe. At this time the lesion is less well defined.

E, body-section radiograph made at the same time as **D**: Revealing a definite mass (**x**) with irregular pseudopods (**a**) along the medial and inferior borders. In addition, a small cavity is present (**arrow**). Eccentric cavities of this nature are not unusual in squamous cell neoplasms.

A 45-year-old woman with a mild cough but no appreciable sputum production complained of considerable fatigue without weight loss. The results of general physical examination and routine laboratory studies were within normal limits. On right upper lobectomy a well-confined lesion was found in the upper lobe. Pathologic diagnosis was cavitating squamous cell carcinoma. No mediastinal extension was demonstrable.

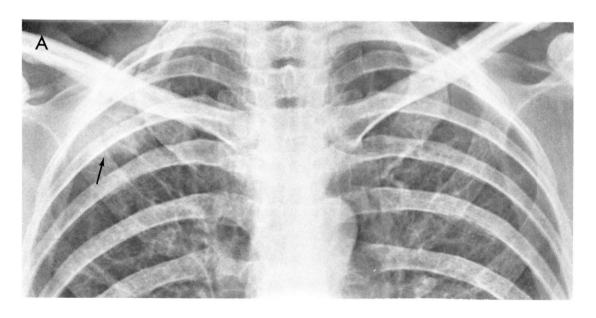

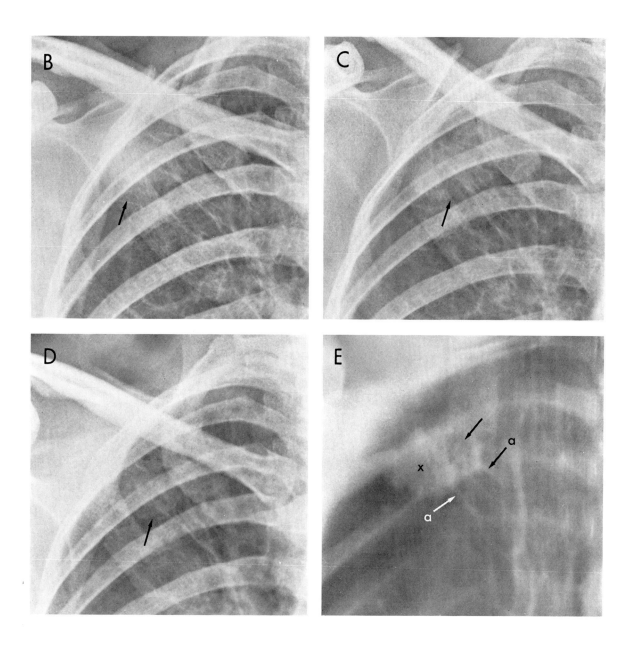

Figure 15 · Squamous Cell Carcinoma: Cavitation / 45

Figure 16.—Squamous cell carcinoma in an emphysematous bleb.

A, posteroanterior radiograph: Revealing emphysematous bullae in both apices (**x**). A sharply marginated soft tissue shadow is present in one of the bullae in the left upper lobe. This was initially considered to be inflammatory. Multiple sputum examinations failed to produce any acid-fast organisms. Empiric drug therapy aimed at broad spectrum coverage was started.

B, close-up of lesion in **A**.

(Continued.)

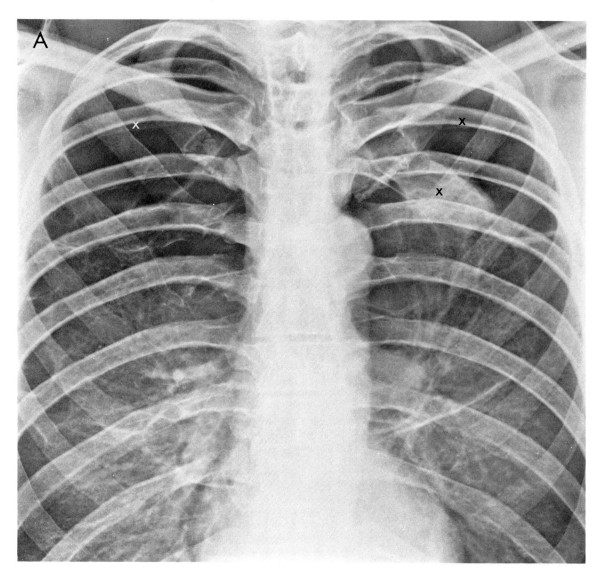

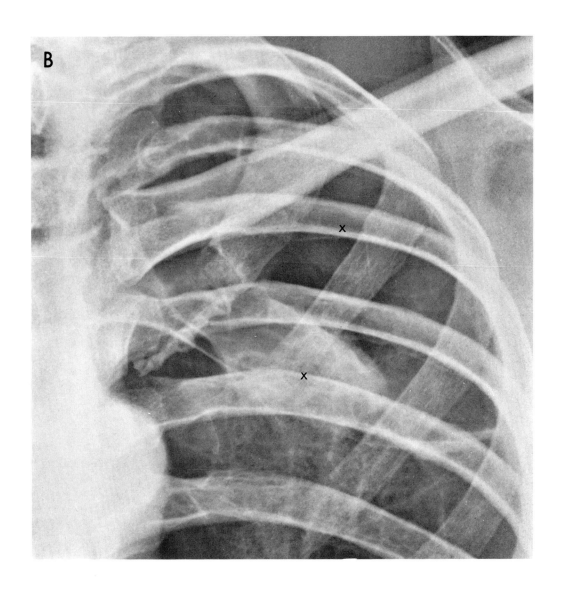

Figure 16 · Squamous Cell Carcinoma / 47

Figure 16 (cont.).—Squamous cell carcinoma in an emphysematous bleb.

C, posteroanterior radiograph, three months later: Demonstrating a distinct air–fluid level (**arrow**) in one of the blebs in the left upper lobe which obscures the ovoid lesion seen previously.

D, lateral projection: Locating the lesion (**x**) in the posterior portion of the left upper lobe (**arrows**). It seems to have increased in size. The solid nature of the shadow (**x**) and its enlargement despite the development of fluid makes one regard this lesion a neoplasm.

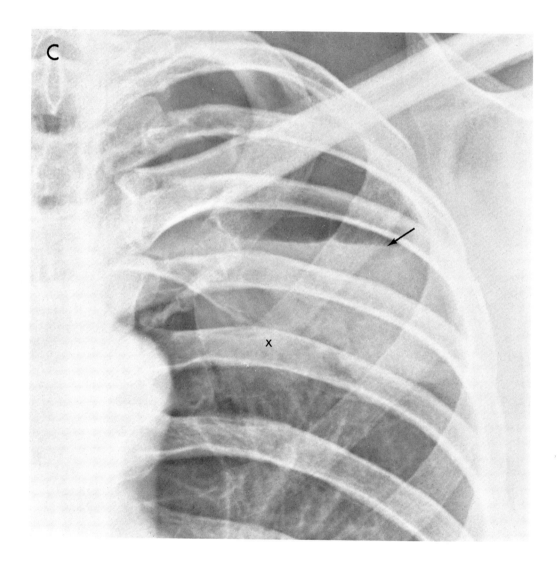

A 45-year-old man was referred by his physician because of an abnormal picture on a tuberculosis chest survey. On initial examination his only complaint was a mild nonproductive cough. No acid-fast organisms were ever detected in the sputum. Left upper lobectomy revealed a squamous cell carcinoma in an emphysematous bulla.

Comment: The initial appearance of the soft tissue mass in the region of the bullae should raise one's suspicion of neoplasm rather than of an inflammatory process. Body-section radiographs, if obtained when the patient was first seen, might have led one to suspect neoplastic disease rather than infection.

Figure 16, courtesy of Dr. Irwin M. Freundlich, Jefferson Medical College, Philadelphia.

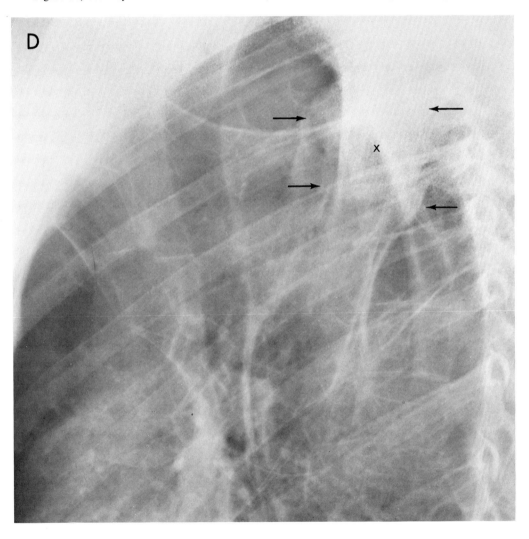

Figure 16 · Squamous Cell Carcinoma / 49

Figure 17.—Squamous cell carcinoma and Klebsiella pneumonia.

A, posteroanterior radiograph: Revealing a large area of consolidation in the right upper lobe. There is some depression of the horizontal interlobar fissure (**a**). Ventilating lung and patches of consolidation in the posterior and apical segments are visible above the mass (**b**).

B, close-up of lesion in **A**: Showing the changes to better advantage.

C, lateral projection: Demonstrating the depressed horizontal fissure (**a**) and the huge consolidation, mainly in the anterior segment but also involving portions of the posterior and apical segments of the right upper lobe.

The density of the mass plus the depression of the horizontal fissure suggest a solid, growing tumor beyond an obstructed bronchus or tumor plus fluid.

A 60-year-old male alcoholic entered the hospital with cough, blood-streaked sputum and high fever. Bronchoscopy revealed a lesion in the right upper lobe bronchus. At the same time, Klebsiellae were identified. Biopsy revealed squamous cell carcinoma. Resection of the right lung revealed a squamous cell carcinoma involving the right upper lobe bronchus with extension to mediastinal nodes.

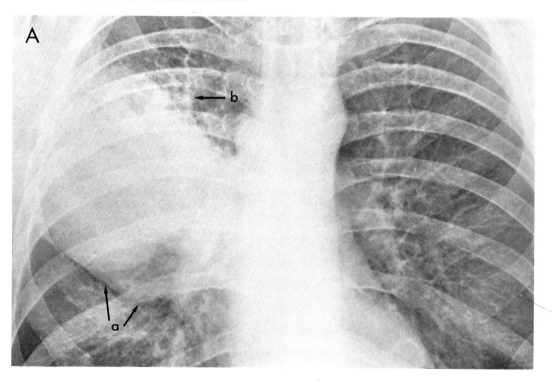

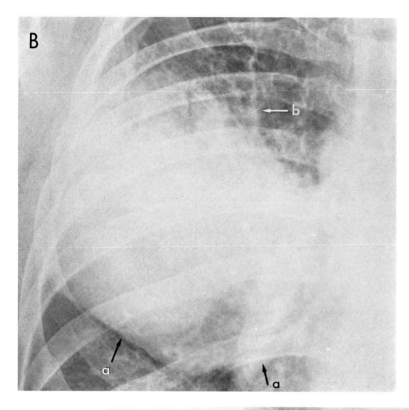

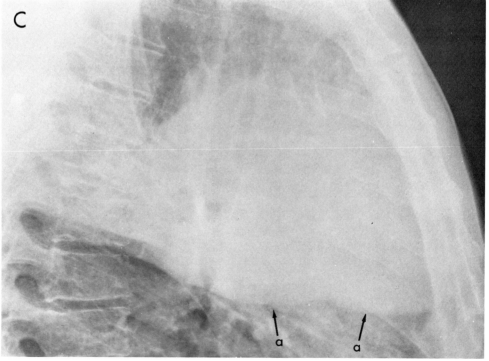

Figure 17 · Squamous Cell Carcinoma & Pneumonia / 51

Figure 18.—Squamous cell carcinoma with a bulging interlobar fissure.

A, posteroanterior radiograph: Showing some displacement of the trachea to the right (a), elevation of a portion of the interlobar fissure (b), plus bulging of its inferior portion (c). The entire mediastinum and heart are displaced to the right.

B, close-up of lesion in A: The tracheal displacement and narrowing are seen at a; the right stem bronchus is compressed (d). The concavity (b) and convexity (c) of the horizontal fissure indicate collapse (b) plus mass (c) due to cancer or fluid.

C, lateral projection: Revealing the collapsed upper lobe (e). The bulging due to mass or fluid at c plus the evidence of bronchial obstruction seen in B are hallmarks of cancer. Expansion of the middle and lower lobes is compensatory.

A 65-year-old man presented himself with an acute onset of chills, fever and cough. Treatment with antibiotics appreciably reduced the bulging fissure and size of the upper lobe. Bronchoscopy revealed a fungating mass obstructing the right upper lobe bronchus. Biopsy diagnosis was squamous cell carcinoma.

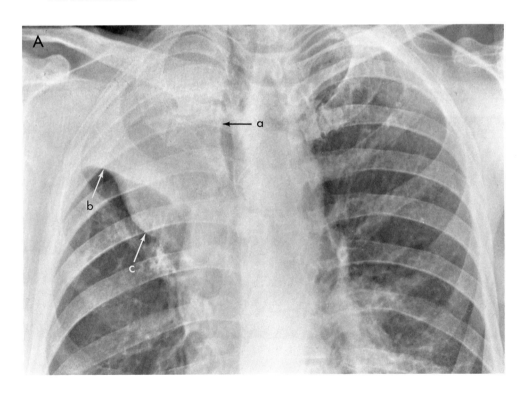

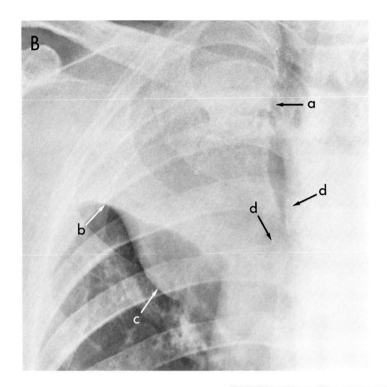

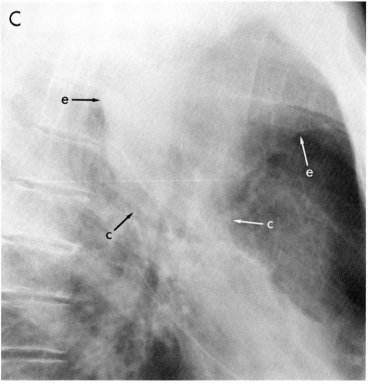

Figure 18 · Squamous Cell Carcinoma / 53

Figure 19.—Squamous cell carcinoma of the left main stem bronchus.

A, posteroanterior radiograph: Revealing a marked shift of the mediastinum to the left (**a**) and a completely opaque left hemithorax. The gastric air bubble (**b**) is not elevated, indicating a normally placed left hemidiaphragm. Note the many old and recent rib fractures in the right hemithorax.

B, lateral projection: An interesting appearance, with the obvious depressed diaphragm and hyperaeration in the right lung representing all the aerating lung present. The tracheal shadow is compressed (**c**), and the normal outline of the left main stem bronchus, which should be demonstrated at

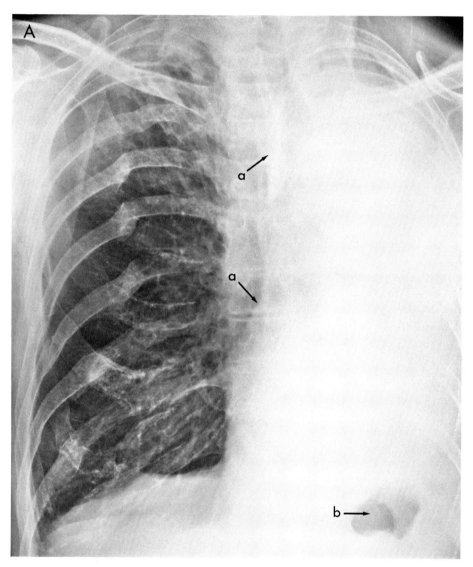

d, is not present. The aortic window is lost and the aortic arch almost indistinguishable. These are indicative of a hilar mass with collapsed lung, mediastinal shift and rotation of the heart and aortic shadows.

A 72-year-old man presented himself because of marked shortness of breath and a long history of intermittent blood-streaked sputum. He was an alcoholic and a most unreliable historian. Clinically there was no question of his dyspnea. Bronchoscopy revealed a fungating tumor completely occluding the region of the left main stem bronchus. Biopsy study of the lesion revealed squamous cell cancer. Severe pulmonary insufficiency precluded any operative procedure.

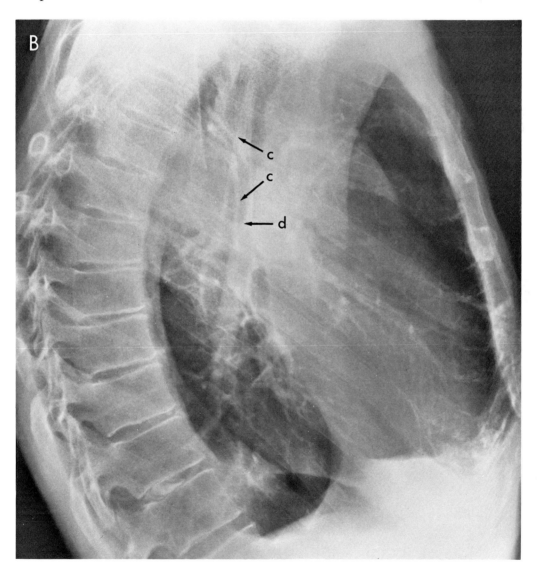

Figure 19 · Squamous Cell Carcinoma of Bronchus / 55

Figure 20.—Squamous cell carcinoma with local extension.

   A, posteroanterior projection: Disclosing a large ill-defined, branching, linear shadow (**x**) which blends into the superior vascular structures above the right hilus and extends to the mediastinum. A segment of the posterior portion of the right seventh rib is missing (**arrow**).

   B, close-up of lesions in **A.**

   (Continued.)

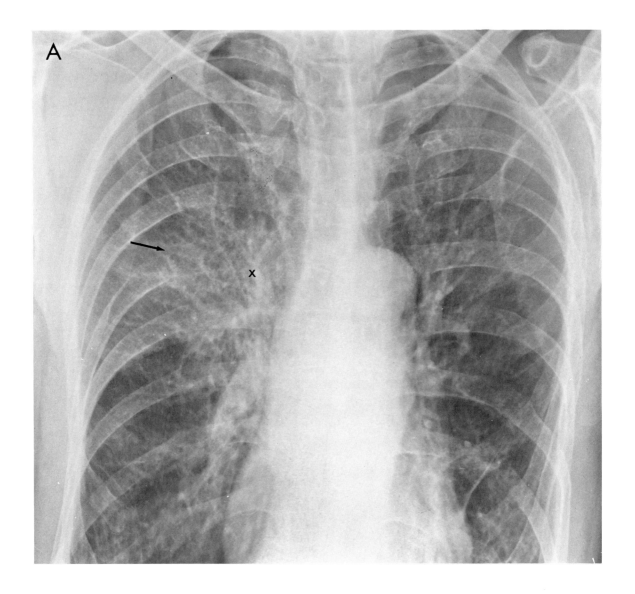

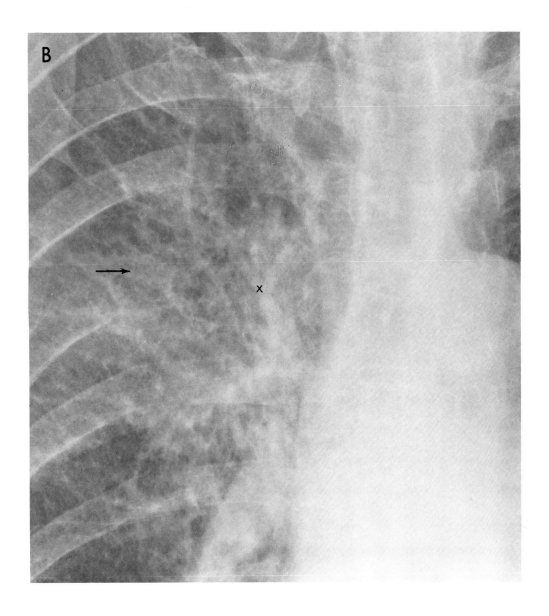

Figure 20 · Squamous Cell Carcinoma Involving a Rib / 57

Figure 20 (cont.).—Squamous cell carcinoma with local extension.

C, lateral radiograph: Showing a more clearly defined mass (**c**). Absence of the rib outline at **d** is in contrast with the shadow of the seventh rib on the opposite side (**e**). An inferior hilar metastatic mass is clearly identified at **y** which is not well appreciated in the posteroanterior view.

D, close-up of lesions in **C.**

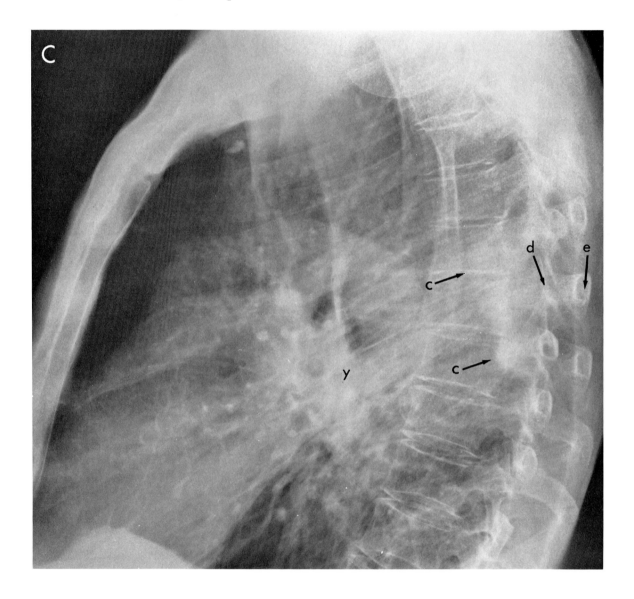

A 65-year-old man was initially seen because of an abscess that developed over the site of a hip-nailing performed five years previously. The abscess was treated. Shortly thereafter he complained of pleuritic pain in the midportion of his chest on the right side. Biopsy of the lesion of the destroyed rib revealed a squamous cell carcinoma.

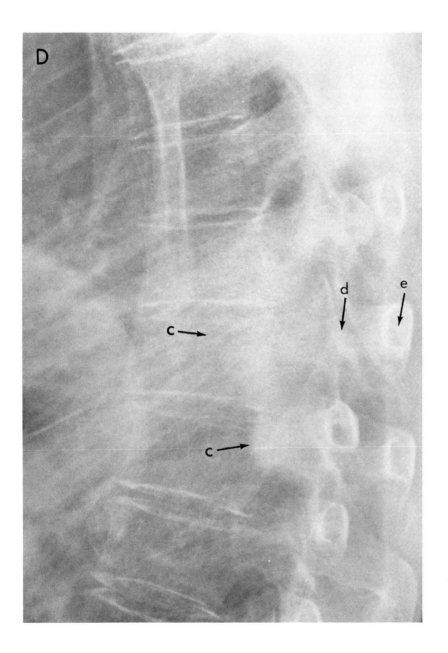

Figure 20 · Squamous Cell Carcinoma Involving a Rib / 59

Figure 21.—Anaplastic bronchogenic carcinoma.

A, posteroanterior radiograph: Revealing a large lobulated rounded mass involving the right hilar area (**arrows**). Note the loss of definition of the vessel margins in the right hilus.

B, lateral projection: More graphically illustrating the bilobed character of the major mass and suggesting ragged extension into the surrounding lung. Normal vascular shadows are completely lost in the mass of neoplastic tissue.

C, supine body-section radiograph: Amplifying the large hilar masses and also showing separation and narrowing of both main stem bronchi (**arrows**) by a mass at **x.**

A 52-year-old woman, a chronic smoker with cough of a long duration, had wheezing of relatively recent onset. Thoracotomy confirmed extensive involvement of the right hilus and lower mediastinum by tumor. Histologic study of biopsy material revealed anaplastic carcinoma.

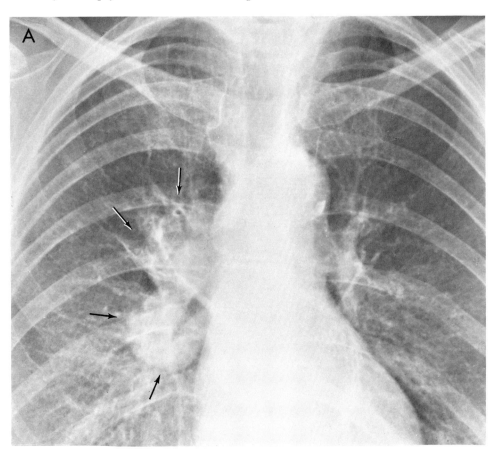

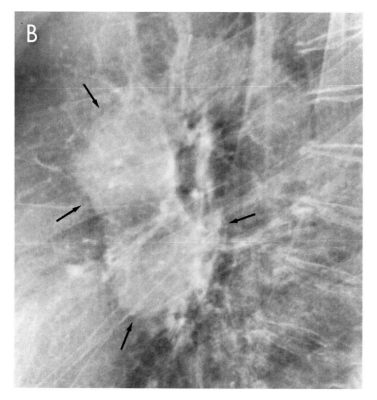

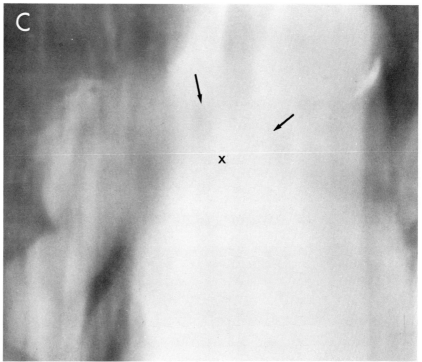

Figure 21 · Anaplastic Carcinoma / 61

Figure 22.—Squamous cell carcinoma of the right upper lobe.

A, posteroanterior radiograph: Revealing a sharply outlined mass in the anterior portion of the right upper lobe near the hilus (**arrow**).

B, close-up view of **A**: Showing obliteration by the mass of the sharp outline of the vessels as they enter the hilus (**a**). Ragged pseudopods (**arrows**) suggest the primary neoplastic origin of the mass.

C, lateral projection: Revealing lobulation of the mass (**b**) with extension into the hilus (**c**), which makes it clear that this is a lung tumor rather than a primary process based in the mediastinum.

A 48-year-old man had vague gastrointestinal complaints but no respiratory symptoms. Thoracotomy revealed a large lobulated mass which began in the right upper lobe and extended to the mediastinum with almost no invasion of adjacent structures. Pathologic analysis revealed a squamous cell carcinoma.

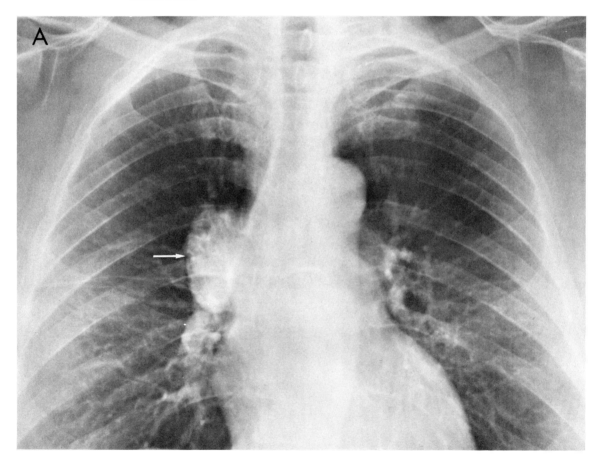

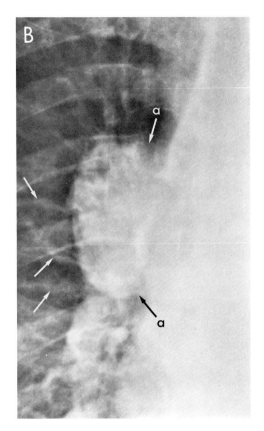

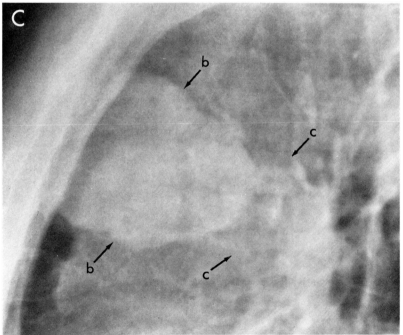

Figure 22 · Squamous Cell Carcinoma: Right Upper Lobe / 63

Figure 23.—Squamous cell carcinoma of the left upper lobe.

A, posteroanterior radiograph: Revealing a wavy-edged left hilar mass (x) adjacent to the mediastinum and loss of visibility of normal left hilar vessels. In addition, vascularity throughout the entire left lung is definitely diminished. Narrowing and irregularity of the left stem bronchus are evident (arrow).

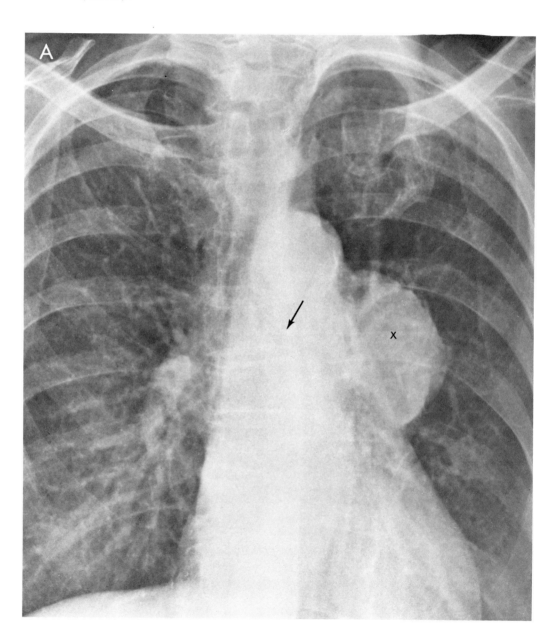

B, lateral projection: Demonstrating upward displacement and curving of at least one large vessel in the left upper lobe (**arrows**). In addition, the major hilar vessels are indistinguishable due to the mass (**x**). The bifurcation of the trachea into the main stem bronchi is displaced posteriorly and distorted (**b**).

A 68-year-old man complained of cough and occasional blood-streaked sputum. Significant weight loss had occurred within the preceding six months. Thoracotomy and biopsy revealed a squamous cell carcinoma.

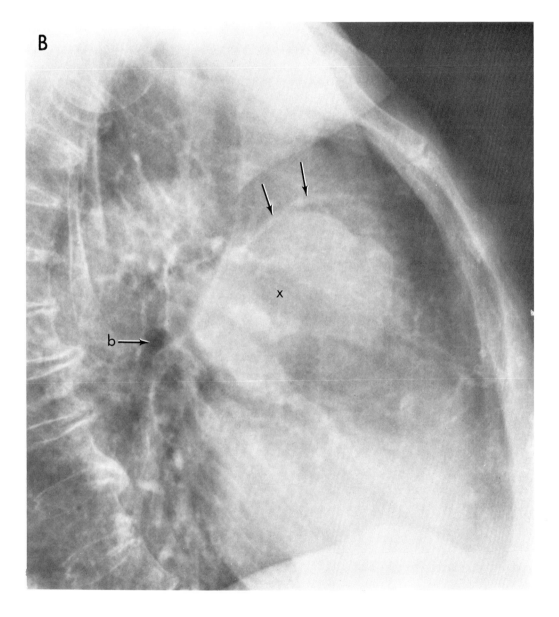

Figure 23 · Squamous Cell Carcinoma: Left Upper Lobe / 65

Figure 24.—Squamous cell carcinoma of the right upper lobe with massive mediastinal invasion.

A, posteroanterior radiograph: Showing a rather ragged upper mediastinum and right hilus. A definite mass (**x**) causes considerable widening of the mediastinum almost to the thoracic inlet on each side (**arrows**). The shadow blends with the superior vessels on the right side.

B, lateral radiograph: Revealing an enormous poorly visualized mass (**arrows**) extending through the entire superior mediastinum with considerable obliteration of the tracheal airway (**a**).

C, body-section study: Delineating the lobulated character of the parenchymal mass in the right upper lobe (**x**) and extension of the mass to the left of the midline (**arrow**), encompassing the entire air-filled trachea.

A 60-year-old man who was a heavy smoker described a change in character of his cough, some blood-streaked sputum and an uncomfortable feeling in his upper chest. Thoracotomy revealed extensive mediastinal and vascular invasion by the lesion. Biopsy study indicated squamous cell carcinoma.

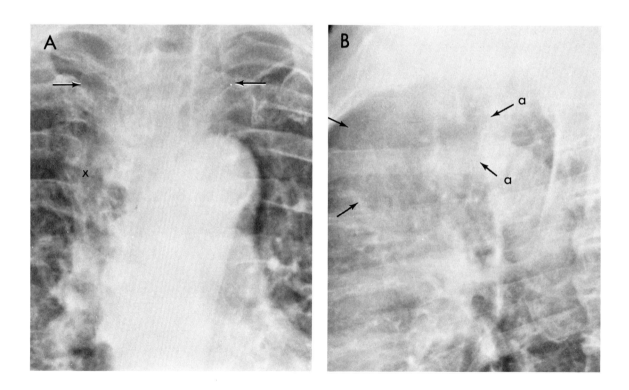

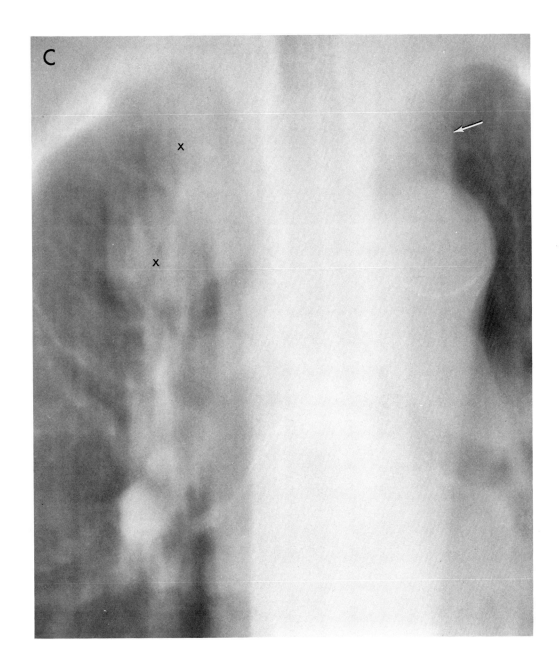

C

Figure 24 · Squamous Cell Carcinoma: Right Upper Lobe / 67

Figure 25.—Anaplastic carcinoma with mediastinal invasion.

A, posteroanterior radiograph: Revealing multiple ragged linear strands (**arrows**) in the right upper lobe extending toward a confluent solid mass near the mediastinum (**x**). The normal outlines of the upper portions of the pulmonary artery and veins blend into the lesion and are lost. In addition, a large, sharp-edged, soft tissue shadow projects to the left of the midline above the aortic knob (**a**).

B, close-up view: More clearly delineating the abnormalities seen in **A.**

(Continued.)

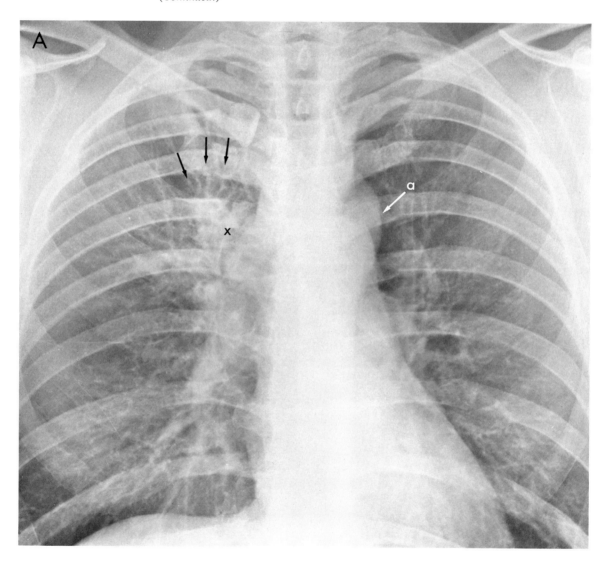

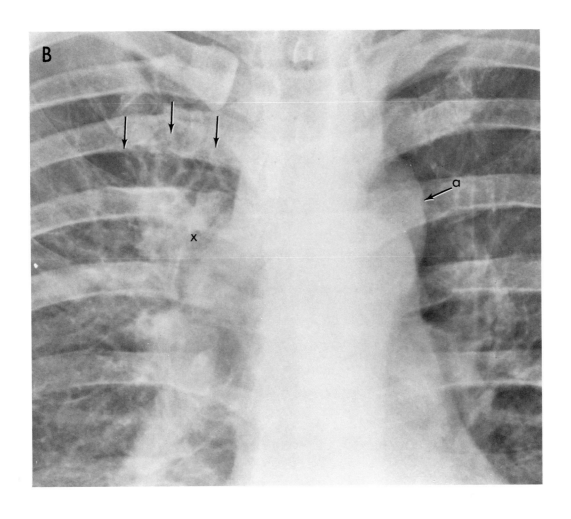

Figure 25 · Anaplastic Carcinoma: Mediastinal Invasion / 69

Figure 25 (cont.).—Anaplastic carcinoma with mediastinal invasion.

C, lateral view: Demonstrating complete loss of the outline of the arch of the aorta and the normal pulmonary vascular structures. Fuzzy linear strandlike shadows are present in the entire mediastinum extending from the superior mediastinum to below the tracheal bifurcation. The massive mediastinal invasion (**y**) surrounds the trachea and distorts it slightly (**arrow**).

A 37-year-old man who was a heavy smoker for many years complained of blood-streaked sputum and an increase in cough for several months. Thoracotomy revealed an inoperable lesion apparently arising in the right upper lobe but extending throughout the major portion of the mediastinum and completely encompassing the major vessels. Biopsy study indicated an anaplastic tumor, most probably of squamous cell origin.

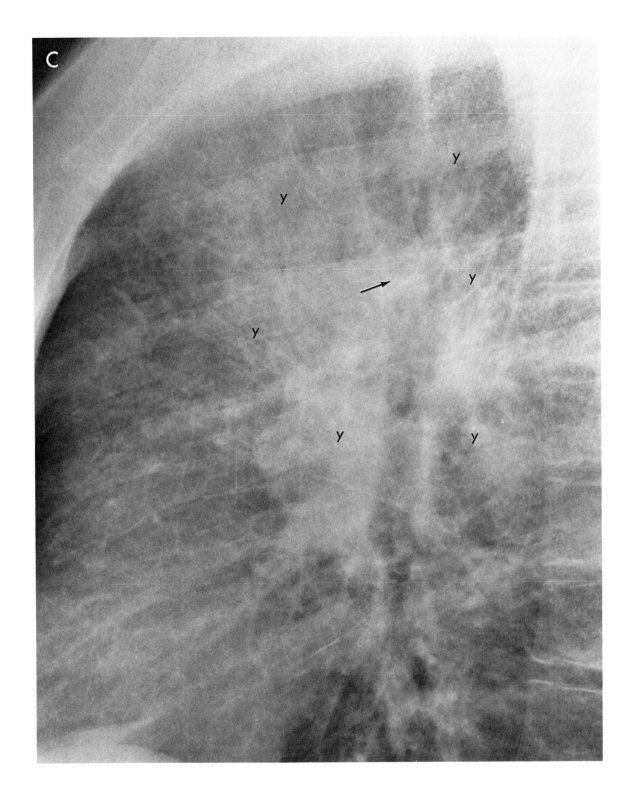

Figure 25 · **Anaplastic Carcinoma: Mediastinal Invasion** / 71

Figure 26.—Squamous cell carcinoma of left lower lobe bronchus with massive mediastinal invasion.

A, initial posteroanterior radiograph: Revealing a barely perceptible soft tissue mass extending laterally to the border of the descending aorta (**arrow**). No other abnormality is visible in this projection.

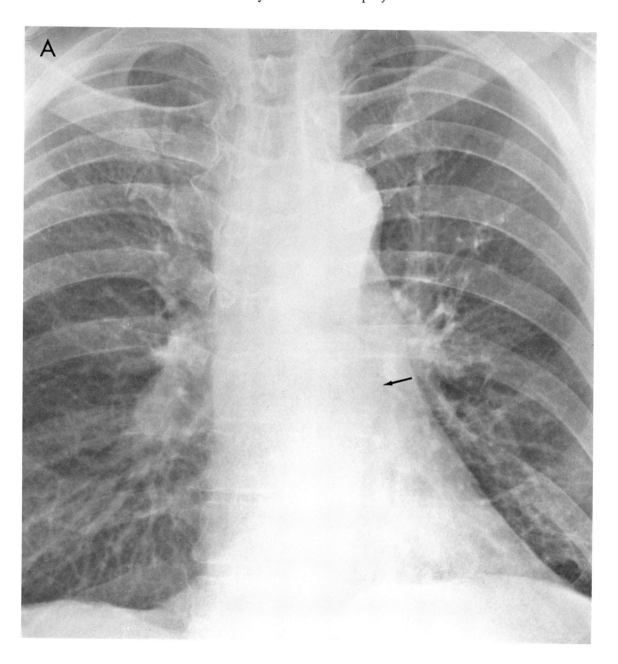

B, lateral projection: Showing a large mass (**arrows**) filling the normal aortic window and obliterating the outline of the distal trachea and its bifurcation (**x**). Normal vascular outlines are completely lost. The patient's physician could not be convinced of the abnormality at this time.

(Continued.)

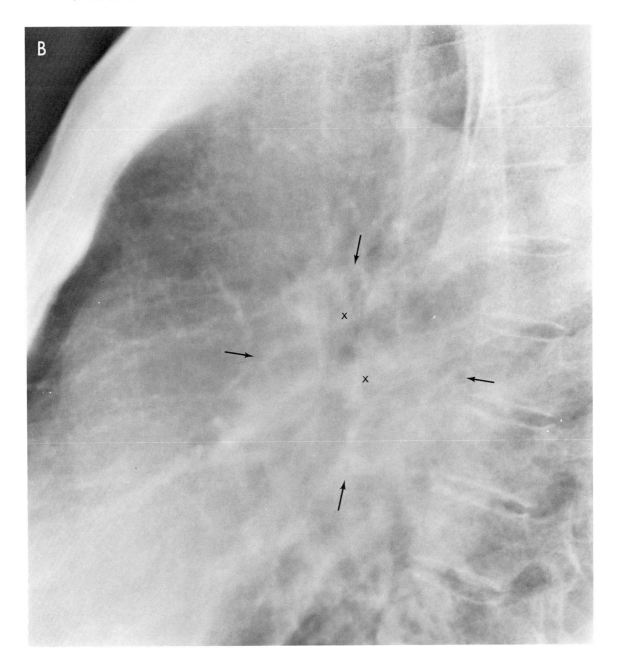

Figure 26 · Squamous Cell Carcinoma with Metastases / 73

Figure 26 (cont.).—Squamous cell carcinoma of left lower lobe bronchus with massive mediastinal invasion.

C, two months later: The lesion is larger and can now be seen through the cardiac shadow (**arrow**). Especially noticeable is a decrease in size of the vessels in the left lung as compared with **A,** and loss of the outlines of the major vessels in the left hilus.

A 65-year-old man saw his physician because of cough, bloody sputum and a wheeze. He had been a heavy smoker for many years. Results of the physical examination, except for a very audible wheeze over the midportion of the chest, were essentially negative. Bronchoscopy and biopsy revealed a squamous cell carcinoma involving the left lower lobe bronchus.

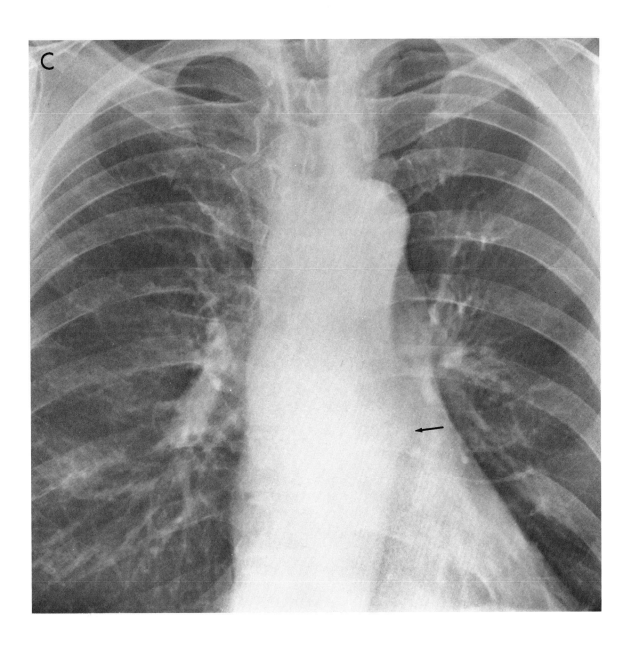

Figure 26 · Squamous Cell Carcinoma with Metastases / 75

Figure 27.—Squamous cell carcinoma with tracheal and superior vena caval invasion.

   A, posteroanterior radiograph: Revealing marked soft tissue widening of the superior mediastinum (**arrows**) and slight narrowing of the trachea at the level of the aortic knob (**a**).

   B, lateral projection: Showing posterior deviation of the esophagus and trachea with irregular narrowing of the trachea (**arrows**) by the mass (**x**).

   C, bilateral subclavian angiogram and superior venacavogram: Delineating considerable narrowing of the superior vena cava (**b**) with irregularities in the lumen (**c**), indicating tumor extension into the vessel.

   Thoracotomy revealed massive mediastinal invasion due to squamous cell carcinoma.

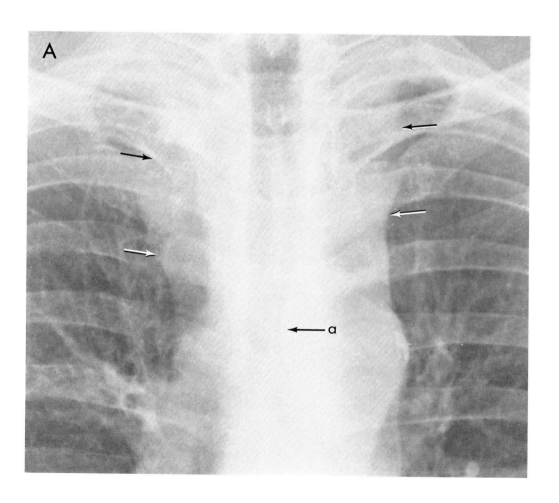

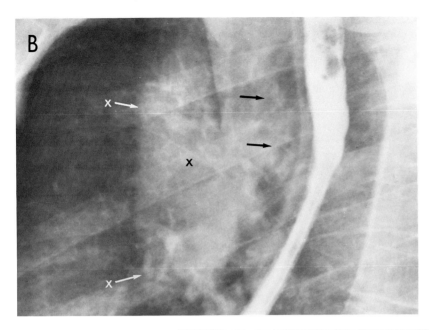

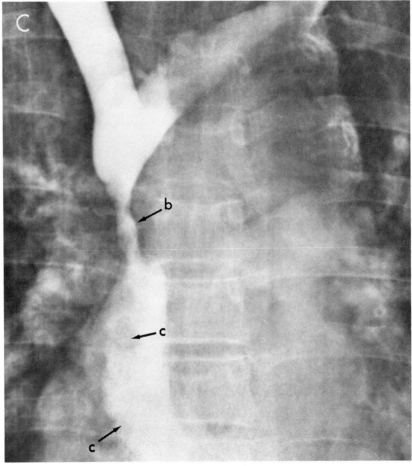

Figure 27 · Squamous Cell Carcinoma with Metastases / 77

Figure 28.—Anaplastic bronchial carcinoma.

A, posteroanterior radiograph: Revealing a nodular mass in the right cardiophrenic angle (**a**). Normal vascular margins in the inferior portion of the left hilus are lost (**b**).

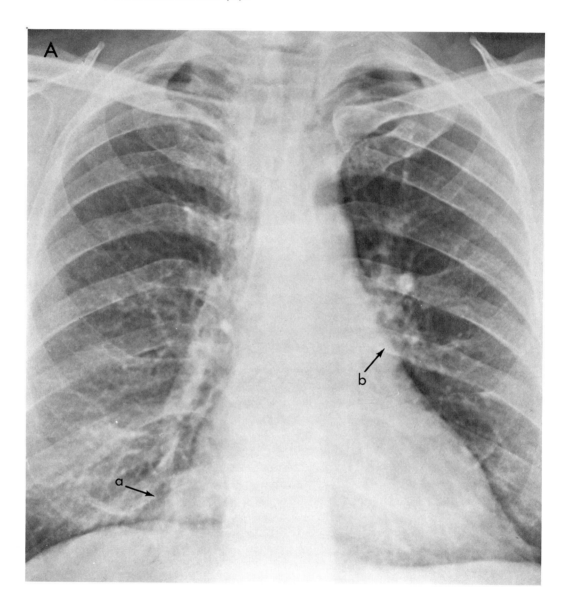

B, lateral projection: Indicating loss of clear visualization of hilar structures. The aortic window, tracheal bifurcation and vessels blend into a huge shaggy mass (**arrows**). The small nodular lesion in the right cardiophrenic angle seen in **A** is not visible.

(*Continued.*)

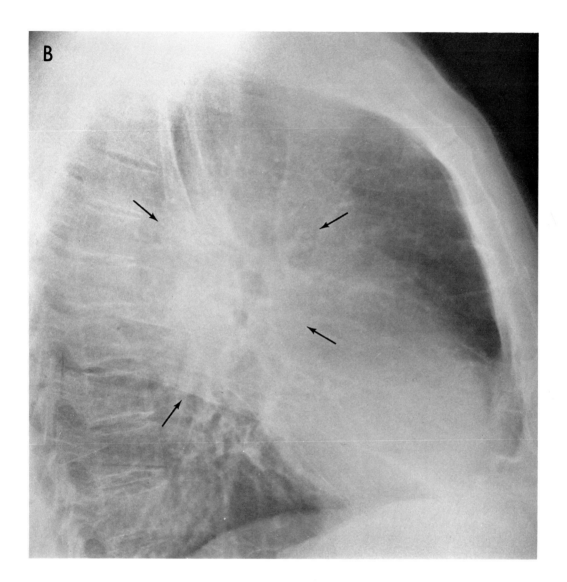

Figure 28 · Anaplastic Bronchial Carcinoma / 79

Figure 28 (cont.).—Anaplastic bronchial carcinoma.

C, body-section study: Revealing spreading of the major bronchi (**arrows**) and appreciable narrowing and irregularity of the left main stem bronchus (**c**). Some distortion of the bronchi to the right lower lobe is also present (**d**).

A 54-year-old man with a chronic cough presented symptoms of myasthenia gravis. The symptoms were believed to be secondary to a bronchogenic neoplasm. Biopsy of the left main stem bronchus revealed squamous cell carcinoma. There was transitory improvement of symptoms following radiation therapy to the mediastinum.

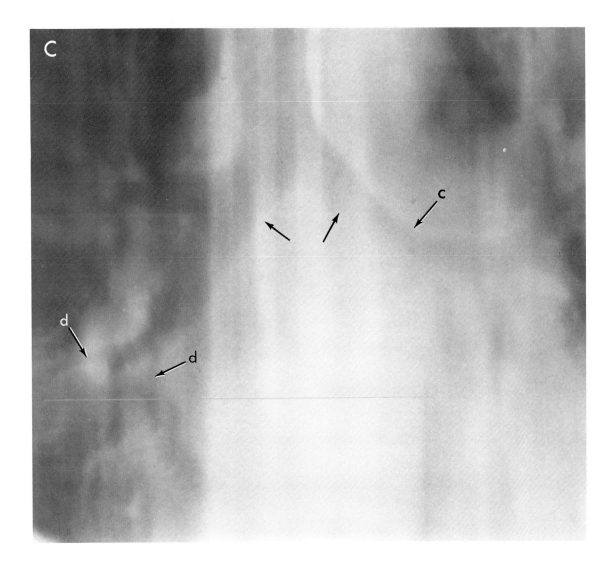

Figure 28 · Anaplastic Bronchial Carcinoma / 81

Figure 29.—Squamous cell carcinoma with mediastinal invasion.

A, initial posteroanterior radiograph: Revealing some blurring of the superior mediastinum bilaterally (**arrows**), especially noticeable along the superior vena cava (**a**). These findings were reported and further studies requested, but the observations were not considered significant enough by the referring physician to warrant further study at this time.

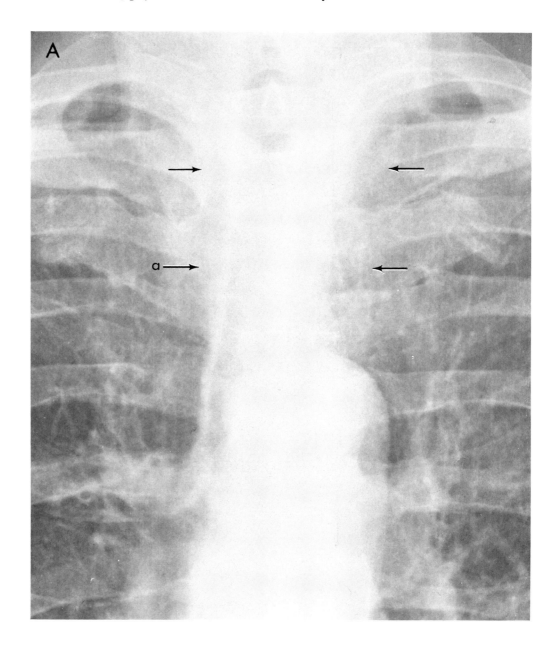

B, a year later: Showing an increase in the width and blurring of the superior mediastinum, especially to the right of the midline (**x**). The vena caval outline is completely lost, as are vascular shadows leading from the upper portion of the hilus to the upper lobe (**b**). In addition, a ragged-edged parenchymal mass is now visible in the right upper lobe (**c**).

(Continued.)

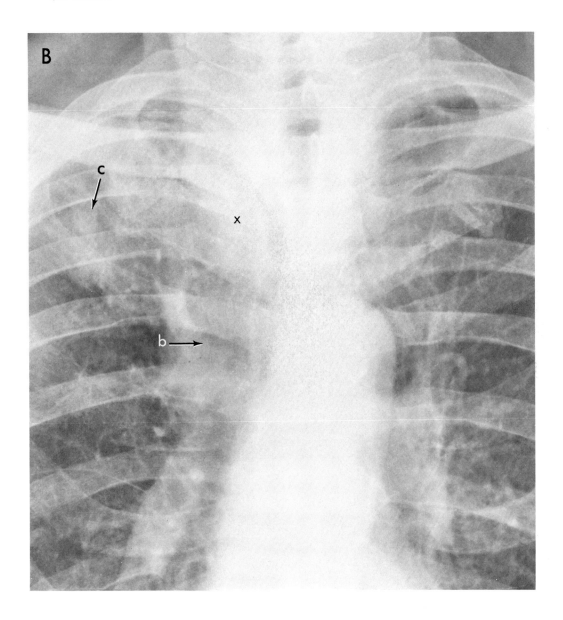

Figure 29 · Squamous Cell Carcinoma with Metastases / 83

Figure 29 (cont.).—Squamous cell carcinoma with mediastinal invasion.

C, lateral projection: Demonstrating a large tumor (**x**) in the superior mediastinum, where one is unable to identify clearly the margins of an air-filled trachea. An obvious soft tissue mass extends anteriorly and adjacent to and slightly behind the trachea and above the arch of the aorta (**d**).

A 55-year-old man who was a chronic smoker presented symptoms of epigastric distress. As part of his study, radiographs of the chest were obtained.

A year later, surgery disclosed a pulmonary parenchymal mass in the right upper lobe with extensive mediastinal invasion. The tumor surrounded a good portion of the superior vena cava on the right side. Examination of the removed material revealed squamous cell carcinoma with direct invasion of the mediastinum and mediastinal nodes. Prognosis was poor and the patient died five months after surgery, having had little benefit from palliative radiation therapy.

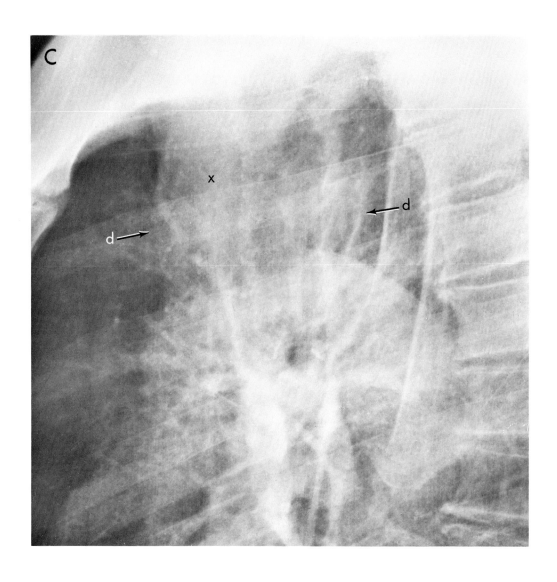

Figure 29 · Squamous Cell Carcinoma with Metastases / 85

Figure 30.—Squamous cell carcinoma of the right upper lobe with mediastinal invasion.

A, posteroanterior projection: Revealing an irregular dense widening of the mediastinum on the right side and a more sharply defined widening of the superior mediastinum on the left, extending to the region of the aortic arch (**arrows**). Several branching pseudopods appear in the right upper lobe where there are emphysematous blebs (**x**). Some upper lobe vascular distortion might be related to the blebs or the growing neoplasm.

B, close-up view of the lesion in **A,** better delineated here.

(*Continued.*)

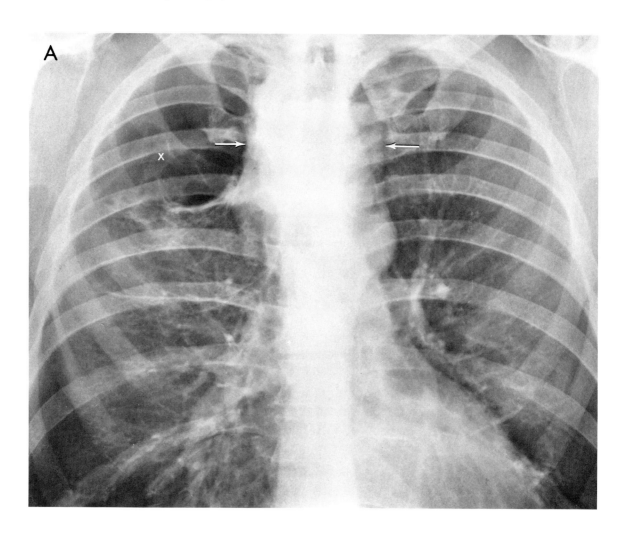

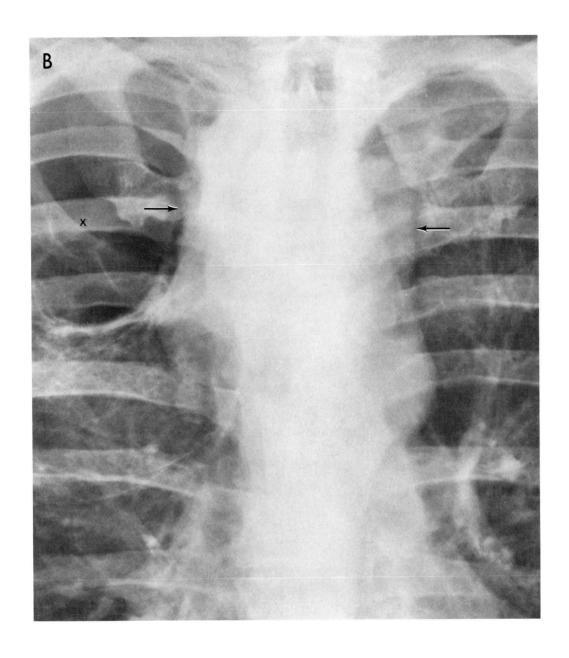

Figure 30 · Squamous Cell Carcinoma with Metastases / 87

Figure 30 (cont.).—Squamous cell carcinoma of the right upper lobe with mediastinal invasion.

C, lateral view: Demonstrating a rather ill-defined mass (**y**) gradually fading into the soft tissues posteriorly and causing anterior displacement of the esophagus and trachea (**a**) without appreciable narrowing.

A 54-year-old man saw his physician because of a wheeze, cough and some dyspnea. In spite of the location and suspected inoperability of the lesion, thoracotomy was performed. Biopsy study revealed a squamous cell carcinoma. Massive mediastinal invasion that encompassed the major vessels was demonstrated.

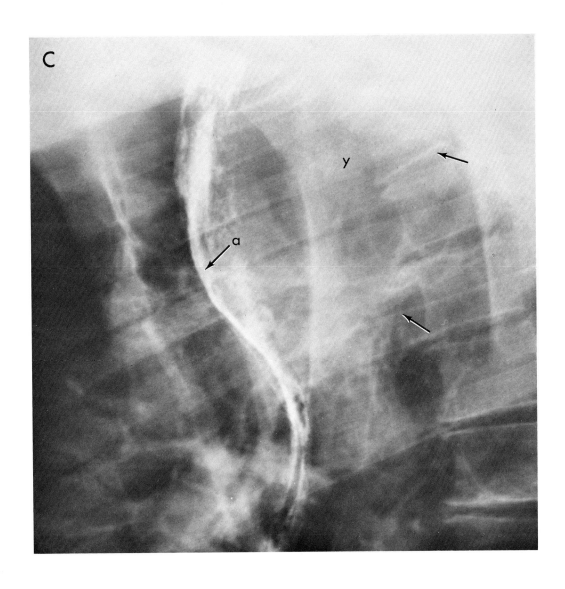

Figure 30 · Squamous Cell Carcinoma with Metastases / 89

Figure 31.—Squamous cell carcinoma of the left upper lobe.

A, posteroanterior radiograph: Revealing widening of the superior mediastinum (**arrows**) and an ill-defined mass in the left upper lobe (**a**).

B, close-up view of changes in **A.**

C, supine body-section radiograph through the mass: Delineating a pulmonary nodule with ragged margins and multiple pseudopods extending into the adjacent lung (**arrows**). The characteristics of the margins are indicative of a malignant process in the lung. The soft tissue widening of the mediastinum is not as apparent in this exposure.

A 66-year-old man who had been a heavy smoker for many years was seen because of a single episode of blood-streaked sputum. He had no other complaints, and results of the physical examination were within normal limits. At lobectomy the mass was found to be limited to the left upper lobe with no mediastinal extension. The pathologic diagnosis was squamous cell carcinoma.

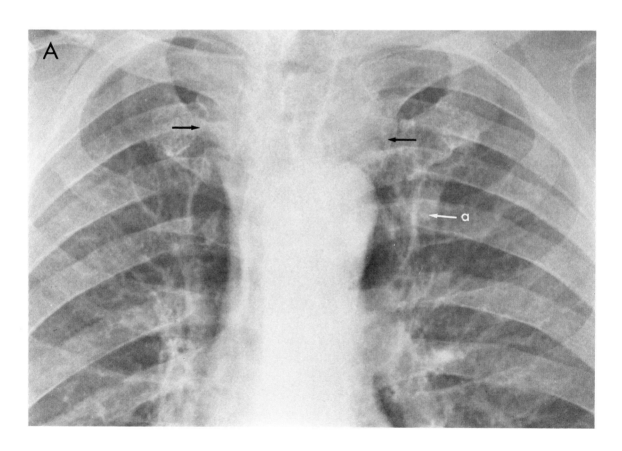

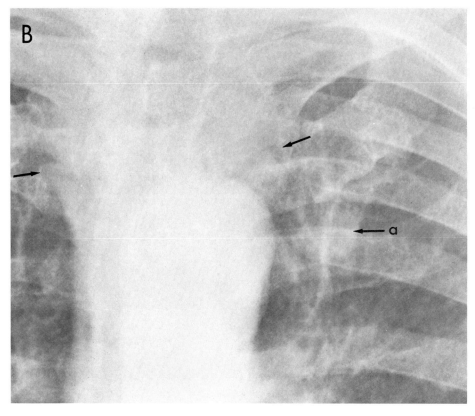

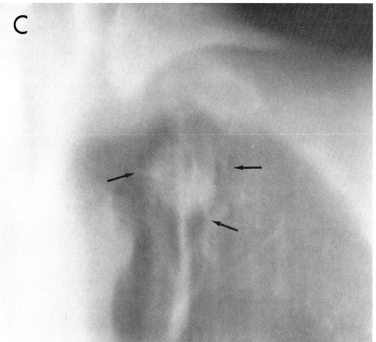

Figure 31 · Squamous Cell Carcinoma: Left Upper Lobe / 91

Figure 32.—Squamous cell carcinoma with extensive nodal metastases.

This patient's original conventional radiographs, not available for reproduction, revealed an apparent mass adjacent to the right hilus. It was uncertain whether this represented a nodal or a pulmonary parenchymal lesion.

A, supine body-section radiograph: Delineating a multilobulated, nodular soft tissue change adjacent to the hilar vessels on the right side (**a**). This contains no calcification. No definite other parenchymal lesion can be identified. **b** indicates the normal azygos vein.

B, bronchial arteriogram: Outlining several fairly large vessels leading to the region of the nodularity. The vessels within the nodular abnormality are

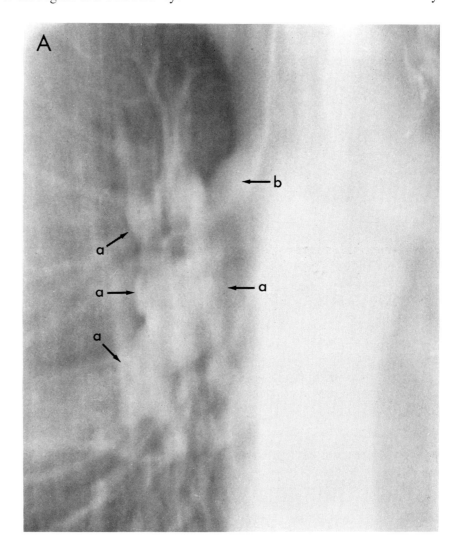

tortuous and irregular and increase somewhat in size as they proceed peripherally. A slight tumor stain is also present (**arrows**). At present, needle biopsy or bronchial brushing would seem to be the diagnostic study of choice to determine the nature of such lesions if the etiology is in question or thoracotomy is refused.

A 56-year-old woman who had been a heavy smoker for many years complained of a change in character of her cough and bloody sputum. A pneumonectomy disclosed a small pulmonary parenchymal mass adjacent to the inferior portion of the right hilus. The major masses seen in the body-section radiograph and arteriogram represent enlarged hilar nodes containing metastatic tumor. The pathologic diagnosis was squamous cell cancer with extensive nodal metastases.

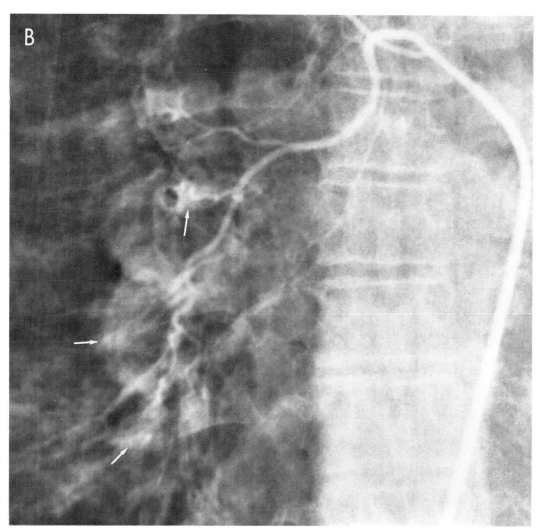

Figure 32 · Squamous Cell Carcinoma with Metastases / 93

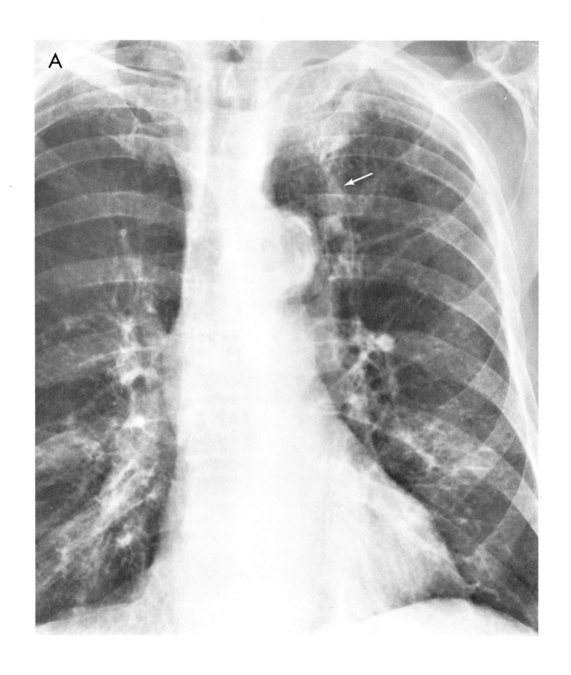

Figure 33.—Squamous cell carcinoma with apical chest wall invasion.

A, posteroanterior radiograph: Demonstrating a difference in aeration in the two lung apices, the left being less well ventilated than the right. Evidence of an ill-defined soft tissue mass extends from the apex into the left hilus (**arrow**).

B and **C,** body-section radiographs through the left apex: Revealing a large tumor (**x**) which extends into the soft tissues in the supraclavicular area.

A 70-year-old man was seen because of increasing dyspnea and a changing cough. His physician was not convinced that the changes represented cancer until it was proved by needle biopsy of the area which revealed squamous cell carcinoma.

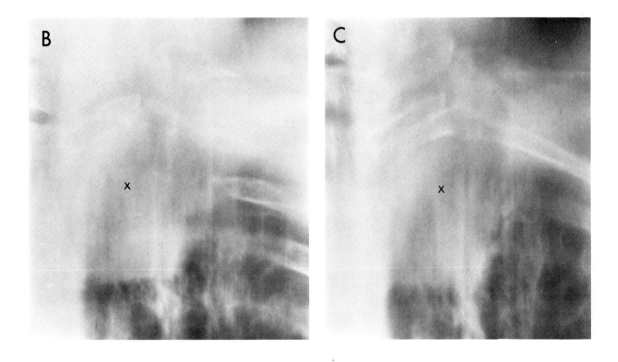

Figure 33 · Squamous Cell Carcinoma with Metastases / 95

Figure 34.—Squamous cell carcinoma of the left lower lobe.

A, posteroanterior radiograph: Revealing a small ill-defined nodule in the left midlung field (**arrow**).

B, supine body-section radiograph: Demonstrating a faint, spiculated ill-defined nodule with a margin characteristic of early cancer.

The patient was a 65-year-old woman who had a routine chest radiograph prior to repair of a cystocele. A left lower lobectomy was performed. Pathologic study revealed a primary squamous cell carcinoma.

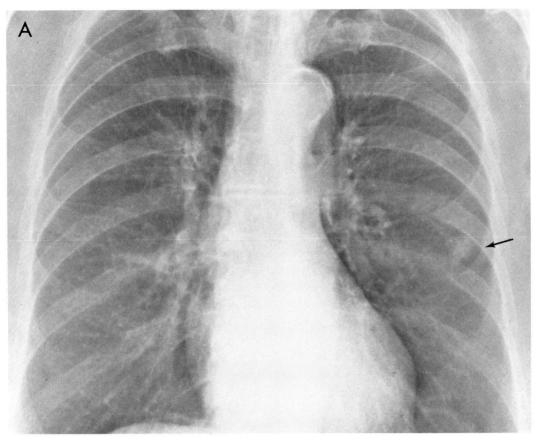

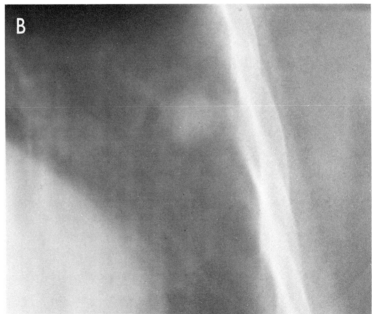

Figure 34 · Squamous Cell Carcinoma: Left Lower Lobe / 97

Figure 35.—Squamous cell carcinoma of the right upper lobe.

A, posteroanterior radiograph: Revealing a small ill-defined hazy lesion in the right first anterior interspace (**arrow**).

B, close-up of lesion in **A.**

C, supine body-section study: Demonstrating the lesion to better advantage as a solid nodular area with the spiculated margins characteristic of a primary neoplasm.

A 53-year-old man who was a heavy smoker with a chronic nonproductive cough sought help because he noted blood-streaked sputum on several occasions. Right upper lobectomy revealed a tumor confined to this area of the lung. Pathologic study revealed squamous cell carcinoma without vascular invasion.

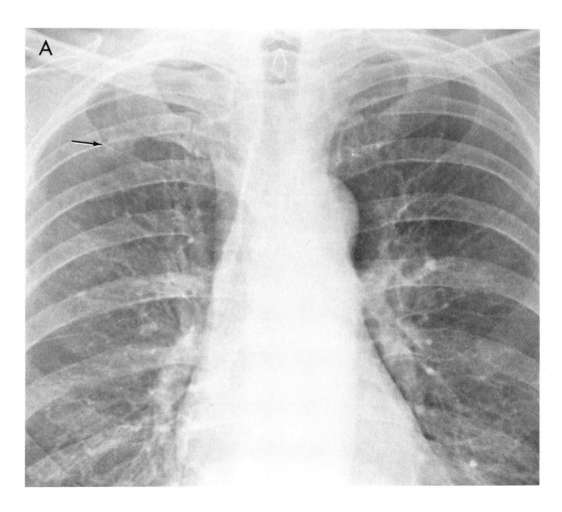

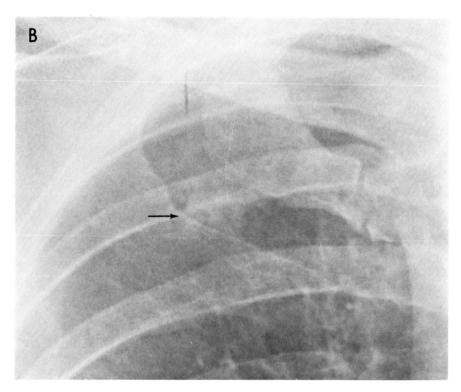

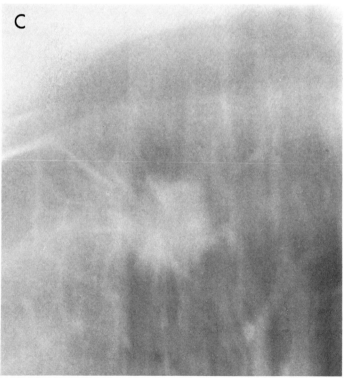

Figure 35 · Squamous Cell Carcinoma: Right Upper Lobe / 99

Figure 36.—Squamous cell carcinoma of the left upper lobe.

A, posteroanterior radiograph: Revealing an ill-defined mass (**arrow**) in the left upper lobe. (This is much better demonstrated in this reproduction than in the original radiographs.) There was considerable discussion between the patient's physician and the radiologists, the latter suspecting a tumor but unable to convince the referring physician.

B, close-up of the lesion in **A,** also better seen here than in the original film.

C, 9 months later: Showing an ill-defined shadow in the interspace between the anterior ends of the left first and second ribs (**arrow**). (In spite of urgings, the significance of the picture still was not appreciated by the patient's physician.)

(*Continued.*)

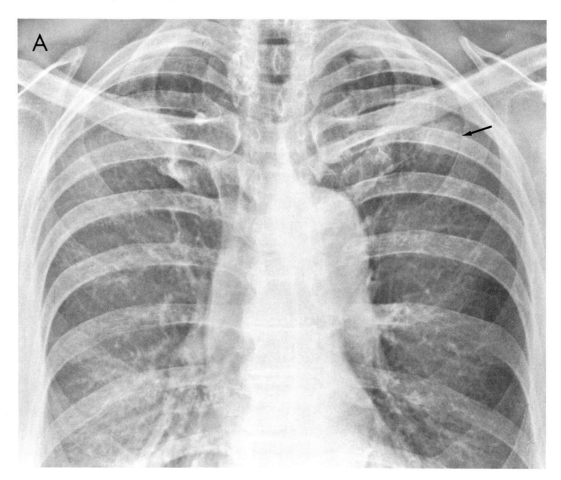

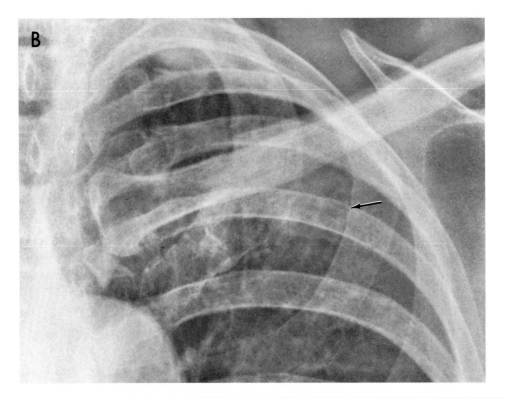

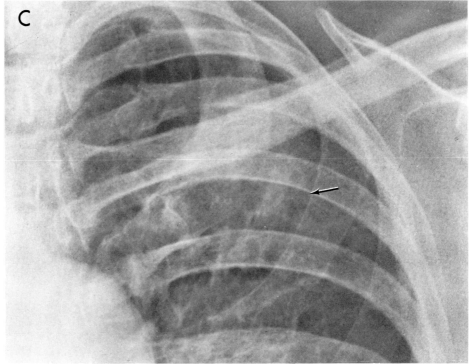

Figure 36 · Squamous Cell Carcinoma: Left Upper Lobe / 101

Figure 36 (cont.).—Squamous cell carcinoma of the left upper lobe.

D, 6 months later (16 months after detection of the original shadow): Now revealing a definite lesion (**arrow**).

E, supine body-section radiographs through the involved area: Demonstrating the irregular margins with pseudopods extending into the adjacent pulmonary parenchyma characteristic of a primary neoplasm.

A 71-year-old woman consulted her physician because of intermittent discomfort in the right upper quadrant. As part of her examination, a chest radiograph was obtained. At left upper lobectomy, a squamous cell neoplasm identified. No mediastinal or nodal extensions were demonstrable.

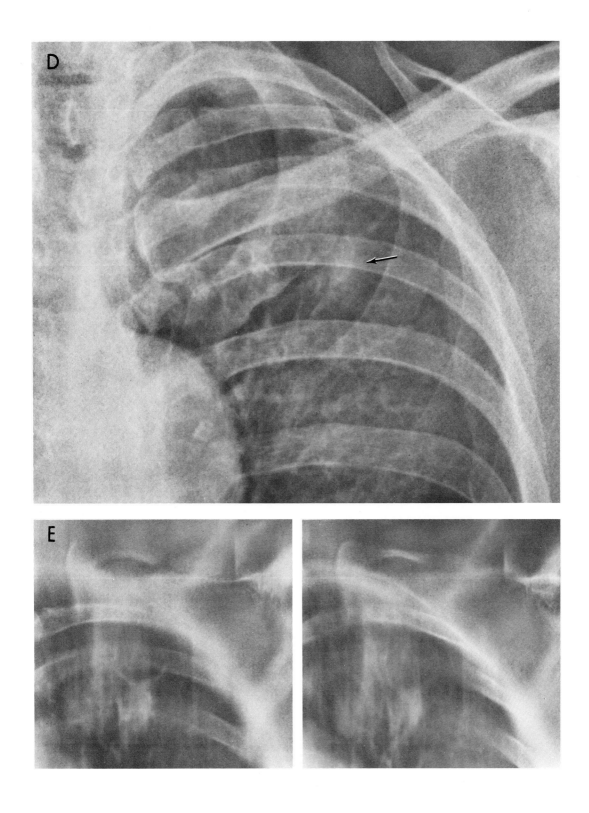

Figure 36 · Squamous Cell Carcinoma: Left Upper Lobe / 103

Figure 37.—Squamous cell carcinoma of the left upper lobe.

Posteroanterior radiograph: Revealing a rounded nodule (**arrow**) with serrations and pseudopodlike extensions into the surrounding pulmonary parenchyma in the left upper lobe.

A 50-year-old heavy smoker with an old history of tuberculosis was seen because of cough and blood-streaked sputum. Left upper lobectomy and pathologic study revealed a squamous cell carcinoma without extension or blood vessel invasion. Prognosis should be good.

Comment: Such lesions should be evaluated when first seen and not passed off simply as an old tuberculous scar. This appearance is most suggestive of a small neoplasm.

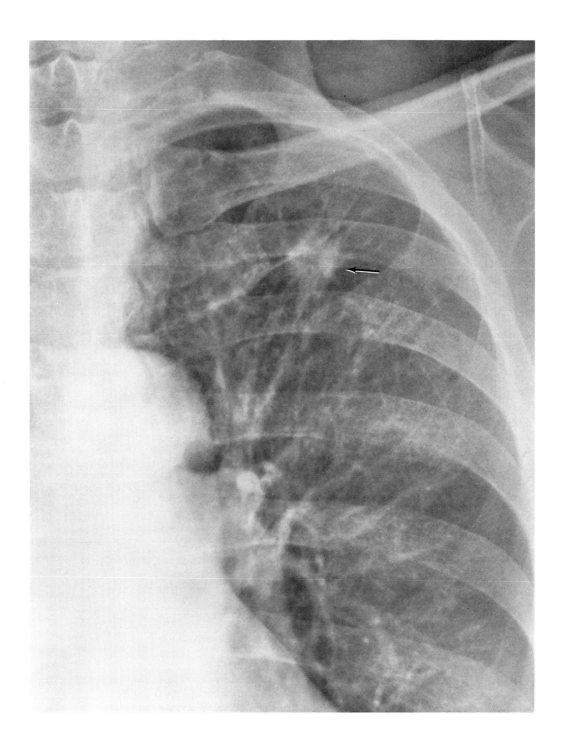

Figure 37 · Squamous Cell Carcinoma: Left Upper Lobe / 105

Figure 38.—Squamous carcinoma of the left upper lobe.

A, posteroanterior radiograph: Revealing a peculiar linear shadow with nodular components (**arrows**) along its course and dendritic extensions into the adjacent lung (**a**). In addition, the upper margin of the pulmonary vessel in the hilus cannot be followed clearly (**b**).

B, lateral projection: Showing the linear (**a**) and nodular (**arrows**) shadows in the posterior inferior portion of the left upper lobe.

A 60-year-old man had had numerous previous bouts of pneumonia. With the most recent episode, clearing was very slow and the linear change persisted for about six weeks. Sputum examination at this time revealed malignant cells. Thoracotomy and left upper lobectomy disclosed a squamous cell neoplasm with some lymphatic extension to the hilar nodes.

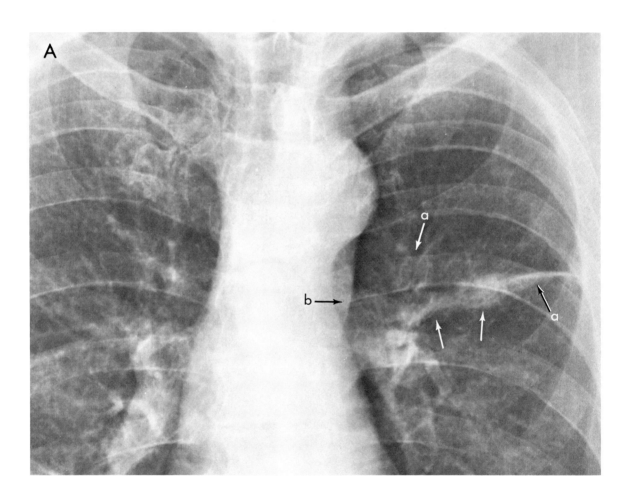

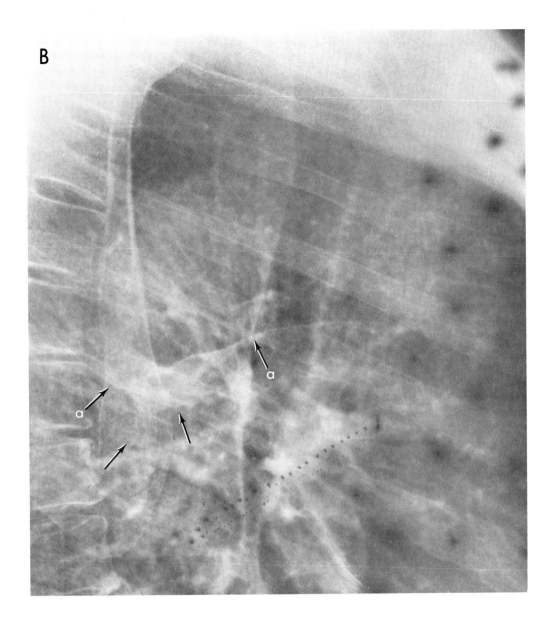

B

Figure 38 · Squamous Cell Carcinoma: Left Upper Lobe / 107

Figure 39.—Squamous cell carcinoma of the right upper lobe.

A, posteroanterior radiograph: Indicating some distortion and enlargement of several vessels leading to the right upper lobe (**arrow**).

B, body-section radiograph: Revealing the multilobed appearance of the lesion (**arrow**) and evidence of some impression upon the segmental upper lobe bronchus (**a**).

A 49-year-old man who was a heavy smoker consulted his physician because of a change in his cough. On right upper lobectomy a lesion was found in the lung without mediastinal or hilar extension. Pathologic analysis revealed squamous cell carcinoma.

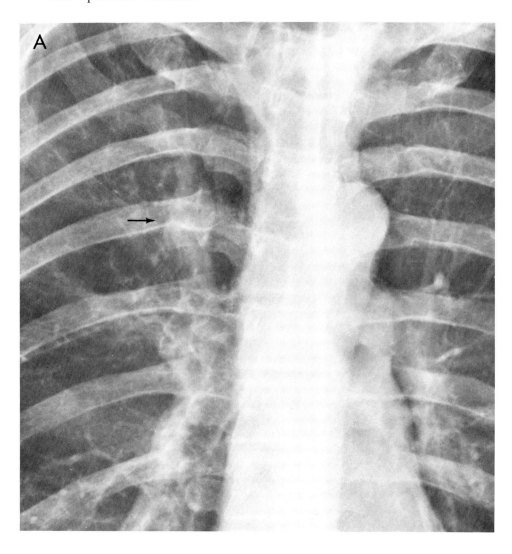

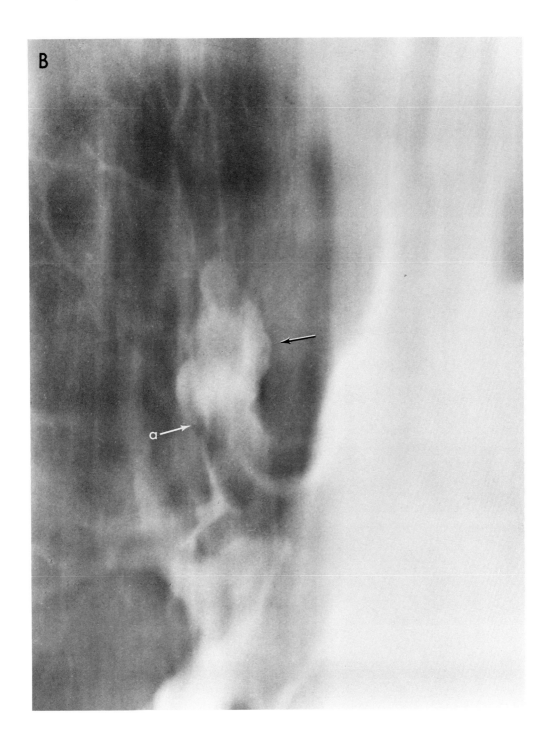

Figure 39 · Squamous Cell Carcinoma: Right Upper Lobe / 109

Figure 40.—Squamous cell carcinoma of the right lower lobe.

A, posteroanterior projection: Revealing loss of the normal pulmonary arterial outlines in the right hilar area (**a**) which extend into adjacent cardiac margins, losing their identity. This soft tissue density blends with clublike processes extending into the lower lobe (**x**). A portion of the right cardiac border is visible (**b**), indicating the posterior location of the lesion.

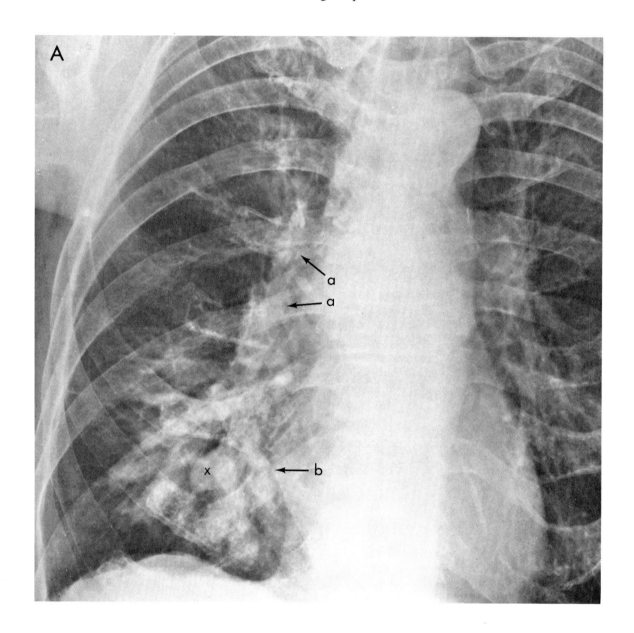

B, lateral view: Demonstrating loss of normal vascular shadows. A large mass with ill-defined margins blends with the hilar shadows (**a**). The club-like shadows (**x**) occupy the posterior portion of the right lower lobe.

(Continued.)

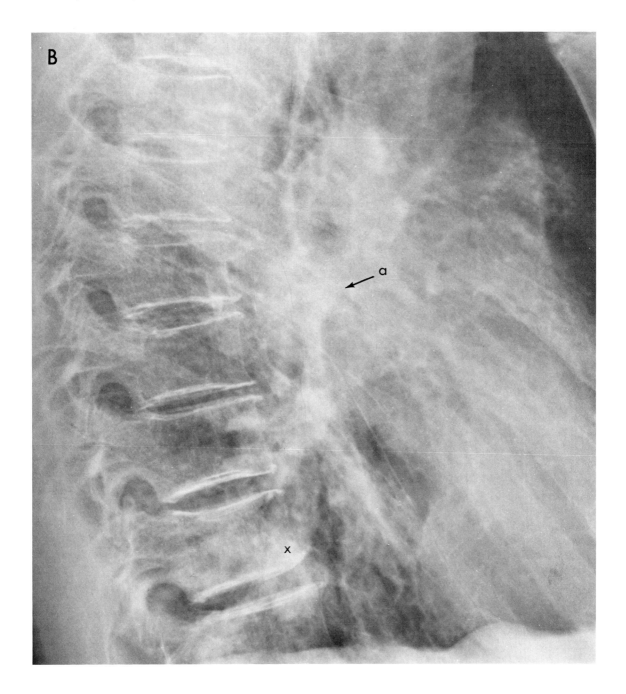

Figure 40 · Squamous Cell Carcinoma: Right Lower Lobe / 111

Figure 40 (cont.).—Squamous cell carcinoma of the right lower lobe.

C and **D,** posteroanterior and oblique projections, barium bronchogram: Revealing an abrupt cut-off of the right lower lobe bronchus (**c**). Although no contrast medium goes beyond this point, air must move in and out because there is only partial collapse of the right lower lobe. Spatial rearrangement of the remaining lung to occupy the volume loss in the right lower lobe has occurred: note the downward shift with slight spread of the right middle lobe

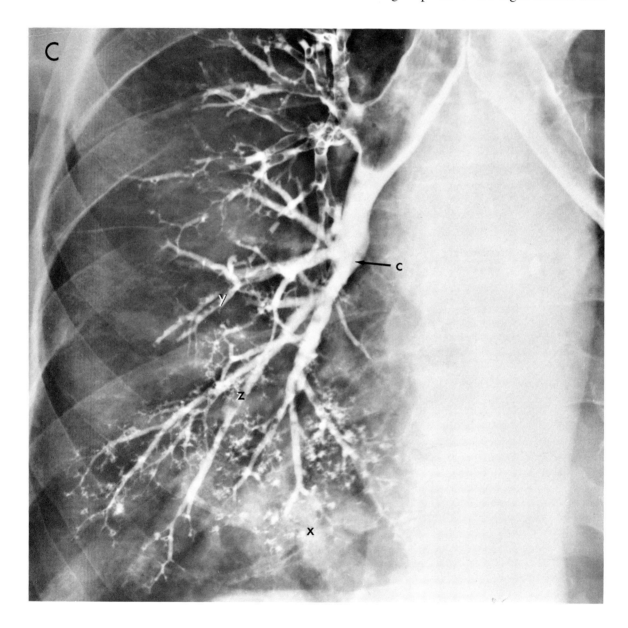

bronchi (**y**) and the superior segmental bronchi of the lower lobe (**z**). **x** indicates the clublike shadows seen in **A** and **B**.

A 58-year-old man had had blood-tingled sputum intermittently for two years and in addition produced ½−1 cup of sputum daily. Bronchoscopy and right pneumonectomy were performed. Pathologic study revealed squamous cell carcinoma with hilar and mediastinal invasion.

Figure 40, courtesy of Dr. Sidney Nelson, Ohio State University, Columbus.

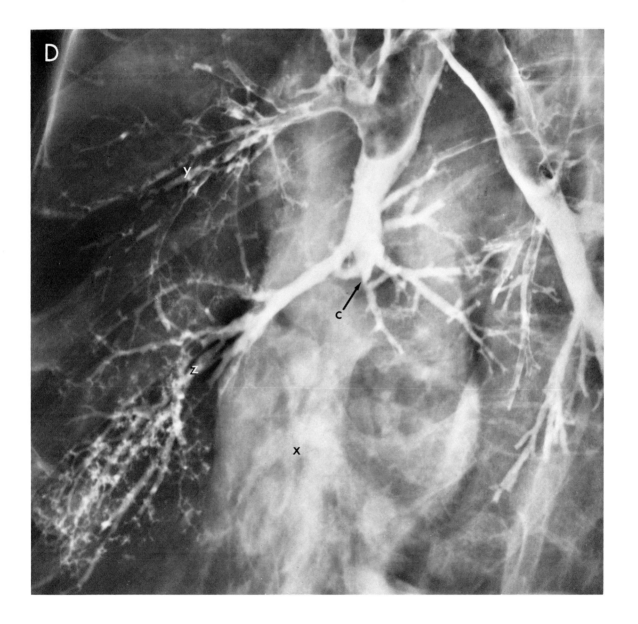

Figure 40 · Squamous Cell Carcinoma: Right Lower Lobe / 113

Figure 41.—Squamous cell carcinoma of the left lower lobe.

A, posteroanterior projection: Indicating a barely discernible linear shadow behind the heart (**arrow**) and loss of normal vessel outlines in the area just adjacent to the cardiac border on the left (**a**).

B, lateral projection: Showing an ill-defined shadow occupying the region of the left lower lobe (**x**). A ragged, more solid appearing shadow blends with the inferior hilar vessels (**c**).

C, left anterior oblique projection, barium bronchogram: Demonstrating rough tapering of the left lower bronchus and proximal lingular segmental branch of the left upper lobe (**arrows**). There is complete occlusion of all but the anterior basal segment of the left lower lobe (**d**).

A 50-year-old man consulted his physician because of an intermittent wheeze. Bronchoscopy and left pneumonectomy were performed. Pathologic diagnosis was squamous cell cancer.

Figure 41, courtesy of Dr. Sidney Nelson, Ohio State University, Columbus.

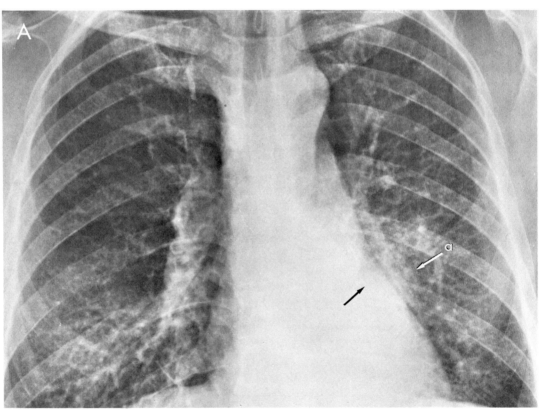

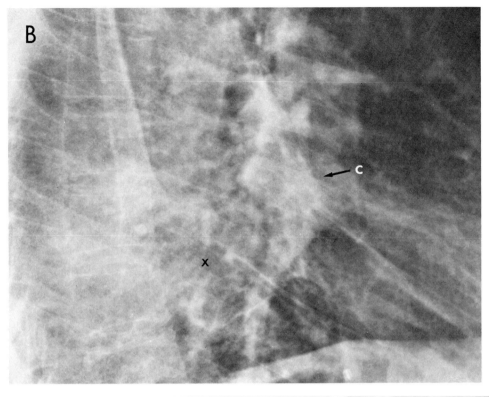

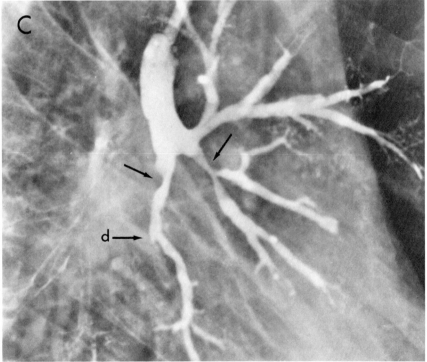

Figure 41 · Squamous Cell Carcinoma: Left Lower Lobe / 115

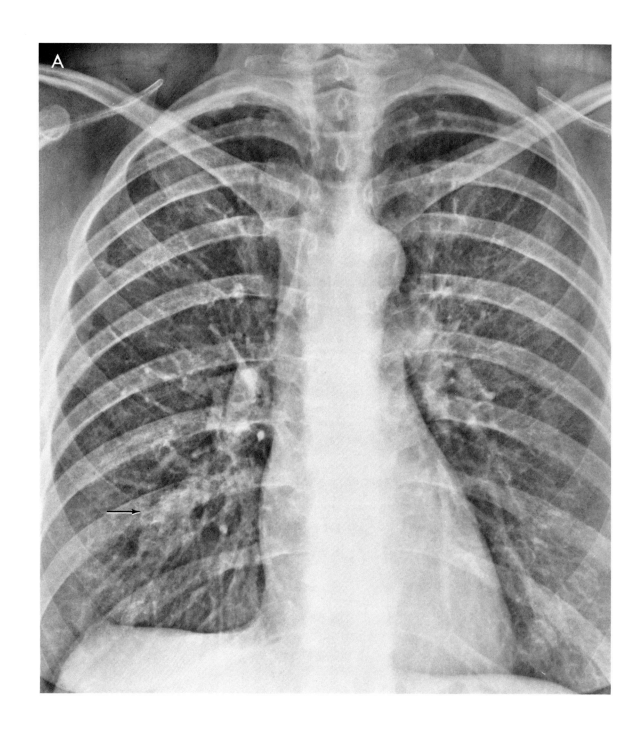

Figure 42.—Squamous cell carcinoma of the right lower lobe.

A, posteroanterior radiograph: Revealing an ill-defined hazy shadow blending with the adjacent vessels in the right lower lobe (**arrow**).

B, close-up of lesion in **A**: Showing it to better advantage.

(*Continued.*)

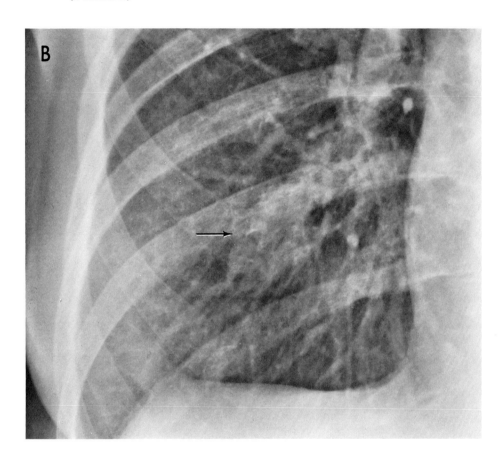

Figure 42 · Squamous Cell Carcinoma: Right Lower Lobe / 117

Figure 42 (cont.).—Squamous cell carcinoma of the right lower lobe.

C, lateral projection, barium bronchogram: Demonstrating an abrupt round cut-off of the anterior segmental bronchus to the right lower lobe (**a**). The vague soft tissue mass is visible just below this area (**x**).

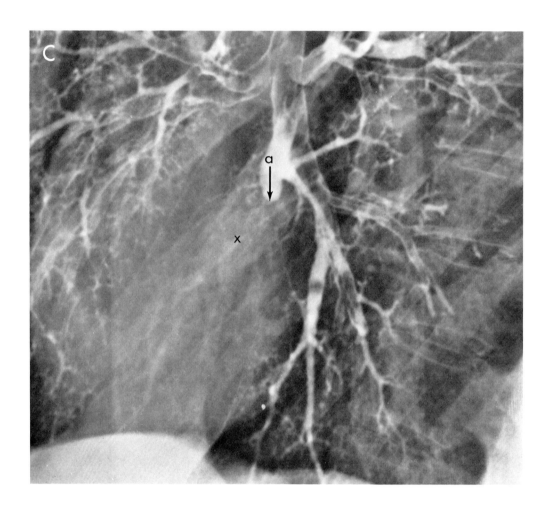

D, left anterior oblique projection: Showing a similar picture of occlusion of the bronchus (**a**). Some superimposition of smaller branching bronchi is present.

A 49-year-old woman reported dyspnea and hemoptysis of about a month's duration. Right lower lobectomy and pathologic study revealed squamous cell cancer.

Figure 42, courtesy of Dr. Sidney Nelson, Ohio State University, Columbus.

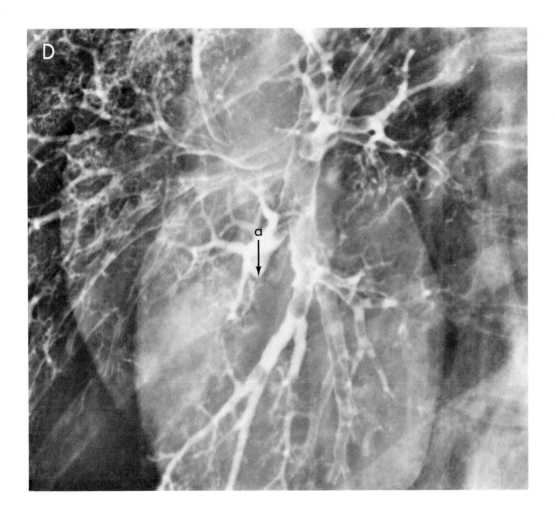

Figure 42 · Squamous Cell Carcinoma: Right Lower Lobe / 119

Figure 43.—Squamous cell carcinoma of the right upper lobe.

A, posteroanterior radiograph: Delineating a large shaggy mass extending to the mediastinum in the right upper lobe and causing narrowing of the right main stem bronchus (**arrow**). Adjacent patchy consolidation of broncho-pneumonia (**x**) is also present. The lesion represents a rather characteristic carcinoma.

B, posteroanterior roentgenogram, exposed 18 months before **A.** At this time a tiny opacification in the parenchyma of the right upper lobe (**a**) was described. Early distortion of the normal vascular markings in the upper lobe (**arrows**), a manifestation of early cancer, was overlooked.

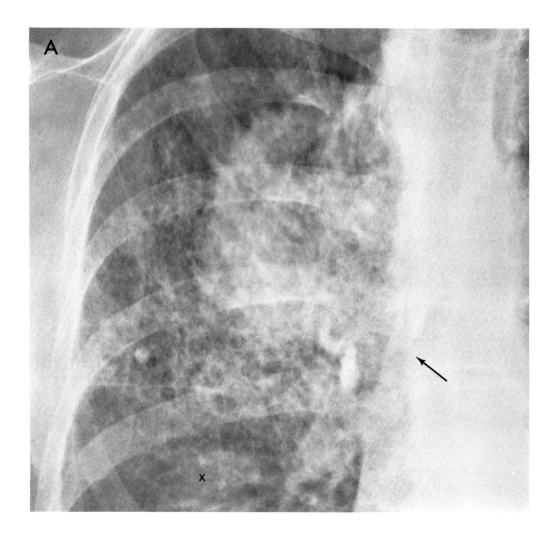

C, posteroanterior exposure, made 2 months after **B** (16 months before **A**): Showing what was considered to be an old scar; but there is an obvious mass (**y**) near the mediastinum. The tiny parenchymal calcification present in **B(a)** is now displaced laterally (**arrow**). At this point it should have been evident that this patient had a neoplasm in the upper lobe. Instead, this was interpreted as being a change in the old inflammatory disease.

This 60-year-old woman was initially seen by the authors at the time **A** was made, when she had chills, fever, cough and blood-streaked sputum. A thoracotomy was performed. Direct mediastinal and nodal invasion was found, necessitating a pneumonectomy. Pathologic diagnosis was squamous cell carcinoma. The prognosis is now poor, but might have been good 16 months earlier.

Comment: The importance of a high index of suspicion with even slight radiographic change cannot be overemphasized.

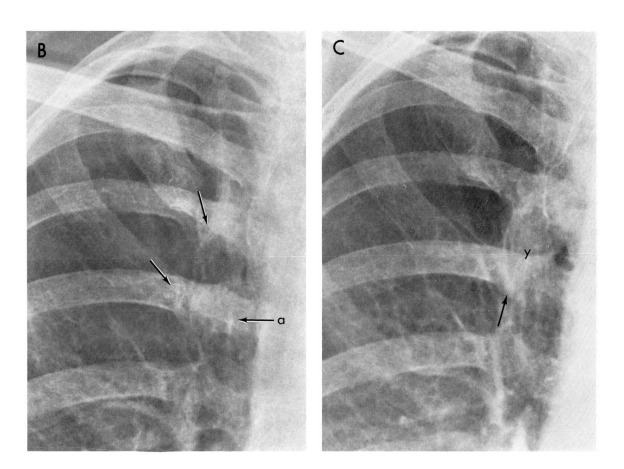

Figure 43 · Squamous Cell Carcinoma: Right Upper Lobe / 121

Figure 44.—Developing squamous cell carcinoma.

A, posteroanterior exposure: Showing several linear streaks and a tiny, barely visible nodular area in the right upper lobe (**a**).

B, posteroanterior projection one year later: Revealing considerable change, with a small amount of pleural tenting (**arrow**) and a little enlargement of the nodular area in the right upper lobe (**a**).

C, posteroanterior projection two years after **A,** one year after **B**: Now revealing an obvious large mass in the right upper lobe (**x**).

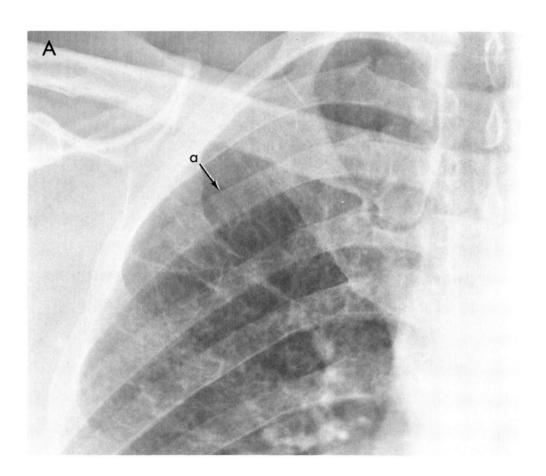

A 60-year-old man with active tuberculosis was treated and apparently cured. He was carefully followed radiographically, but the slight changes in the first of this series of radiographs (**A**) were not appreciated. On numerous repeat studies, each radiographic picture was compared with the one obtained three months previously; thus the very slight changes between each new study and that immediately preceding were not deemed significant. Attempted resection disclosed considerable invasion of the chest wall, and pathologic analysis of biopsy material revealed squamous cell carcinoma.

Comment: This case demonstrates again the absolute need to compare the current radiographic picture with the *earliest* studies in order to distinguish subtle changes.

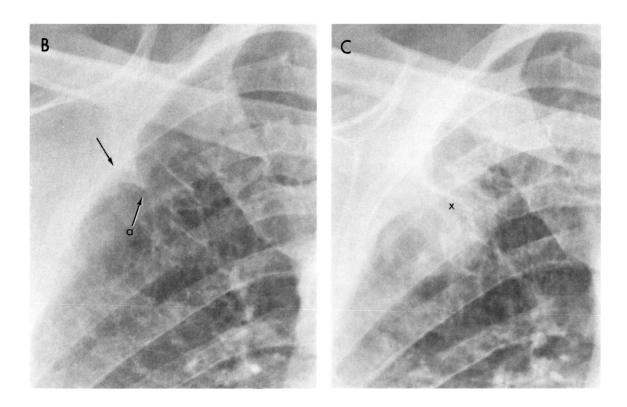

Figure 44 · Developing Squamous Cell Carcinoma / 123

Figure 45.—Primary squamous cell carcinoma of the trachea.

A, posteroanterior radiograph: Indicating an ill-defined widening of the superior mediastinum (**arrows**).

B, lateral projection: Demonstrating a soft tissue mass (**arrows**) that blurs the normal sharp outlines between the trachea and adjacent lung.

C, body-section radiograph, with patient supine: Revealing narrowing of the trachea with irregular rough margins (**arrows**). The paratracheal soft tissue mass is obvious on the left side (**x**).

D, with contrast material in the trachea: Accentuating the irregularity of the long involved midportion of the trachea (**arrows**).

A 45-year-old man consulted his physician because of repeated bouts of hemoptysis. Physical examination and laboratory studies were not contributory. Bronchoscopy revealed a friable long lesion in the trachea. Pathologic diagnosis of tissue from the lesion was primary squamous cell carcinoma.

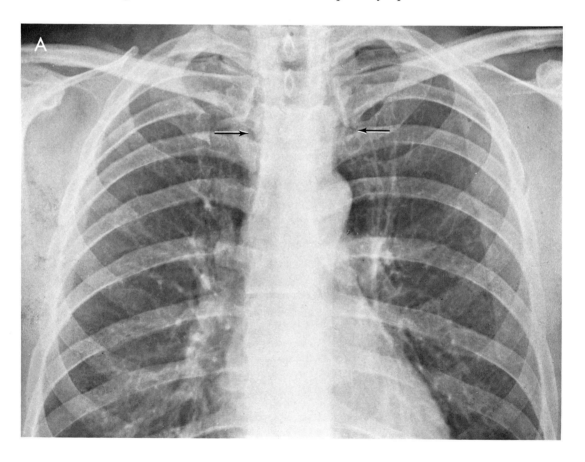

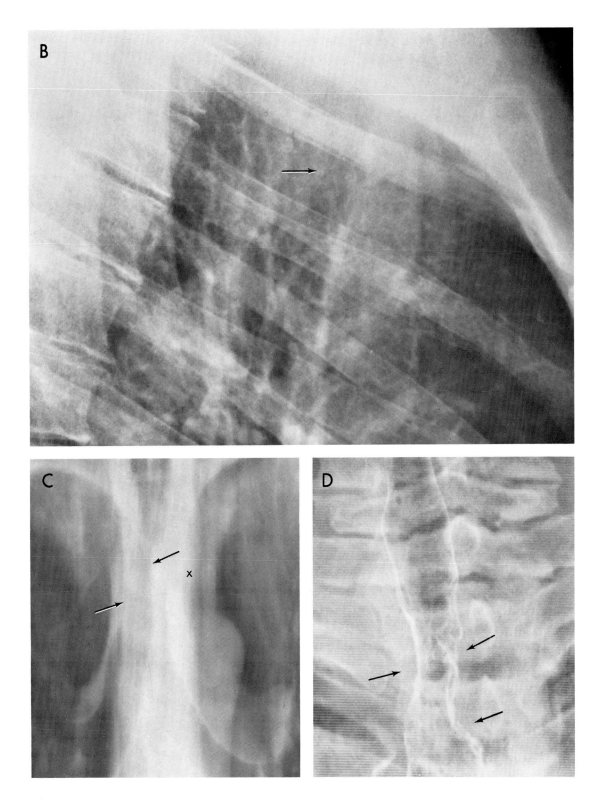

Figure 45 · Squamous Cell Carcinoma of Trachea / 125

Figure 46.—Developing squamous cell carcinoma.

    A, posteroanterior radiograph: Revealing a large mass (**x**), fluffy and having shaggy margins, in the left upper lobe. The outlines of the major hilar vessels (**y**) are ill-defined. Because of a history of tuberculosis, antituberculous therapy was instituted.

    (Continued.)

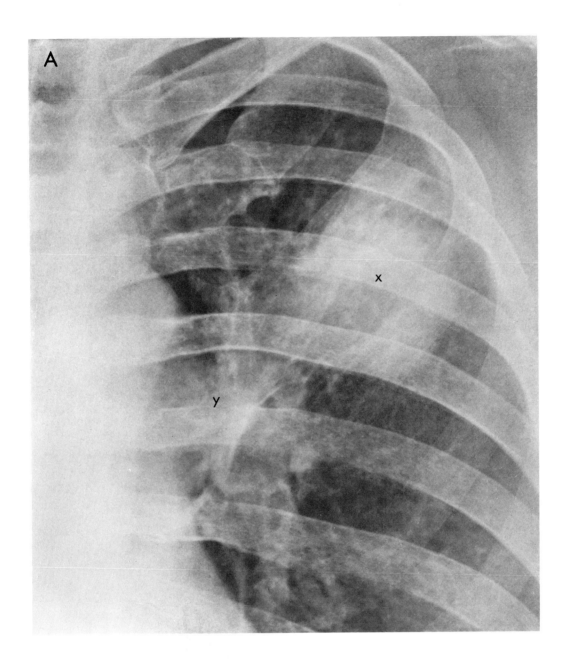

Figure 46 · Developing Squamous Cell Carcinoma / 127

Figure 46 (cont.).—Developing squamous cell carcinoma.

B, after two weeks of antituberculous therapy: Showing remarkable regression of the massive parenchymal lesion (**x**). Again, however, the margins and borders of the hilar vessels cannot be seen (**y**). Aerating lung (**z**) is present in the area which should be filled by normal vascular structures.

C, posteroanterior projection six months after **B**: Demonstrating continued failure to define the major vessels, but now they are obscured by a huge mass extending into the pulmonary parenchyma. Several small, barely visible

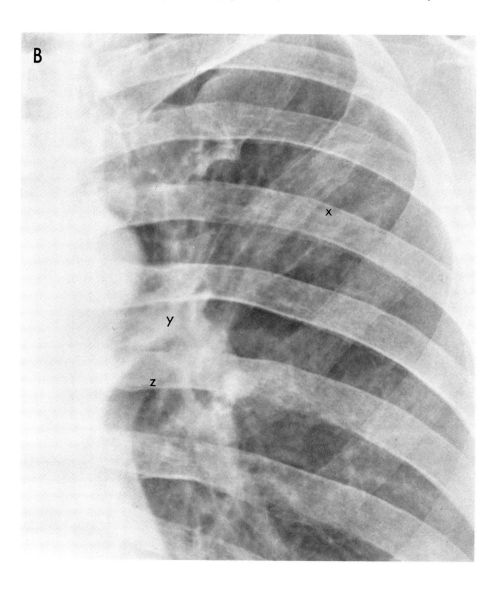

calcifications, not previously demonstrable, are now present in the mass (**arrow**); these were probably carried laterally with growth of the mass.

A 50-year-old man had been previously treated for tuberculosis. At the time of the initial study (**A**) he was seen because of an episode of chills, fever and hemoptysis: He was immediately placed on antituberculous therapy, which was continued in spite of inability to recover acid-fast organisms from the sputum. For some reason, after the initial clearing (**B**) subsequent radiographic study was delayed for six months. Thoracotomy disclosed massive hilar invasion. Pathologic study of biopsy material revealed squamous cell cancer.

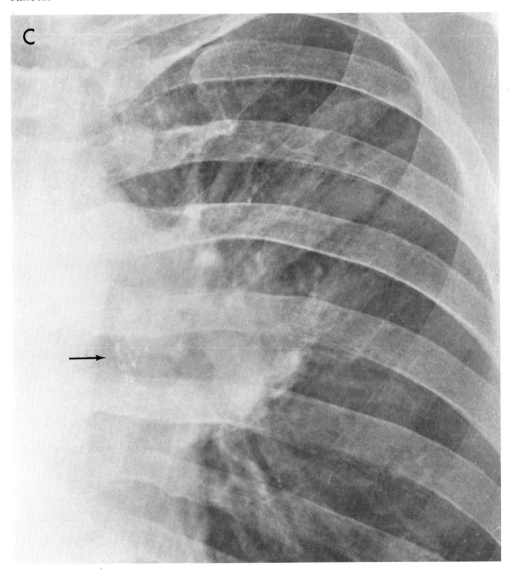

Figure 46 · Developing Squamous Cell Carcinoma / 129

Figure 47.—Squamous cell carcinoma developing adjacent to an old granuloma.

   A, posteroanterior projection: Revealing a fibrotic scar with calcific debris within and adjacent to it in the apex of the left upper lobe (**a**). Inferior to this is a larger, ill-defined soft-tissue mass with overlying fibrotic changes and speckled calcifications (**b**). Some distortion and elevation of the vessels from the left upper lobe leading to the hilus are also present.

   B, lateral projection: Showing portions of the calcification and linear streakings (**a**) in the apical and posterior segments of the left upper lobe. The ovoid mass (**b**) with several pseudopods extending from its margins overlies the midportion of the trachea.

   (*Continued.*)

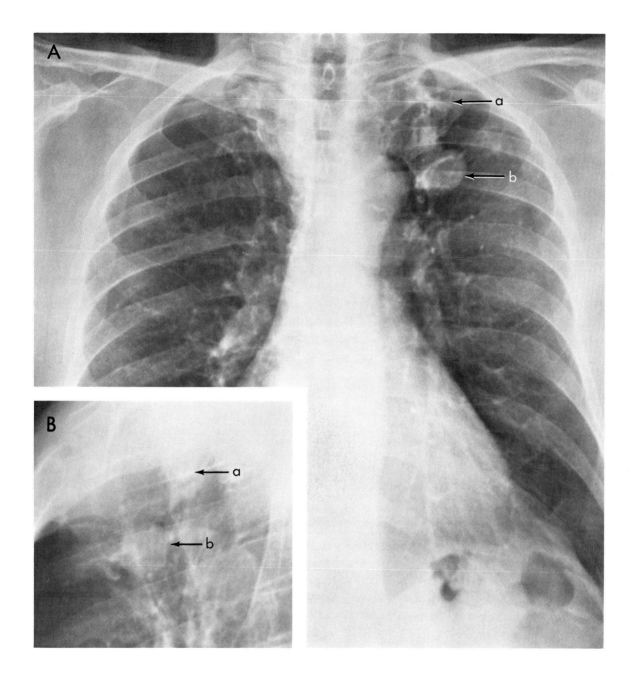

Figure 47 · Squamous Cell Carcinoma and Granuloma / 131

Figure 47 (cont.).—Squamous cell carcinoma developing adjacent to an old granuloma.

C, magnification of involved area in **A,** seen to better advantage.

D, body-section radiograph: Revealing faint calcifications (**c**) above the major portion of the mass (**x**) with a taillike extension (**d**) leading to the main body of the mass (**x**). The upper changes most certainly represent an old granuloma; however, the eccentric nature of the calcification and development of a new mass should make one reasonably certain of the presence of a neoplasm rather than reactivation of an old tuberculous focus.

E, body-section exposure made behind **D**: Revealing the old calcified granuloma (**c**) to better advantage. The mass (**x**) and its extension from above (**d**) are now out of the focal plane level. The eccentric nature of the calcification (**c**) plus development of the mass (**x**) are hallmarks of cancer developing in the scar of an old infection.

A 60-year-old man had been treated for tuberculosis many years before and had had repeated chest radiographs for follow-up study of that old infection. He was asymptomatic at the time of the present study, which was a three-year follow-up examination. At this time the mass was discovered. Thoracotomy and left upper lobectomy revealed an old granulomatous process with squamous cell carcinoma in the inferior mass.

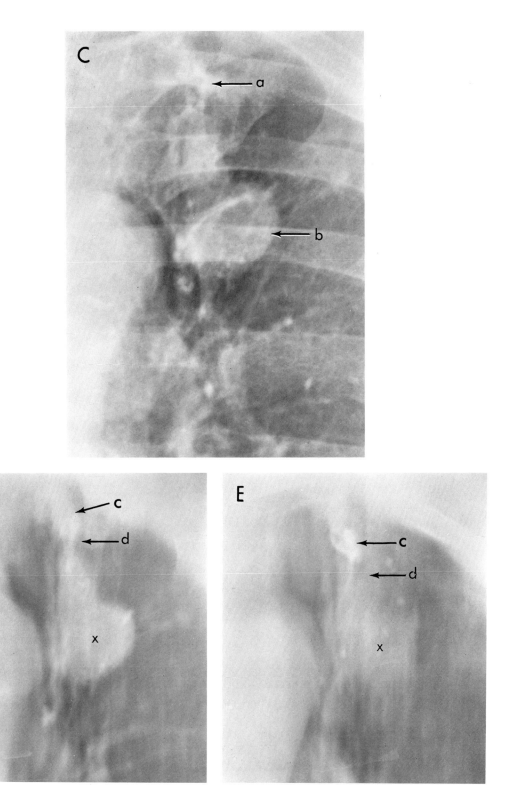

Figure 47 · Squamous Cell Carcinoma and Granuloma / 133

Figure 48.—Early squamous cell carcinoma of the right upper lobe.

A, posteroanterior radiograph: Demonstrating an obvious fibrotic and calcific lesion in the right upper lobe, most certainly representing scarring from an earlier disease due to acid-fast organisms. A peculiar irregular density (**arrow**) was viewed with suspicion because it looks different from the linear scars above it.

(Continued.)

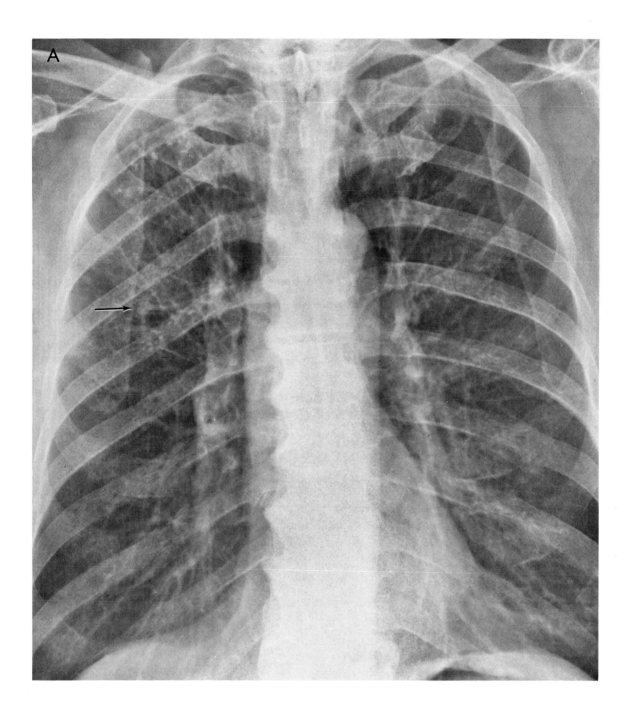

Figure 48 · Early Squamous Cell Carcinoma / 135

Figure 48 (cont.).—Early squamous cell carcinoma of the right upper lobe.

B, magnification of the questioned site in **A**: Revealing an unusual confluence of shadows (**arrow**). Because this raised the suspicion of early neoplasm, body-section studies were recommended.

C, supine body-section radiograph through the right upper lobe: Clearly delineating the calcifications in the upper portions of the lobe with linear fibrotic changes extending into the hilus. Again, in the inferior margin is a

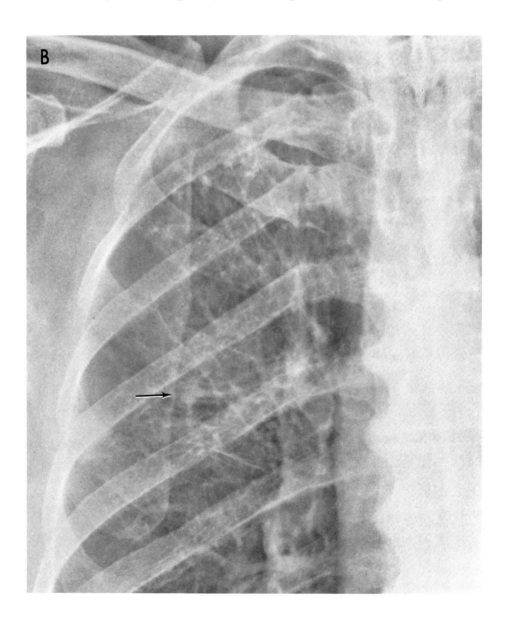

single small, ill-defined, irregular soft tissue shadow with pseudopods extending into the adjacent pulmonary parenchyma (**arrow**). In spite of the obvious old, fibrotic and calcific disease, this confluent soft tissue change with its pseudopods must be regarded as neoplastic.

A 68-year-old man was seen because of vague upper gastrointestinal complaints. Because he had been a heavy smoker, his chest was examined. Subsequent right upper lobectomy disclosed a 3 mm squamous cell carcinoma developing in the inferior portion of an extensively scarred right upper lobe.

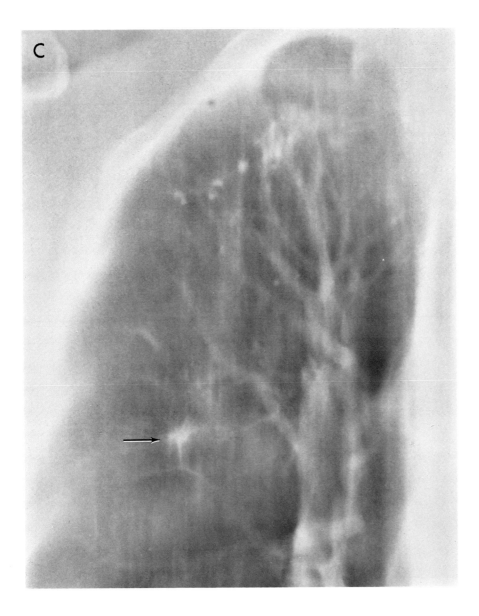

Figure 48 · Early Squamous Cell Carcinoma / 137

Figure 49.—Squamous cell carcinoma of the left lower lobe.

A, posteroanterior radiograph: Showing irregular fibrous change with multiple emphysematous blebs in the posterior portion of the right upper lobe. In addition there is a more solid area with ill-defined margins in the upper portion of this lesion (**a**). No significant calcification is evident in this process. The shadow of greater concern is an ill-defined soft tissue lesion overlying the anterior end of the left fifth rib (**arrows**). Its margins are irregular, with pseudopods that gradually fade into the adjacent surrounding lung.

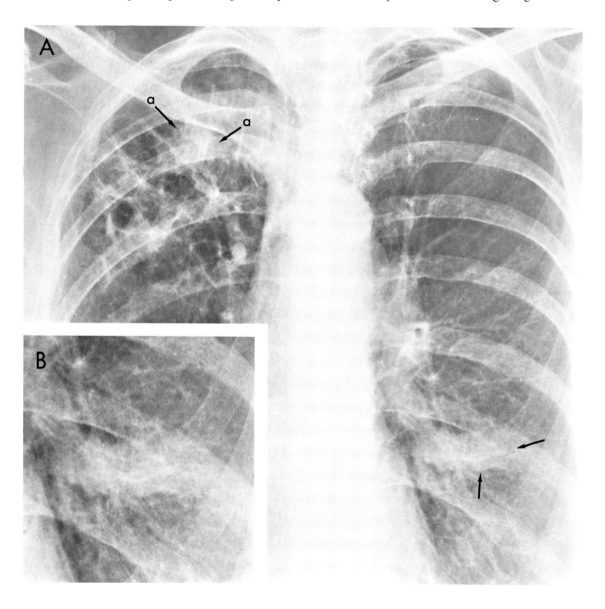

B, magnification of the lesion in the left lower lobe: Revealing its irregular outline.

C, lateral projection: Demonstrating the right-sided lesion in the posterior portion of the right upper lobe (**a**). The lesion on the lower left lies in the posterior segment of the left lower lobe (**arrow**).

A 57-year-old woman with cough, blood-streaked sputum and a history of successfully treated tuberculosis was referred for study. Repeated sputum examinations failed to recover acid-fast organisms. It was believed that the patient had two lesions which were probably unrelated. The left lower lobe was removed, and a squamous cell carcinoma was found in the posterior segment. A subsequent right upper lobectomy revealed scars of an earlier disease due to acid-fast organisms but no neoplasm.

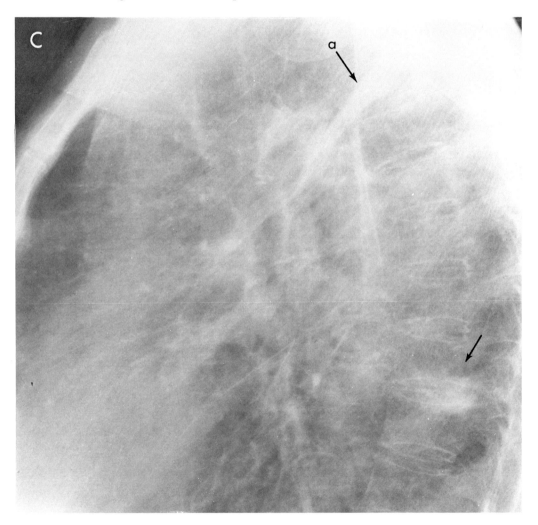

Figure 49 · Squamous Cell Carcinoma: Left Lower Lobe / 139

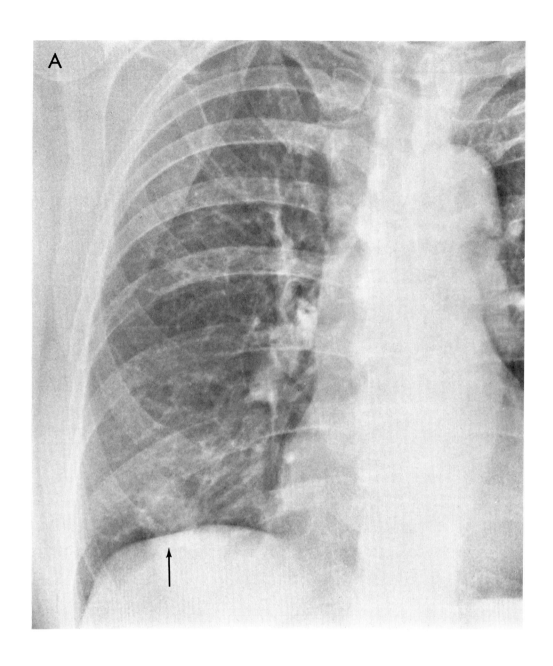

Figure 50.—Granuloma and primary squamous cell carcinoma of the right lower lobe.

A, posteroanterior radiograph: Revealing a multilobed lesion in the right lower lobe of the lung (**arrow**). Adjacent vessels appear to be normal.

B and **C,** body-section radiographs through the mass: Demonstrating its lobulated character and a central nidus of calcification in the lower lobule. The upper margins are less distinct, with pseudopods extending into the adjacent lung (**arrows**). The presence of calcification suggests granuloma; but it is eccentric, and this plus the lobulation and pseudopods makes cancer highly probable.

A 50-year-old woman was hospitalized because of recurrent uterine bleeding. The chest study was part of the routine examination. Right lower lobectomy was performed, and a granulomatous process as well as an adjacent squamous cell carcinoma incorporating the granuloma were found.

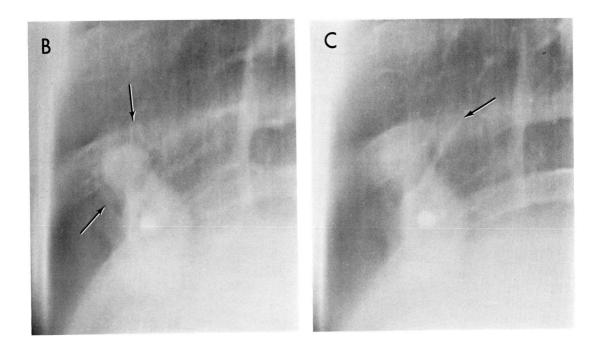

Figure 50 · **Squamous Cell Carcinoma and Granuloma** / 141

Figure 51.—Granuloma and squamous cell carcinoma of the left hilus.

A, posteroanterior projection: Demonstrating an irregular nodule (**arrow**) in the left lower lobe. The left hilus is enlarged (**x**) and its normal vascular outlines are lost.

B, body section radiographs of the nodule in the left lower lobe: Indicating its ill-defined dendric margins (**arrows**). Its general increased density and spotted calcification make the diagnosis uncertain.

(Continued.)

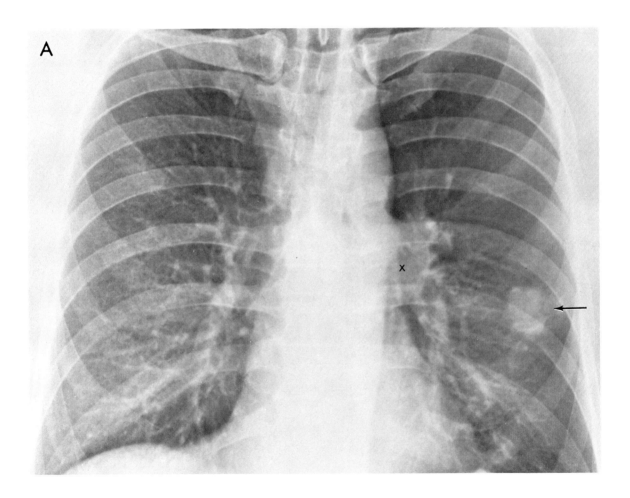

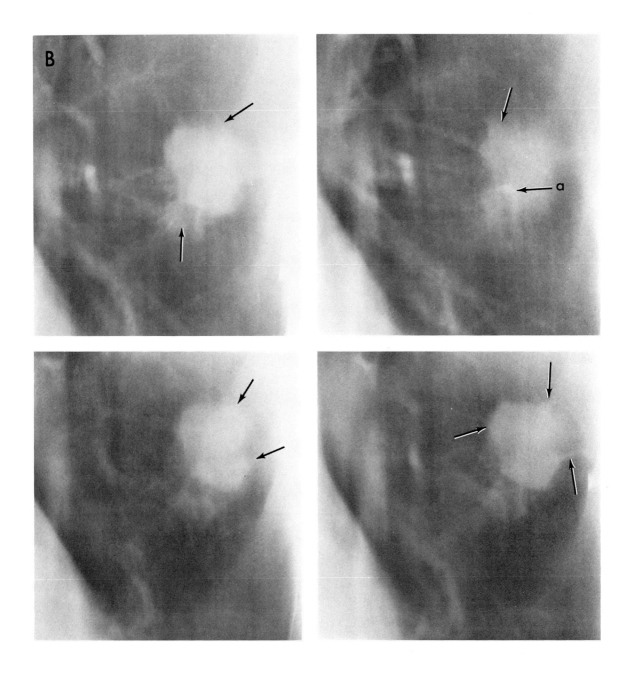

Figure 51 · Granuloma and Squamous Cell Carcinoma / 143

Figure 51 (cont.).—Granuloma and squamous cell carcinoma of the left hilus.

C, body-section radiograph, anteroposterior view, through the left hilar area: Revealing an abrupt cut-off and narrowing of the left main stem bronchus (**a**) and loss of normal vascular outlines in the hilus (**x**) suggesting a neoplasm.

A 55-year-old man was seen because of blood-streaked sputum and changing cough. He was one of a group being studied by fluorodensitometry to evaluate ventilation. The ventilation in the left lower lobe was markedly diminished. Bronchoscopy revealed a squamous cell lesion of the left lower lobe. At surgery, extensive involvement of the left hilar area was found. The peripheral lesion was a granuloma.

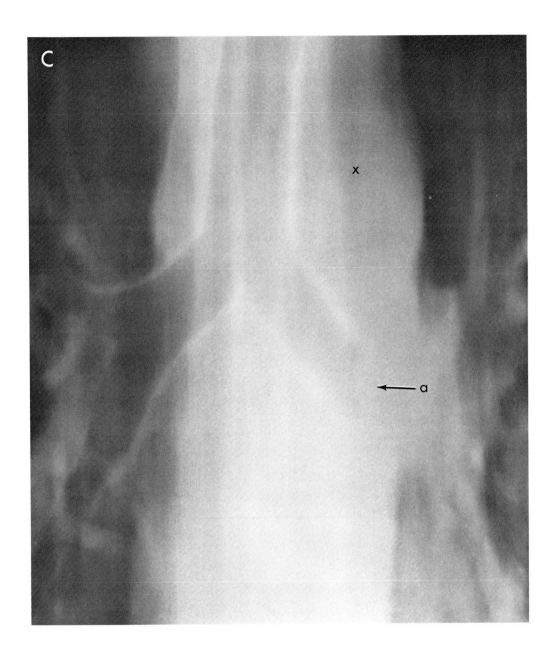

Figure 51 · Granuloma and Squamous Cell Carcinoma / 145

Figure 52.—Squamous cell carcinoma and a conglomerate mass of silicosis.

A, posteroanterior radiograph: Revealing two adjacent rounded masses of different size in the left lower lobe (**arrows**). Some distorted vessels are seen below the hilus (**a**). Faint, scattered fine nodules are present in the remaining portions of the lung, especially noticeable overlying the masses.

B, posteroanterior exposure of the right forearm and wrist: Disclosing periosteal proliferation (**arrows**) and osteoporosis compatible with pulmonary osteoarthropathy.

A 55-year-old hard coal miner complained of pain in the right forearm, wrist and hand. On the basis of the periosteal reaction noted in the forearm indicative of hypertrophic pulmonary osteoarthropathy, the chest was examined radiographically. Left lower lobectomy was performed. The small upper lesion represented a conglomerate mass of silicosis; the lower larger mass was a squamous cell carcinoma. The pains in the forearm disappeared after thoracotomy, and on subsequent radiographic study of the forearm the pulmonary osteoarthropathic changes had disappeared.

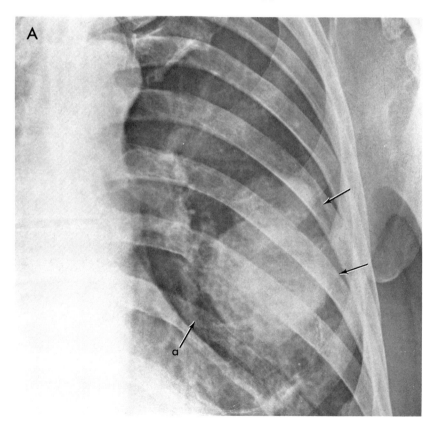

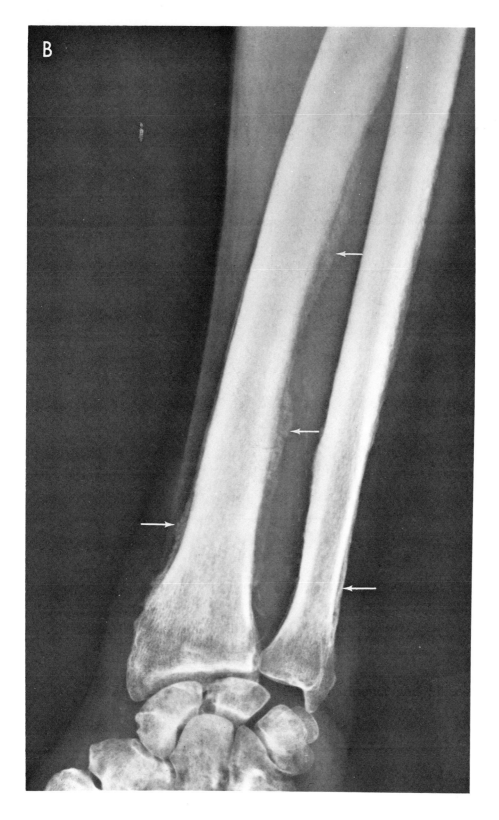

Figure 52 · Squamous Cell Carcinoma and Silicosis / 147

Figure 53.—Hamartoma and squamous cell carcinoma.

A, posteroanterior projection: Revealing a somewhat undulating ovoid mass (**x**) with smooth margins in the right upper lobe. A characteristic stellate calcification (**arrow**) within the mass suggests hamartoma. Note the character of the vessels in the right hilus and compare with **B.**

B, four years after **A**: Demonstrating no change in the appearance of the ovoid mass in the right upper lobe (**x**). Now, however, below and lateral to it is a second ill-defined mass (**y**). In addition, the smooth margins of the upper pulmonary vessels in the hilar region noted four years previously (**A**) are now blurred and have changed in shape (**a**).

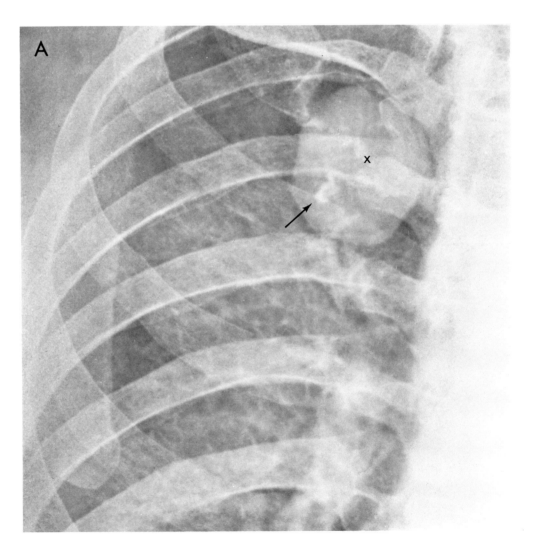

A 35-year-old man was seen initially for repair of an inguinal hernia. The mass (**A**) was discovered incidentally during a routine chest survey at this time. Its characteristics were considered to be classic for hamartoma, and because the patient was reluctant to have a second operative procedure, it was not removed. He failed to return for four years, until he had some cough and streaks of blood in the sputum on several occasions. At this time the lower mass and vascular changes were discovered. Its appearance and the hilar distortion seemed clear evidence of a second neoplasm. Thoracotomy required a right pneumonectomy. The superior lesion was proved microscopically to be a hamartoma. The lower one was squamous cell carcinoma with invasion of the hilar lymph nodes.

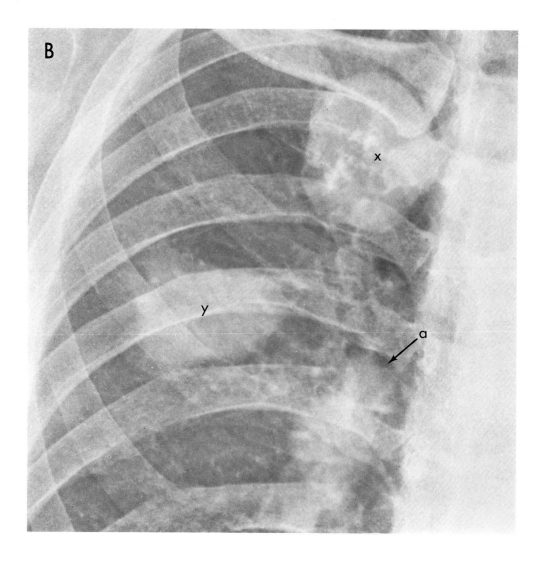

Figure 53 · Squamous Cell Carcinoma and Hamartoma / 149

PART 3

Lymphomas

Characteristics of Lymphomas
in the Thorax

UNDER LYMPHOMAS we have included Hodgkin's disease, lymphosarcoma, reticulum cell sarcoma, Burkitt's lymphoma and pseudolymphoma. Because of the extensive diffuse lymphatic tissues normally present in the thorax, an endless variety of possible intrathoracic manifestations of lymphomas can be found. Advanced knowledge of the protean pictures of these diseases allows the skilled physician to arrive at a proper diagnosis early.

All too often the first indication of a lymphoma is found in the radiographs of the chest of a young person with vague, nonspecific systemic complaints. Usually the first changes are enlargements of either or both mediastinal and hilar nodes. Enlargement of the hilar and/or paratracheal nodes on one or both sides may herald the disease. The subcarinal nodes too may thus be affected. Any single group of nodes or variations in groups may be involved. If one carefully evaluates the nodal margins and their relationship to one another and to adjacent tissues and structures, the correct differentiation from diseases of similar appearance, such as sarcoid, can be made with certainty most of the time.

HODGKIN'S DISEASE.—This is the type of lymphoma most often found in the thorax. As a rule the cervical and supraclavicular nodes are involved first, but at some time during the course of the disease mediastinal or hilar nodes, or both, are invaded (Figs. 54, 55, 58 and 59). About one-third of patients with Hodgkin's disease eventually have parenchymal lesions (Figs. 60 and 61), usually late in the course. The disease is two or three times more frequent in males than in females. It may occur at any age, but is most common between 20 and 40 years. Of all lymphomas it has the best prognosis.

The roentgen appearance in the chest is not pathognomonic, but the experienced viewer usually can distinguish the lesions of Hodgkin's disease from those of other lymphomas and diseases that cause nodal enlargements, such as sarcoid and certain allergic conditions. Characteristic are mediastinal or hilar nodal enlargements with sharply marginated wavy edges extending into one or both sides of the chest (Figs. 55 and 56). The *nodes tend to be matted* (Figs. 59, 60 and 63) and not discrete masses, as seen with lymphosarcoma (Fig. 65) and the inflammatory processes.

Rarely is a patient seen initially with a primary parenchymal lesion; if such is present, the appearance is similar to that late in the disease, with a predilection for the upper lobes. A branching, rough-edged expanding mass with margins fading into the adjacent lung is the usual appearance of very early or very late parenchymal lesions (Figs. 60 and 61). Most often, hilar and mediastinal nodes are also implicated, although in a patient who has had radiation therapy to the mediastinum, such enlargements may not be present (Fig. 61). Usually, parenchymal lesions are a poor prognostic sign. Cavitations may develop; when they do, the cavities are shaggy and thick-walled, resembling other neoplastic cavitating masses. In such circumstances Reed-Sternberg cells may be found in the sputum.

Primary pulmonary lesions in Hodgkin's disease are rare; when they do occur, an endobronchial site of origin is more common than the parenchymal one. Most cases have been discovered because of lobar collapse, with adjacent local nodal enlargement completely mimicking a bronchial neoplasm.

LYMPHOSARCOMA.—The clinical course of lymphosarcoma differs from that of Hodgkin's disease and is invariably fatal. In general the progress is more rapid and, although initial response to therapy may be excellent, relapses are usual. The roentgen patterns are of two major types. One is characterized mainly by nodal disease with enlargement of bilateral paratracheal nodes, frequently symmetrical (Figs. 65 and 70). These lesions closely resemble the changes of sarcoid (Fig. 60), and differentiation between the two may be impossible without biopsy. Lymphosarcoma usually does not cause bronchial obstruction; when it does, the lesions are endobronchial with distal atelectasis and infection. The second type is characterized by large parenchymal masses and may be asymptomatic for a long time. The microscopic appearance is the same in the two types and they have a similar prognosis. They usually occur in the age group from 40–60 and about equally between the sexes.

Giant follicular lymphoma has no distinguishing roentgen characteristics that allow one to separate it from lymphosarcoma and Hodgkin's disease. Reticulum cell sarcoma (Fig. 73) also may mimic the roentgen pattern of the former.

LYMPHATIC LEUKEMIA.—This condition may be manifested by enlarged hilar and mediastinal lymph nodes in any node-bearing areas (Fig. 71). The roentgen appearance may be identical with that of lymphosarcoma or giant follicular lymphoma. Whereas all may produce tiny diffuse pulmonary parenchymal shadows, such shadows are more common with the leukemias. Early in the disease these neoplasms are very sensitive to radiation. Chest fluoroscopy alone has been well documented as producing a remission and disappearance of the tiny pulmonary parenchymal nodules in 12–24 hours.

A patient with small diffuse pulmonary parenchymal nodules and hilar nodal enlargement should be suspected of having lymphatic leukemia. Rarely, diffuse parenchymal nodules are seen with myeloid or monocytic leukemia.

BURKITT'S LYMPHOMA.—This is the name given a multifocal lymphomatous tumor in children who have multiple tumors of the jaw or viscera, or both. The microscopic appearance is of a poorly differentiated lymphocytic lymphoma containing nonmalignant histiocytes (Fig. 75).

The radiographic appearance in the jaw is essentially that of a medullary osteolytic lesion which may begin around the tooth roots. The tumor may progress to extrabony extension with soft tissue masses around the mandible and may involve one or both sides. Other bones are occasionally affected.

Associated visceral lymphomatous change may involve the chest or abdomen. When in the chest, the lesions are mainly mediastinal, as with other lymphomas. The association of a lobulated mediastinal mass and soft tissue lumps around the mandible and bony osteolytic lesions suggests the diagnosis of Burkitt's tumor.[4,12]

PSEUDOLYMPHOMA.—A number of reported parenchymal lesions without nodal enlargement (Fig. 74) but with the histologic appearance of lymphoma have been described as pseudolymphoma. The concept of this lesion should be appreciated by the physician concerned with chest disease because the prognosis is excellent and further therapy after removal is unnecessary. We are dependent on histologic diagnosis for the final answer; such lesions are, however, extranodal, without lymphomatous change in regional nodes but sometimes showing a degree of hyperplasia. Pseudolymphomatous masses microscopically may show preservation of nodal architecture, a follicular pattern and some remnant of germinal centers. Focal granulomas, fibroblastic proliferation and polymorphic cells may be found throughout, but no Reed-Sternberg cells are present. Occasionally the entire appearance may be that of a lymph node.

BIBLIOGRAPHY

1. Abel, M. R.: Lymphoid hamartoma, Radiol. Clin. North America 6:15, 1968.
2. Baron, M. G., and Whitehouse, W. M.: Primary lymphosarcoma of the lung, Am. J. Roentgenol. 85:294, 1961.
3. Berne, A. S., et al.: Diagnostic carbon dioxide pneumomediastinography, New England J. Med. 267:225, 1962.
4. Davidson, J. W., and Renouf, J. H. P.: Radiographic findings in "Burkitt type" lymphoma, J. Canad. A. Radiologists 19:121, 1968.
5. Del Regato, J. A.: Reflections on the so-called lymphomas, Radiol. Clin. North America 6:3, 1968.
6. Foyos, J. V.: Extrapulmonary intrathoracic manifestations of Hodgkin's disease, Radiol. Clin. North America 6:131, 1968.

7. Hoakins, E. O. L.: Unusual manifestations of Hodgkin's disease, Proc. Roy. Soc. Med. 60:729, 1967.

8. Miller, W. T., *et al.*: Lymphangiomatosis, Am. J. Roentgenol. 109:565, 1971.

9. Robbins, R.: Pseudolymphomas, Am. J. Roentgenol. 108:149, 1970.

10. Sheimel, A., *et al.*: Hodgkin's disease of the lung: Roentgen appearance and therapeutic management, Radiology 54:165, 1950.

11. Strickland, B.: Hodgkin's disease: Peripheral pulmonary manifestations, Proc. Roy. Soc. Med. 60:739, 1967.

12. Whittaker, L. R.: The radiological appearance of Burkitt's tumor involving bone, Australasian Radiol. 13:307, 1969.

Figure 54.—Hodgkin's disease.

A, posteroanterior radiograph: Revealing marked widening of the mediastinum caused by a large mass. Note the lobulation along the left border (**a**) and straighter margin along the right (**arrow**).

B, lateral projection: Demonstrating the anterior location of the mass (**x**) with somewhat ill-defined margins.

C, close-up of the mediastinal area in **A.**

A 40-year-old man had malaise and slight chest discomfort, but no abnormal physical findings except fever. A small thoracotomy incision and biopsy of the mass revealed a lymphoma consistent with a diagnosis of Hodgkin's disease.

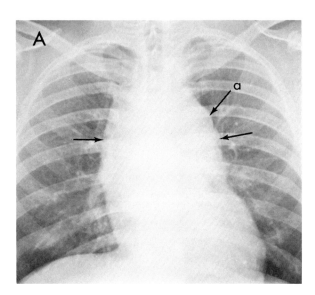
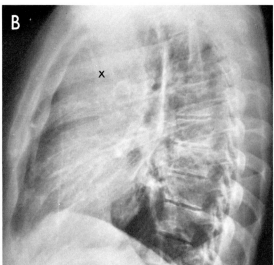

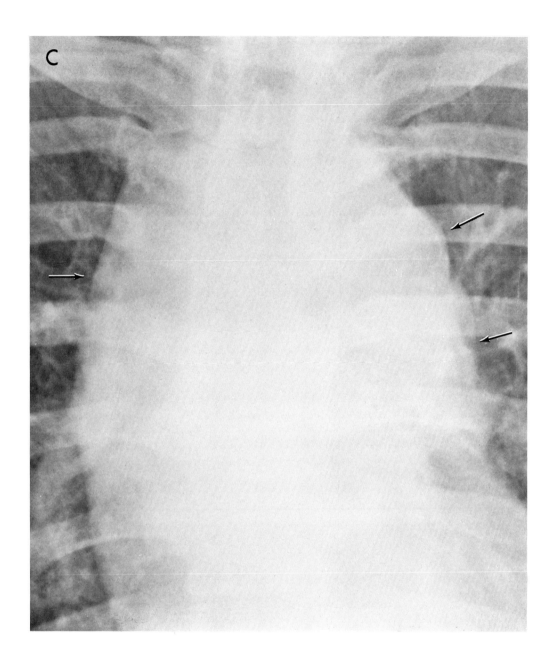

Figure 54 · Hodgkin's Disease / 157

Figure 55.—Hodgkin's disease.

A, posteroanterior radiograph: Revealing a wide superior mediastinum with undulating margins on both sides extending into and blending with the cardiac shadow. The density of the mass is similar to the cardiac outline. The normal vascular outlines in both hili are obliterated by the overlying mass.

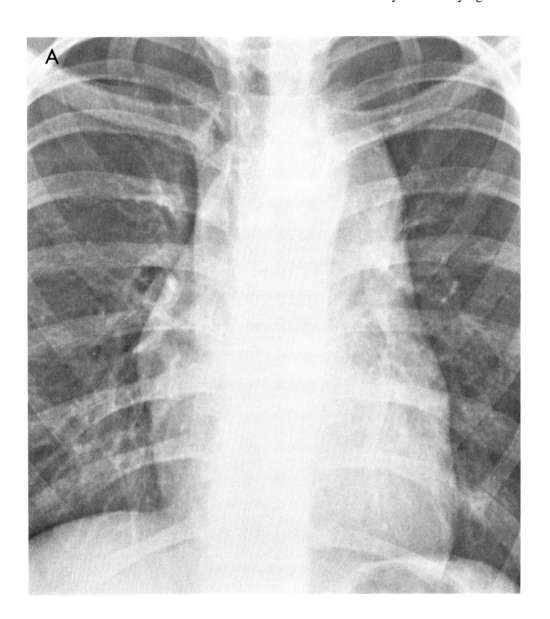

B, lateral projection: Demonstrating obliteration of the normal retrosternal air space (**x**) plus loss of the definitive hilar vascular shadows (**y**). In the superior mediastinum the tracheal outlines (**a**) are faintly visible. The bifurcation of the trachea is in the normal location and quite clear (**b**). The inferior border of the lymphomatous mass overlies the heart (**arrow**).

A 19-year-old youth complained of easy fatigability. His physician found low-grade fever and anemia. Biopsy of the chest mass revealed Hodgkin's disease.

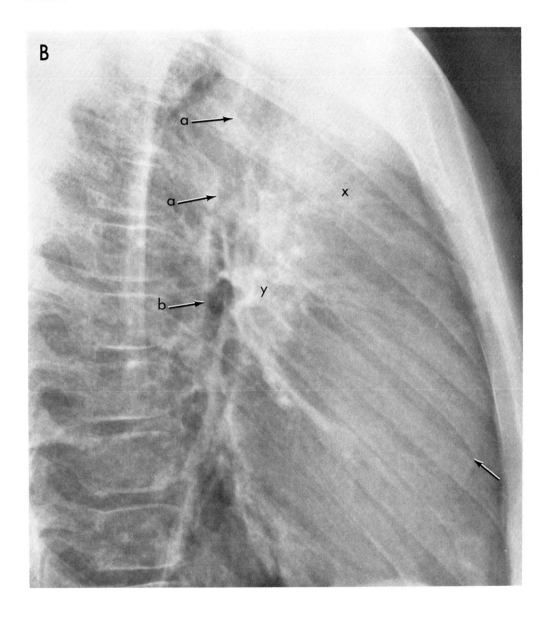

Figure 55 · Hodgkin's Disease / 159

Figure 56.—Hodgkin's disease.

A, posteroanterior radiograph: Delineating a teardrop-shaped mass (**x**) extending from the mediastinum into the right upper lobe. The upper margin is convex (**arrow**). The normal outline of the right hilar vessels blends with the inferior margin of the mass. The lesion extends into the left hemithorax, crosses the shadow of the arch of the aorta (**a**) and blends with the proximal portion of the superior margin of the left hilar vessels (**y**).

B, lateral view: Showing the large ovoid mass to occupy the anterior segment of the superior mediastinum (**x**) with a large portion superimposed on the tracheal airway (**b**). Both walls of the trachea are sharp and clearly outlined. The inferior margin blends with the superior portion of the hilar pulmonary vascular shadows.

C, close-up of superior mediastinal mass seen in **A.**

A 25-year-old man complained of fatigue and cough. No peripheral adenopathy was discovered. Some afternoon fever was detected. A portion of the mass was removed, and histologic diagnosis was Hodgkin's disease.

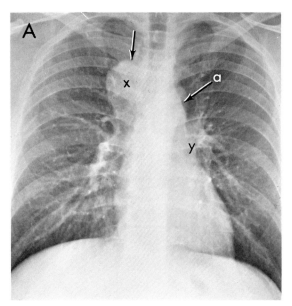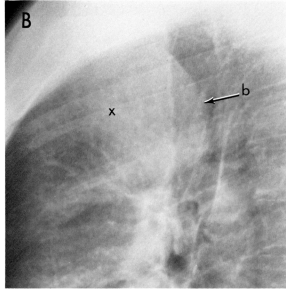

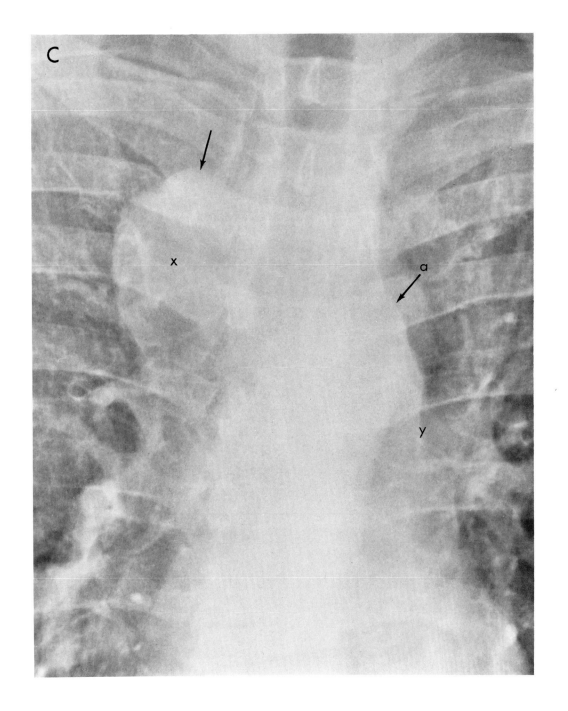

Figure 56 · Hodgkin's Disease / 161

Figure 57.—Hodgkin's disease.

A, posteroanterior radiograph: Revealing a mass in the superior mediastinum (**arrows**) on both sides of the midline. On the left side the mass overlies the aorta (**x**).

B, lateral view: Showing the mass (**arrows**), with rather ill-defined margins, in the anterior mediastinum.

C, close-up of the mass in **A.**

A 26-year-old man was seen because of malaise and slight weight loss. The radiographic picture three months previously had been interpeted as being within normal limits. Continued follow-up led to the radiographic study shown here. No peripheral nodes were palpable. Biopsy examination of the mass revealed Hodgkin's disease.

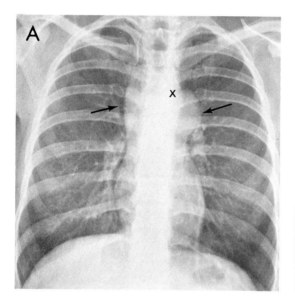
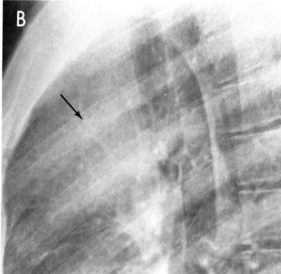

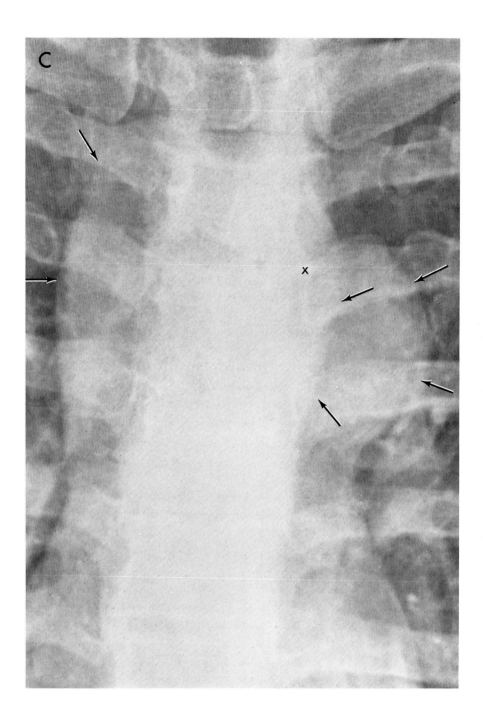

Figure 57 · Hodgkin's Disease / 163

Figure 58.—Hodgkin's disease.

This study was made with a cobalt-60 therapy unit eliminating some of the bony thoracic cage in its portrayal. The photographic reproduction increases the contrast of visible bony structures. In spite of this, the visibility of all the air-containing lung, trachea, and main stem bronchi is enhanced. Fine detail in the outlines of the pulmonary parenchymal vascular structures may be somewhat impaired by this technique.

A, posteroanterior radiograph: Revealing a sharply bordered superior mediastinal mass on the right (**x**) which displaces but produces only barely

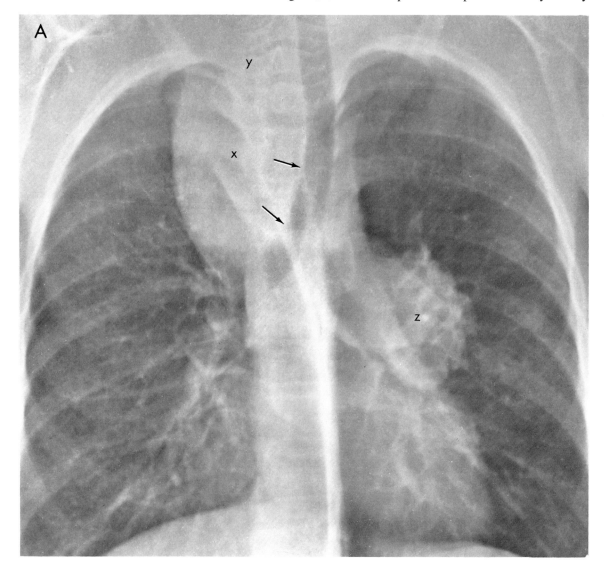

appreciable narrowing of the trachea and right main stem bronchus (**arrows**). This mass seems continuous with the soft tissues of the neck (**y**) but did not move with swallowing, and therefore was not thought to be part of the thyroid. Enlarged, sharp-edged left hilar nodes obscure the pulmonary vascular structures in this region (**z**).

B, close-up of mass seen in **A.**

This patient was a 26-year-old man undergoing radiation therapy for Hodgkin's disease. At the time of initiation of therapy, this study was made using the ^{60}Co unit.

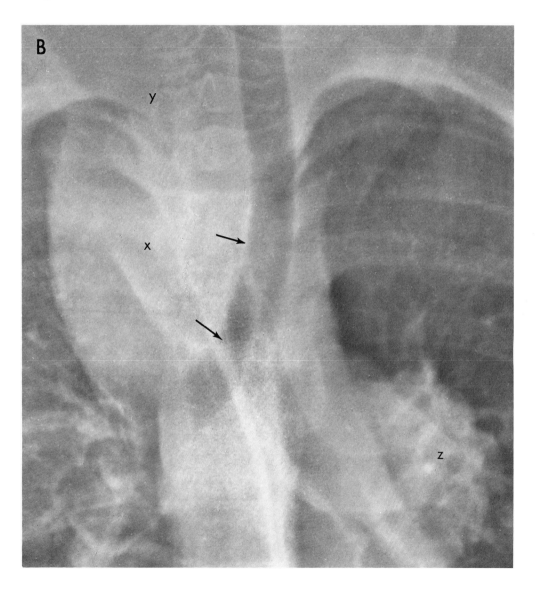

Figure 58 · Hodgkin's Disease / 165

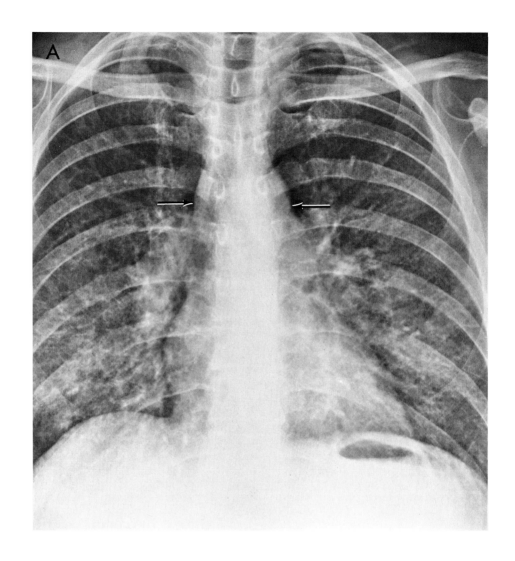

Figure 59.—Hodgkin's disease involving the lungs and mediastinum.

A, posteroanterior radiograph: Disclosing bilateral minor mediastinal adenopathy (**arrows**). On the left the aortic knob is partially obscured by the nodal enlargement. Normal hilar vascular outlines are completely obscured by the enlargement in both hilar areas. Diffuse parenchymal lesions involve the inferior two-thirds of each lung. Normal vessels are obscured by the fuzzy outlines of the interstitial lesions.

B, close-up study of the nodular irregularities that obscure the blood vessels in the right lower lobe. Note the characteristic "interstitial" pattern.

(*Continued.*)

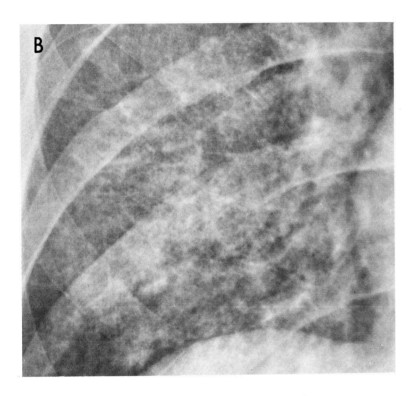

Figure 59 · Hodgkin's Disease / 167

Figure 59 (cont.).—Hodgkin's disease involving the lungs and mediastinum.

C, lateral view: Demonstrating the enlarged paratracheal and hilar nodes obscuring the normal vascular outlines in the central mediastinum (**arrows**). In addition, the normal outline of the tracheal bifurcation is obscured by the enlarged nodes.

A 52-year-old man complained of fever, cough and considerable shortness of breath. There was bilateral supraclavicular node enlargement. Biopsy study of the supraclavicular nodes revealed classic Hodgkin's disease.

Figure 59, courtesy of Dr. Gerald D. Dodd, M. D. Anderson Hospital, Houston, Tex.

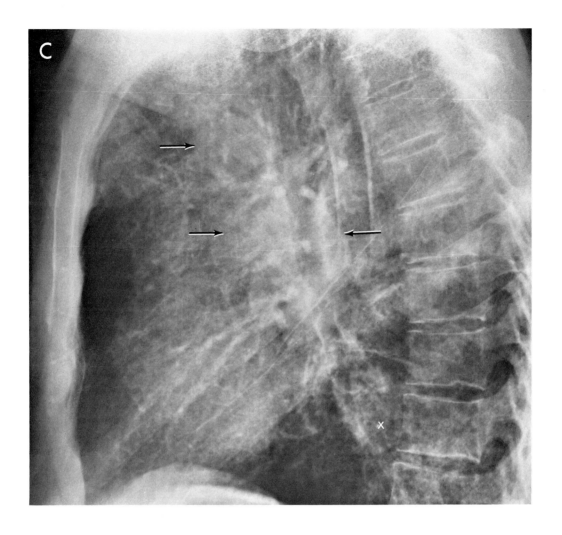

Figure 59 · Hodgkin's Disease / 169

Figure 60.—Hodgkin's disease of the mediastinum with parenchymal extension.

A, posteroanterior radiograph: Demonstrating bilateral large hilar nodes which extend more laterally than the usual hilar enlargement. Aerating lung is visible between the enlarged nodes and the mediastinum (**arrows**). No normal vascular margins can be seen in either hilus. Prominent parenchymal markings, which are bilateral, indicate diffuse extension of the disease.

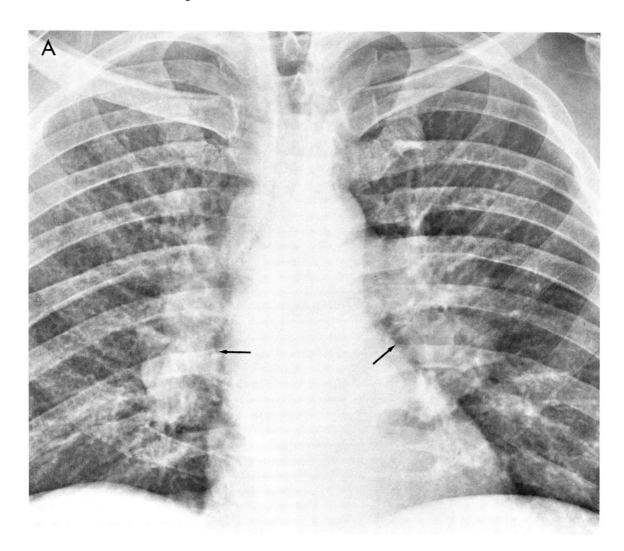

B, lateral study: Revealing a mass of enlarged nodes with smooth margins (**arrows**) that completely obscures hilar vascular structures. The normal trachea and its bifurcation are hidden by the overlying mass of nodes.

The appearance of the enlarged hilar nodes may be confused with that of the enlarged nodes due to sarcoid. However, in Hodgkin's disease the lateral margins of the nodes fade into the surrounding lung, as seen in **A.** Also, the margins of adjacent nodes seem matted together and are not as discrete as the nodes usually described in sarcoid.

This 42-year-old man had fever and weight loss. Biopsy diagnosis of enlarged supraclavicular nodes was Hodgkin's disease.

Figure 60, courtesy of Dr. Gerald D. Dodd, M. D. Anderson Hospital, Houston, Tex.

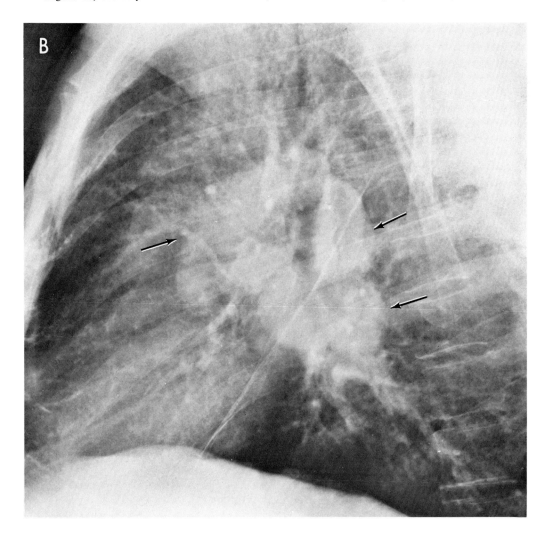

Figure 60 · Hodgkin's Disease / 171

Figure 61.—Hodgkin's disease with pulmonary extension.

A, posteroanterior radiograph: Showing enlargement of the peripheral nodular groups in each hilar area (**x**) with some aerating lung (**arrows**) between these nodes and the mediastinum. The major pulmonary arteries and veins are obscured by the large nodes. There are also bilateral enlargements of the paratracheal nodes (**a**). The normal aortic knob is obscured by the nodule enlargement in the region of the azygos vein on the right (**b**). There are some ill-defined nodular and linear parenchymal extensions in both lungs.

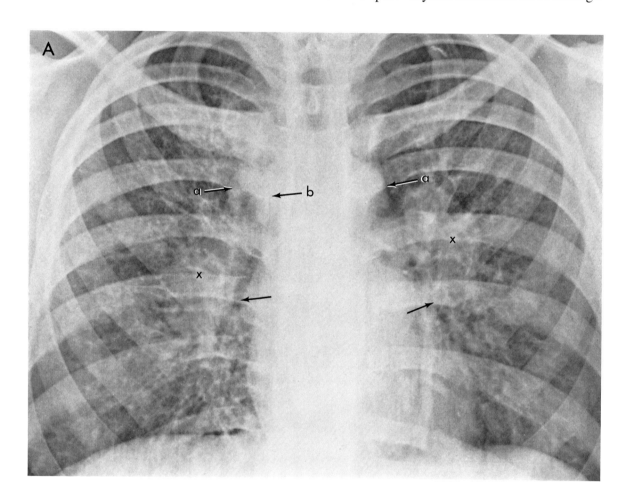

B, posteroanterior view following chemotherapy: Whereas the right hilar mass has decreased in size, there is a marked increase in the right paratracheal nodal mass (**y**) with pronounced increase in the diffuse parenchymal lesions in the right lung.

(Continued.)

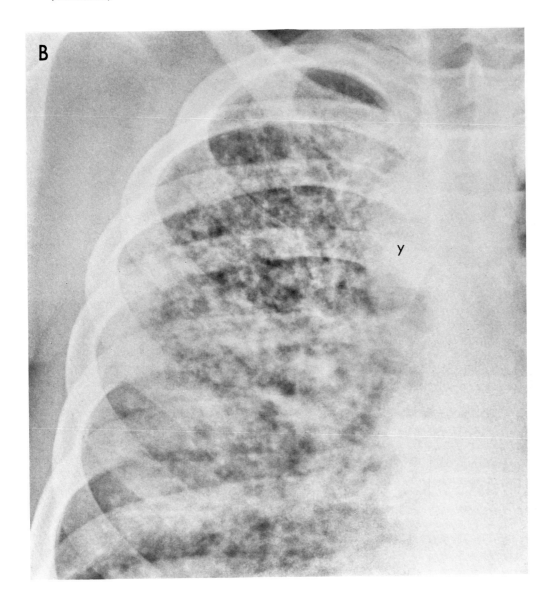

Figure 61 · Hodgkin's Disease / 173

Figure 61 (cont.).—Hodgkin's disease with pulmonary extension.

C, six months later: In spite of additional chemotherapy and irradiation, there is evidence of progressive disease in the right lung. The mediastinal and hilar nodal masses have diminished. There is considerable increase in the parenchymal involvement of the right lung with an air–fluid level in the mid-portion of this lung (**c**). In addition, there is evidence of extensive pleural involvement by the lymphomatous disease (**d**).

A 13-year-old boy was seen because of fatigue, weakness and fever. Biopsy of a supraclavicular node revealed Hodgkin's disease. In spite of various forms of therapy, the boy died soon after **C** was obtained.

Figure 61, courtesy of Dr. Gerald D. Dodd, M. D. Anderson Hospital, Houston, Tex.

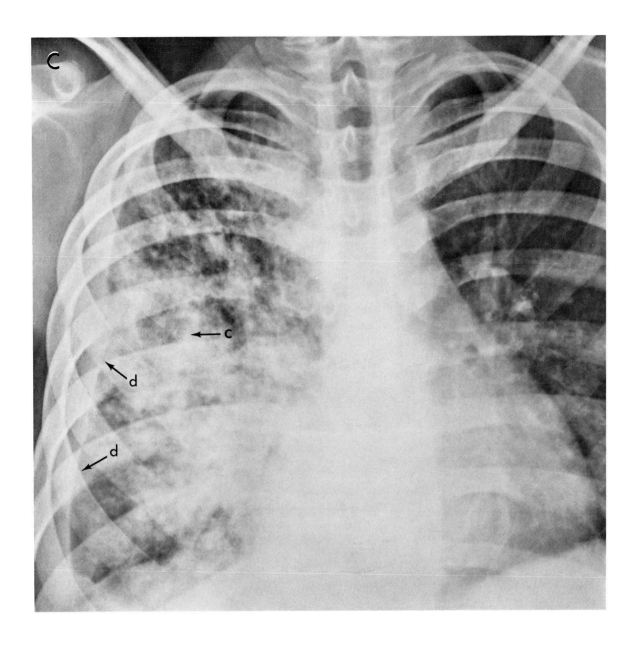

Figure 61 · Hodgkin's Disease / 175

Figure 62.—Hodgkin's disease.

Posteroanterior radiograph: Revealing soft tissue masses in the right paraspinal areas (**arrows**). In addition, the superior mediastinum is wide and the aortic arch obliterated by soft tissue masses.

A 19-year-old youth was examined because of chills, fever, weight loss and inguinal adenopathy. Lymphangiography delineated extensive lymphomatous involvement of the abdominal nodes. Biopsy of an inguinal node revealed Hodgkin's disease.

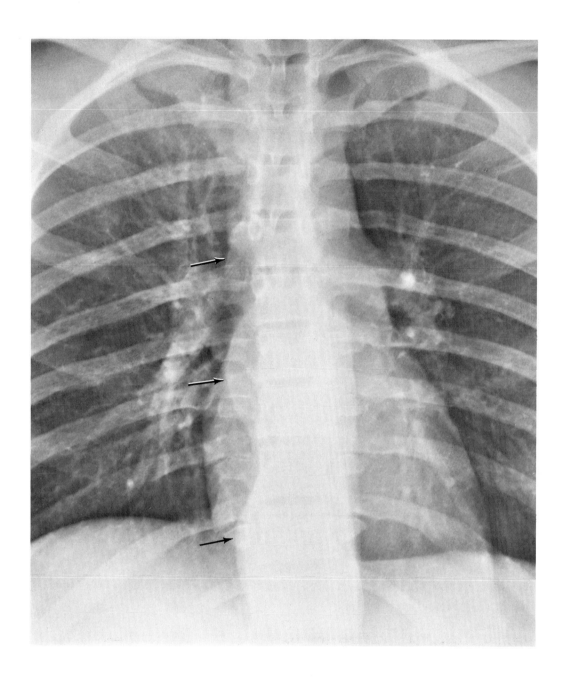

Figure 62 · Hodgkin's Disease / 177

Figure 63.—Hodgkin's disease.

A, posteroanterior radiograph: Revealing a vague, ill-defined density extending to each side of the mediastinum (**a**), more marked on the left, and gradually fading as it extends laterally. The margin on the right blends into the ascending aorta. (Note the similarity to the frontal view of metastatic breast carcinoma to the sternum in Figure 170.) No discrete adenopathy is present in the hilar areas.

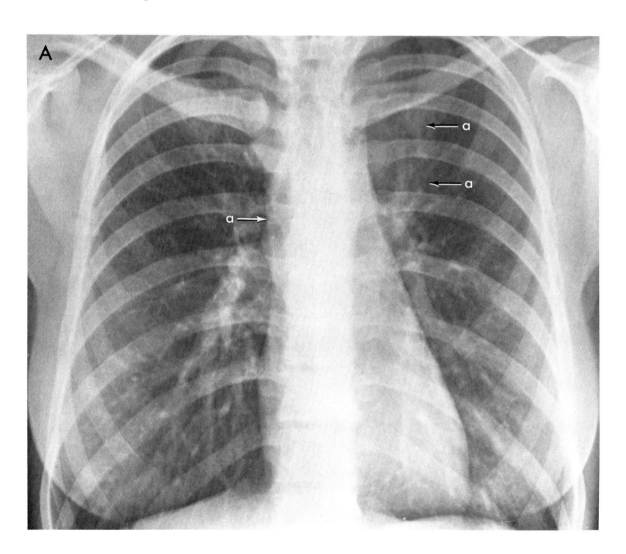

B, lateral projection: Indicating the retrosternal nature of the undulating soft tissue mass, but no bone destruction is present (**b**).

A 22-year-old woman had a node removed from the left axilla. This was interpreted as representing Hodgkin's disease. No other nodes, including those observed on abdominal lymphangiography, were thought to be abnormal. The involved retrosternal nodes regressed after radiation therapy.

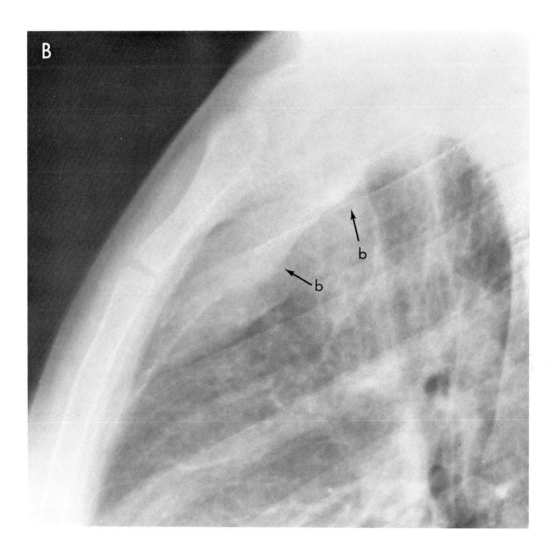

Figure 63 · Hodgkin's Disease / 179

Figure 64.—Hodgkin's disease.

   A, posteroanterior projection: Revealing superior mediastinal widening which is sharply marginated and extends into both sides of the midline (**arrows**). The aortic arch is slightly obscured by the mass (**a**).

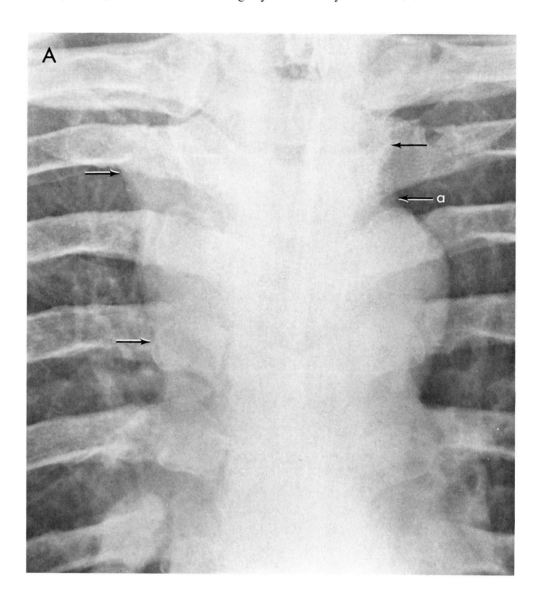

B, lateral exposure: Showing a soft tissue mass in the anterior portion of the mediastinum adjacent to the aortic shadow (**arrows**). Whereas lesions at this site may be extremely difficult to evaluate, the changes in **A** are rather representative of nodular enlargement of the superior mediastinum.

A 20-year-old college student felt unusually tired during his fall semester in school. The entire physical examination yielded negative results. There were no palpable lymph nodes. The blood count was also normal. Thoracotomy and biopsy examination of the enlarged nodes revealed Hodgkin's disease.

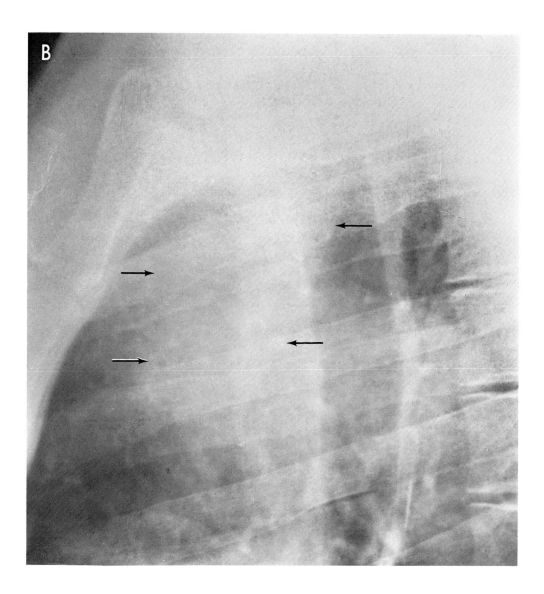

Figure 64 · Hodgkin's Disease / 181

Figure 65.—Hodgkin's disease.

A, posteroanterior study: Revealing an ill-defined mass in the left upper lobe (**x**) with hilar and mediastinal enlargement on the left. The mass also blends with the superior vascular portion of the right hilus (**arrow**). An air bronchogram is visible within the mass (**a**).

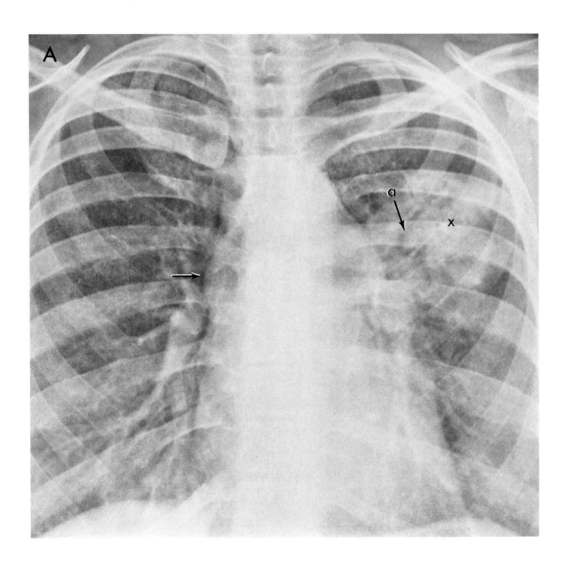

B, body-section radiograph of the lesion in **A:** Delineating a shaggy, irregular, superior border of the mass (**arrow**), a hallmark of malignancy. Note the involvement of the hilar nodes (**y**), air in the bronchi and small cavities within the mass (**b**). Rounded hilar nodal enlargement is present just below the mass and in the paratracheal area, obscuring the aortic knob.

A 24-year-old woman was seen because of rather sudden onset of chills, fever and rusty sputum. Her physician suspected an acute pneumonic process. The radiographic evidence suggested a neoplasm, most likely a lymphoma. Removal of several peripheral nodes revealed Hodgkin's disease. The thoracic portions responded very well to radiation therapy initially.

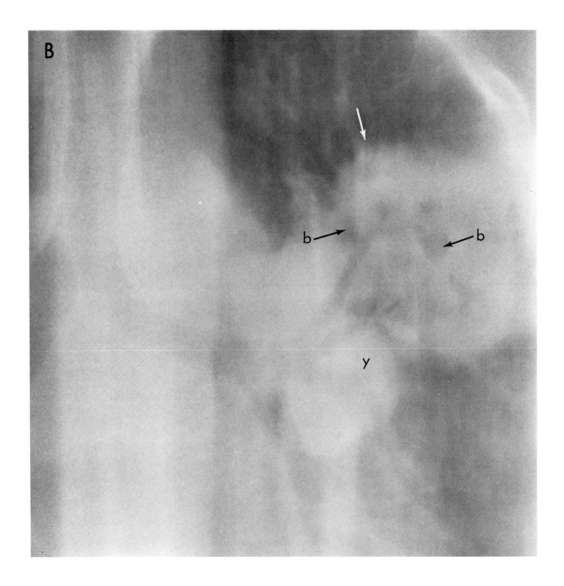

Figure 65 · Hodgkin's Disease / 183

Figure 66.—Hodgkin's disease.

A, posteroanterior projection: Revealing an ill-defined shadow occupying a large portion of the anterior segment of the right upper lobe (**x**) and slight adjacent hilar nodal enlargement and vascular obliteration (**arrow**).

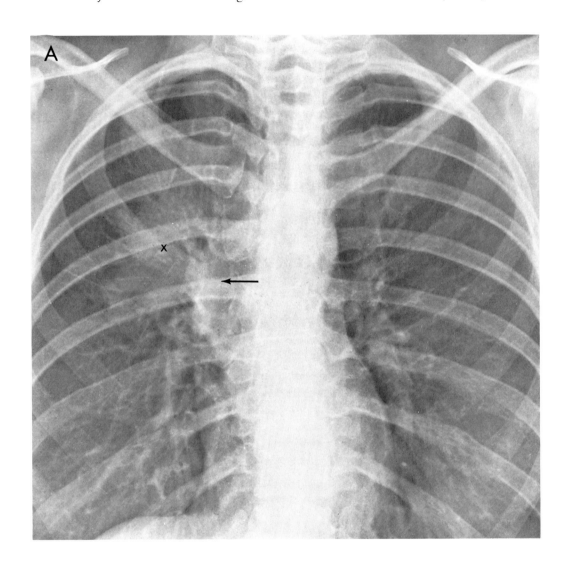

B, body-section radiograph through the midportion of the mass: Delineating its true size more realistically than **A.** Note the shagginess of its entire outline. Hilar and pulmonary vessels are incorporated in the mass (**y**).

A 21-year-old woman complained of an annoying, nagging cough and weight loss. The cough was nonproductive but constant. The general physical examination as well as routine laboratory studies revealed no further abnormality. Thoracotomy disclosed the neoplasm extensively involving the mediastinum and a considerable portion of the pulmonary parenchyma in the anterior segment of the right upper lobe. Examination of biopsy material confirmed the diagnosis of Hodgkin's disease.

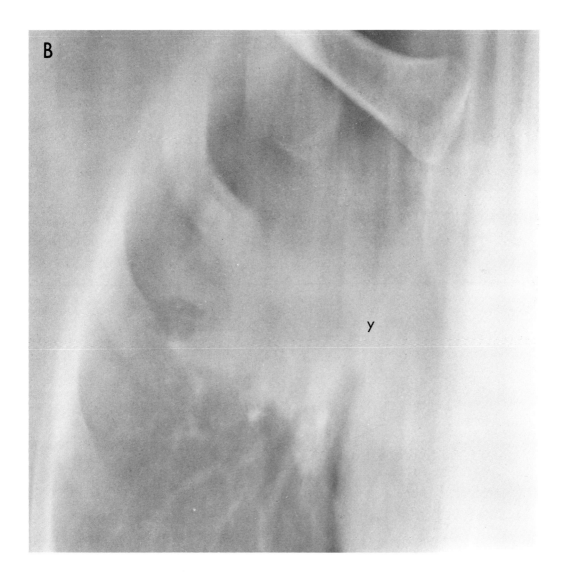

Figure 66 · Hodgkin's Disease / 185

Figure 67.—Pulmonary interstitial Hodgkin's disease.

A, posteroanterior radiograph: Disclosing no evident abnormalities. The pulmonary parenchyma appears to be normal, as do the mediastinal structures. Lateral projections at this time revealed nothing abnormal.

B, posteroanterior chest study three months after **A:** Revealing bilateral interstitial and vascular changes, more pronounced in the right lung.

(Continued.)

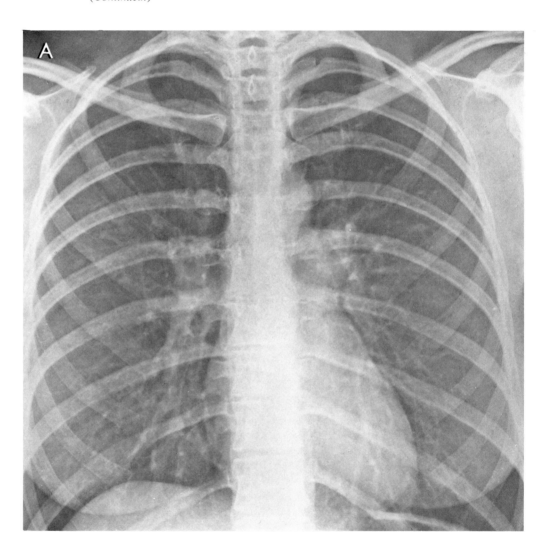

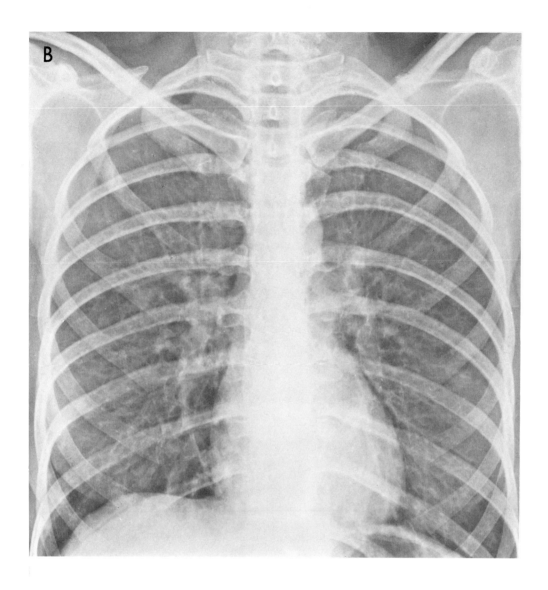

Figure 67 · Pulmonary Interstitial Hodgkin's Disease / 187

Figure 67 (**cont.**).—Pulmonary interstitial Hodgkin's disease.

C, close-up of the healthy right midlung field in **A.**

D, close-up of the abnormal right midlung field in **B:** Demonstrating interstitial and vascular changes with early coalescent mottling.

A 20-year-old girl was examined because of cervical lymphadenopathy and fever. Biopsy revealed Hodgkin's disease. Her condition rapidly deteriorated, with increasingly severe dyspnea, and in spite of various forms of treatment she died a week after this study.

At autopsy, the lungs remained distended in the thoracic cage when the chest was opened. A gritty, sandy sensation was experienced on sectioning of the lungs, and the cut surface revealed extensive tumor throughout the interstitial areas. Pathologic diagnosis was diffuse interstitial Hodgkin's disease.

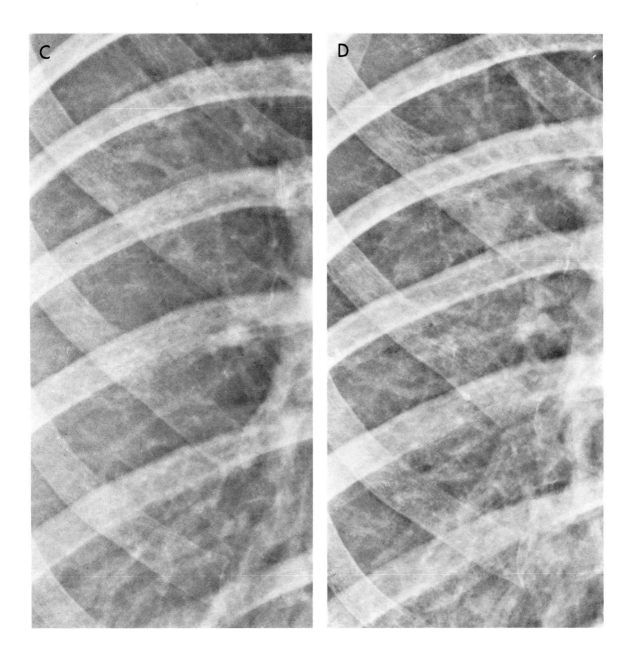

Figure 67 · Pulmonary Interstitial Hodgkin's Disease / 189

Figure 68.—Lymphosarcoma.

A, posteroanterior radiograph: Demonstrating a huge, smooth-margined anterior mediastinal mass occupying mainly the right hemithorax but extending to the left in the region of the pulmonary outflow tract of the right ventricle (**arrow**). The pulmonary hilar vessel shadows are lost on both sides.

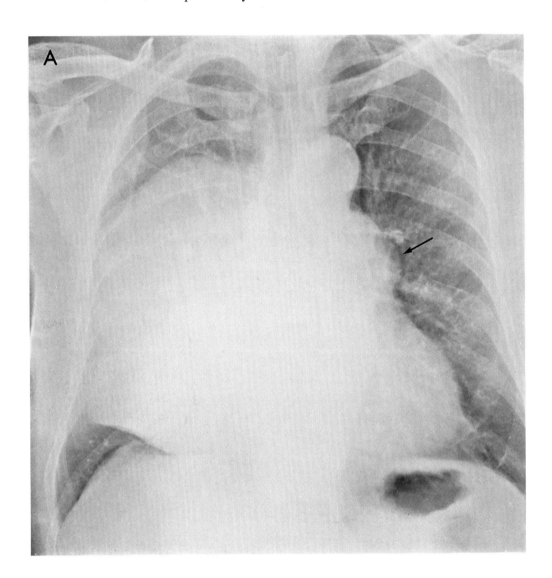

B, lateral view: Showing the mass occupying the anterior one-half of the chest, obscuring cardiac outlines and vascular structures and impinging on the normal air-filled structures.

A 72-year-old man had a chronic nonproductive cough and severe dyspnea. No nodes were palpable. The mass was totally removed at operation. Pathologic study revealed a lymphosarcoma.

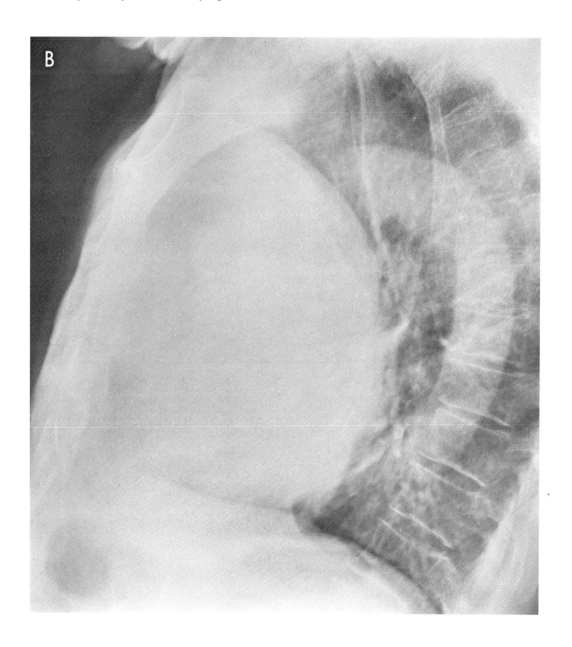

Figure 68 · Lymphosarcoma / 191

Figure 69.—Lymphosarcoma.

A, posteroanterior radiograph: Revealing a large mass filling the upper two-thirds of the right hemithorax with extension across the midline of the mediastinum, obliterating the aortic arch. There is also some shift of the cardiac silhouette to the left. A diagnostic pneumothorax (**arrow**) had been

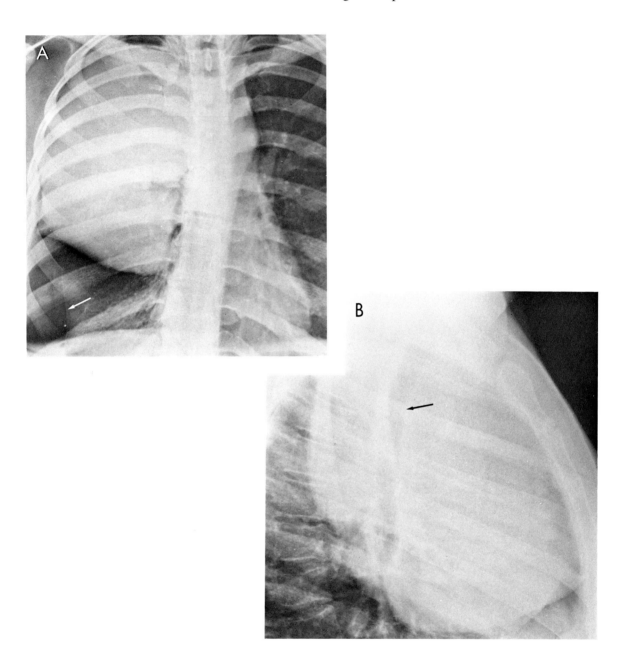

performed because the initial radiographs revealed a completely opacified right hemithorax due to a pleural effusion as well as the tumor.

B, lateral exposure: Showing the mass occupying the midportion and anterior segment of the mediastinum. The trachea is bowed slightly posteriorly (**arrow**).

C, right subclavian venogram: Demonstrating occlusion (**a**) of the right subclavian vein and multiple collateral channels.

D, left subclavian injection: Showing tumor invasion of the right innominate vein (**b**) and the lateral margin of the superior vena cava (**c**).

A 21-year-old woman was examined because of signs of superior vena caval obstruction and marked dyspnea. Surgical removal of the mass was attempted but had to be abandoned because of the extensive invasion of the major vessels and adjacent structures. Pathologic study revealed a lymphosarcoma. Radiation therapy led to complete disappearance of the mass.

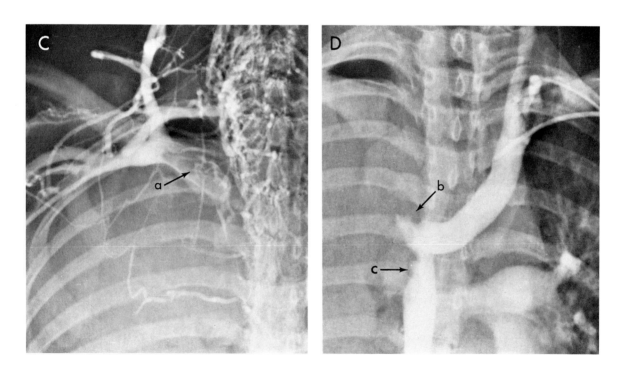

Figure 69 · Lymphosarcoma / 193

Figure 70.—Diffuse pulmonary lymphoma closely resembling Hodgkin's disease.

A, routine posteroanterior radiograph made at the time of the patient's initial complaint: Showing an essentially normal appearance.

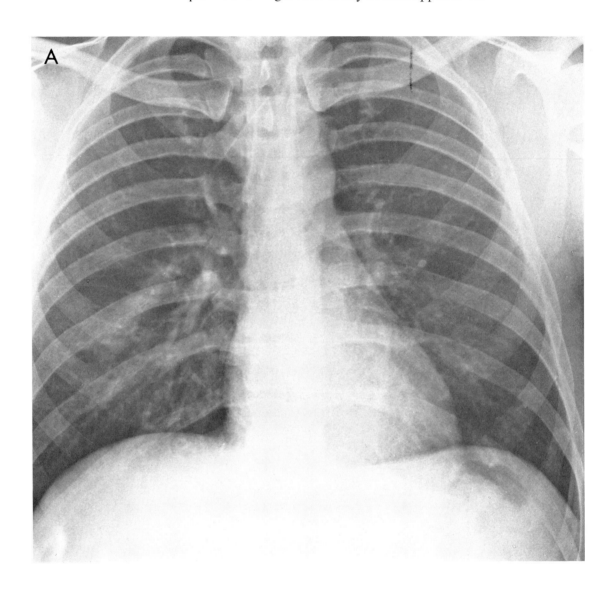

B, posteroanterior exposure 1 week after **A** and 24 hours after onset of symptoms: Revealing a dramatic change in the appearance of the chest. A few shaggy densities now obscure the normal vascular outlines in both lungs. The change is most striking in the lower lobes. Wires overlying the right base are in postoperative dressings.

(Continued.)

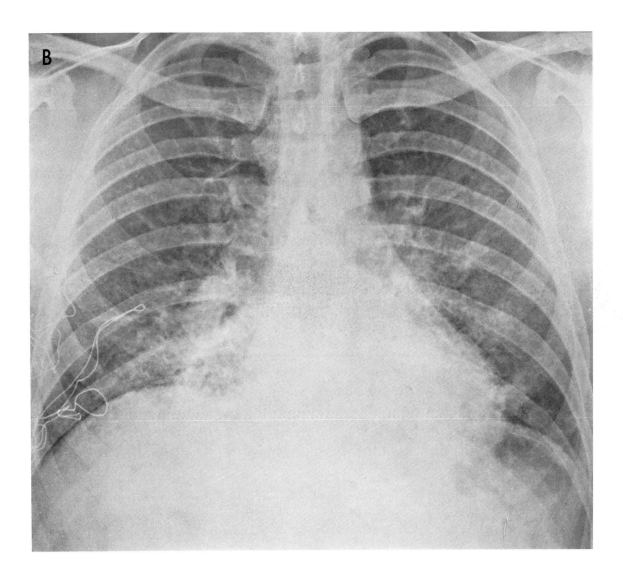

Figure 70 · Lymphoma Resembling Hodgkin's Disease / 195

C, close-up of the right lower lobe in **B.**

D, close-up of the left lower lobe in **B.**

A 20-year-old sailor presented with a large, hot, swollen, tender, painful right axillary mass which had appeared about five days previously and was gradually increasing in size. This was thought to be an abscess, but an incision disclosed no pus. A larger incision then revealed a large solid mass, which was excised. This proved to be a very cellular lymphoma with some characteristics of Hodgkin's disease. The patient became increasingly short of breath and died five days after the biopsy despite radiation therapy. At autopsy the lungs remained hyperinflated; diffuse tiny, granular, nodular changes were present which, on microscopic study, were found to resemble those in the axillary mass. Final diagnosis was "a very anaplastic lymphoma."

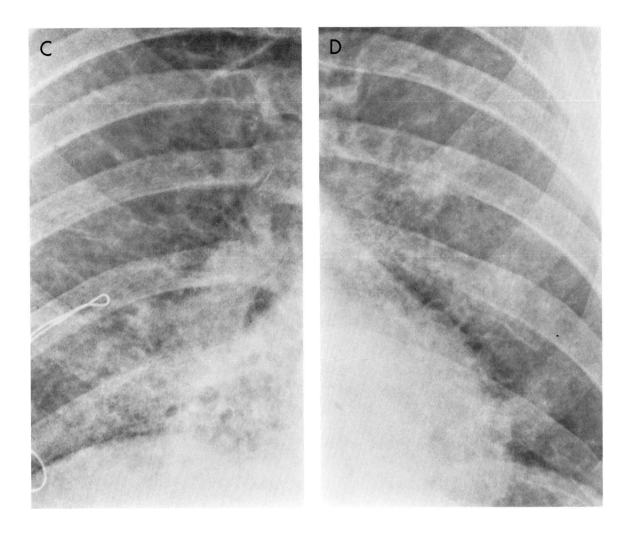

Figure 70 · Lymphoma Resembling Hodgkin's Disease / 197

Figure 71.—Acute lymphatic leukemia.

A, posteroanterior radiograph: Revealing diffuse tiny nodular lesions in both lungs, slightly more marked in the bases and hilar areas. The apices are relatively free of visible nodules.

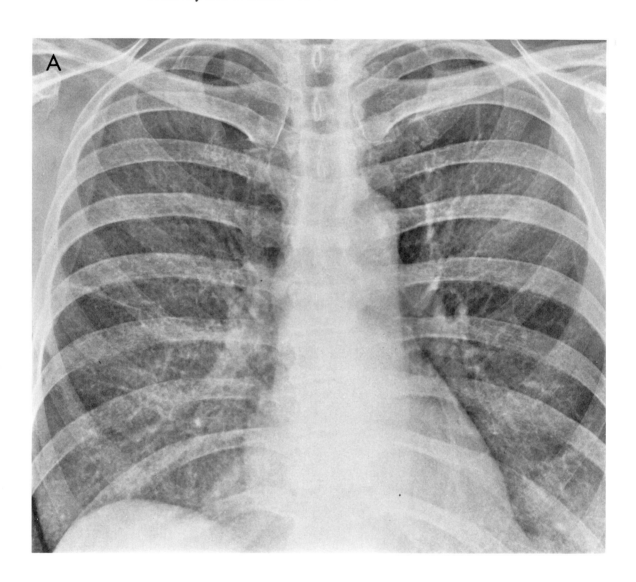

B, close-up of the right lower lobe in **A:** Delineating the thickening and nodularity adjacent to the small vessels (**arrows**) indicative of the interstitial nature of the pulmonary changes. No enlarged nodes are identifiable.

A 28-year-old woman was examined because of weakness, fever, and night sweats. Peripheral blood and bone marrow studies revealed acute lymphatic leukemia. Chemotherapy caused rapid disappearance of the nodular lesions; within 48 hours the chest appeared to be normal radiographically.

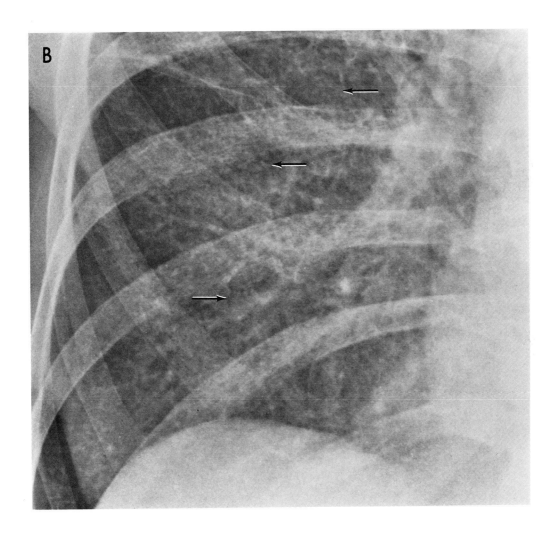

Figure 71 · Acute Lymphatic Leukemia / 199

Figure 72.—Acute myeloid leukemia.

A, posteroanterior radiograph: Demonstrating prominent pulmonary markings throughout both lungs with fluffy, soft, ill-defined nodular lesions immediately adjacent to the vessels. One cannot be certain whether these are alveolar or interstitial, but the latter seems more likely.

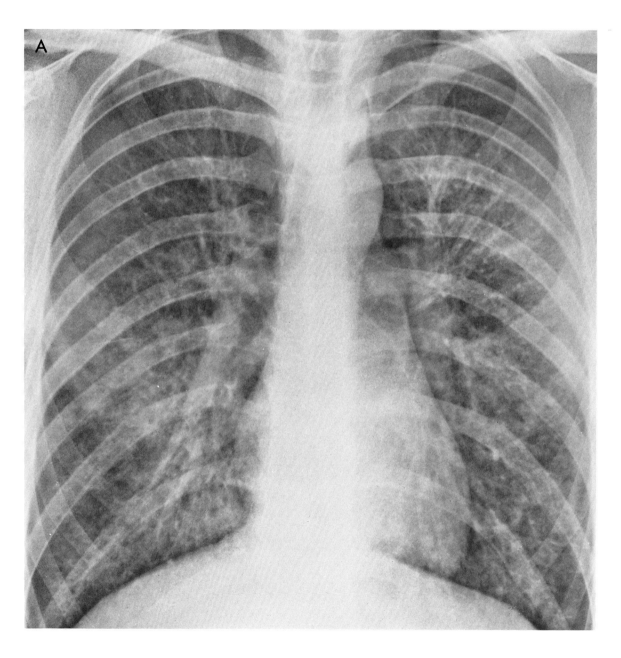

B, close-up of the left lower lobe in **A:** Revealing abnormal vascular structures to better advantage.

A 23-year-old man consulted his physician because of rapidly progressing fatigue, fever, cough and dyspnea of about 10 days' duration. Blood studies revealed acute myeloid leukemia. Chemotherapy was of some help, with the pulmonary parenchymal disease disapppearing 24 hours after therapy was started, but he died 3 months after these studies.

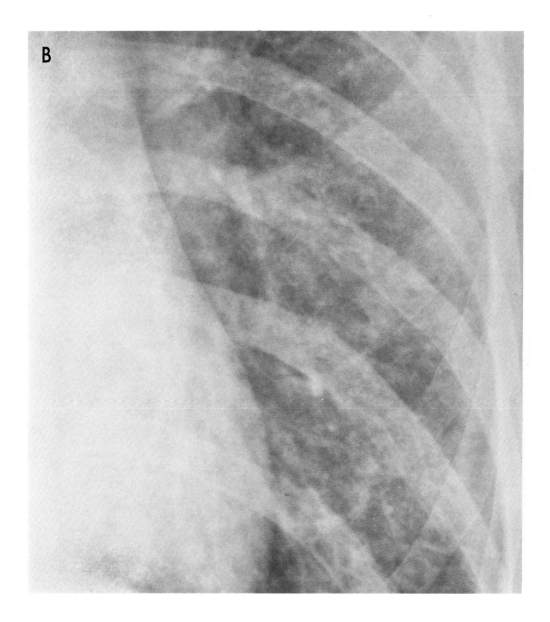

Figure 72 · Acute Myeloid Leukemia / 201

Figure 73.—Reticulum cell sarcoma of the lung.

A, posteroanterior projection: Showing a solitary pulmonary nodule in the right lower lobe (**arrow**). Except for this nodule, the chest is normal.

B, magnification of the nodule in the right lower lobe in **A:** Demonstrating the slightly spiculated borders of the nodule which suggest malignancy. There are no calcifications within or adjacent to the nodule.

A 54-year-old woman was in the hospital for pelvic surgery. Results of the physical examination and standard laboratory studies were within normal limits except for pelvic floor relaxation and the nodule found on the routine chest examination. Pathologic study revealed a primary reticulum cell sarcoma of the lung. Prognosis was considered guarded. At the end of five years, no recurrence or extension of the neoplasm was detected.

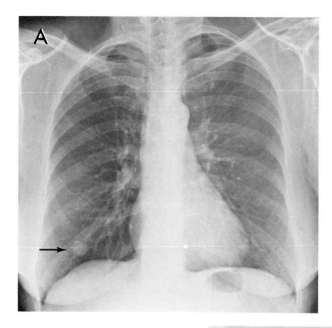

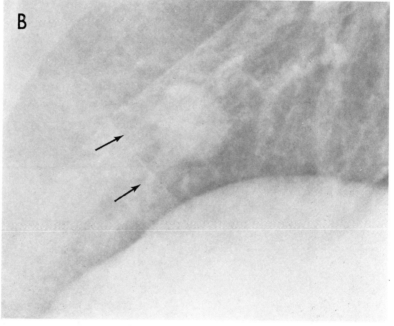

Figure 73 · Reticulum Cell Sarcoma / 203

Figure 74.—Primary lymphosarcoma of the lung (pseudolymphoma).

A, posteroanterior radiograph: Revealing scattered calcifications in both lungs, unrelated to the smooth, round, sharply outlined mass adjacent to the right hilus (**x**).

B, lateral view: Delineating the sharply circumscribed mass (**x**) that lies in the right middle lobe. Just posterior to it are some enlarged hilar lymph nodes (**y**) that deform the esophagus (**arrow**).

C, close-up of right hilar mass (**x**) in **A:** Showing loss of the normal hilar vascular outline (**arrow**).

A 40-year-old man entered the hospital for repair of a right inguinal hernia. Results of the physical examination, except for the hernia, were essentially negative. No enlarged lymph nodes were found; the blood count and ultimately the bone marrow studies were normal. The chest mass was thought to be more important than the inguinal hernia and was removed. Microscopic study revealed tissue resembling lymphosarcoma arising in the lung. One enlarged right hilar node adjacent to the mass showed lymphoid hyperplasia. The patient was well without evident of additional or recurrent disease five years later. The prognosis still appears to be excellent.

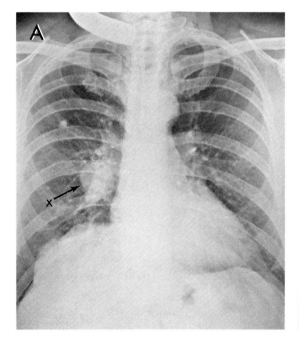
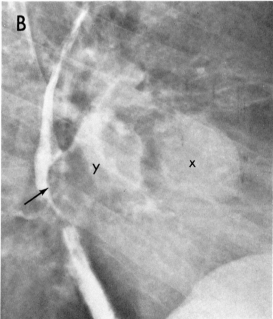

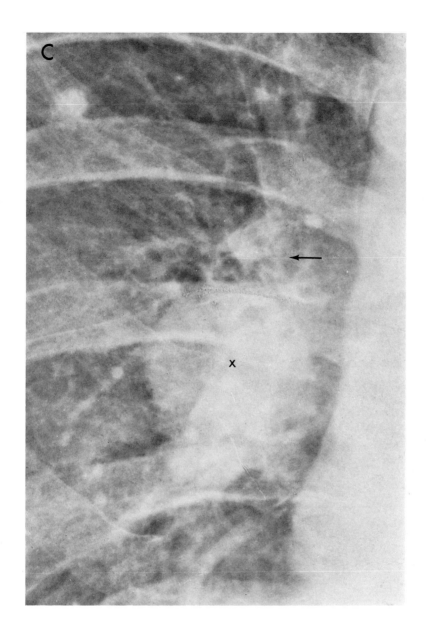

Figure 74 · Pseudolymphoma / 205

Figure 75.—Burkitt's lymphoma (lymphoreticular tumor).

A, posteroanterior radiograph: Showing a large, undulating, smooth-edged extracardiac mass extending from the mediastinum into the right hemithorax (**arrows**). The pulmonary vasculature in the right hilar area is obscured by the mass (**x**); however, the right cardiac border blends with the outline of the mass, indicating its anterior mediastinal location.

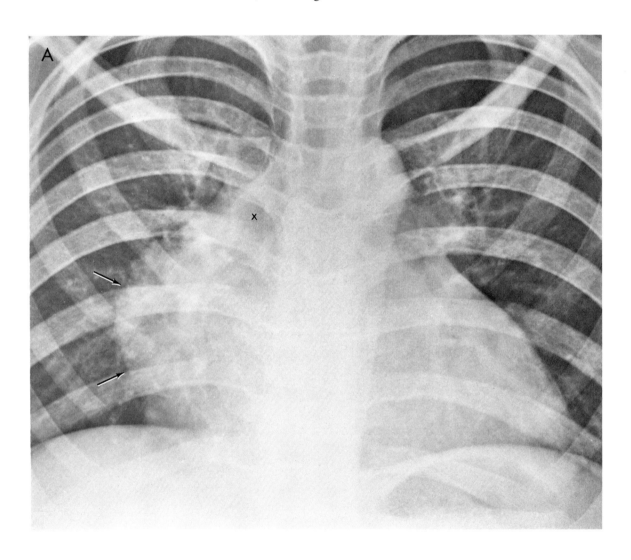

B, roentgen kymogram: Demonstrating poor pulsations along the right margin of the mass, attesting to its solidity (**arrow**). Excellent cardiac pulsations are defined along the left cardiac border (**a**).

(Continued.)

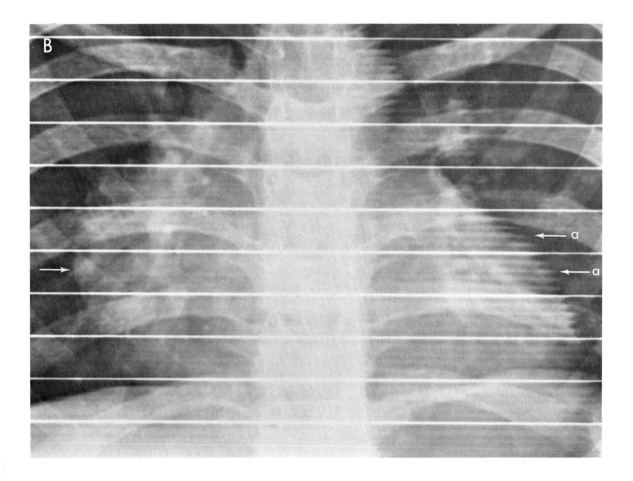

Figure 75 · Burkitt's Lymphoma / 207

Figure 75 (cont.).—Burkitt's lymphoma (lymphoreticular tumor).

C, body-section radiograph: Revealing marked narrowing and displacement of the right lower and middle lobe bronchi (**arrows**). The undulating nature of the lateral margins of the mass (**b**) is more apparent in this radiograph.

D, posteroanterior radiograph of the mandible: Revealing a destructive lesion of the mandible (**arrows**) characteristic of this multifocal lymphomatous tumor.

Figure 75, courtesy of Dr. Leslie R. Whittaker, Kenyatta National Hospital, Nairobi, Kenya.

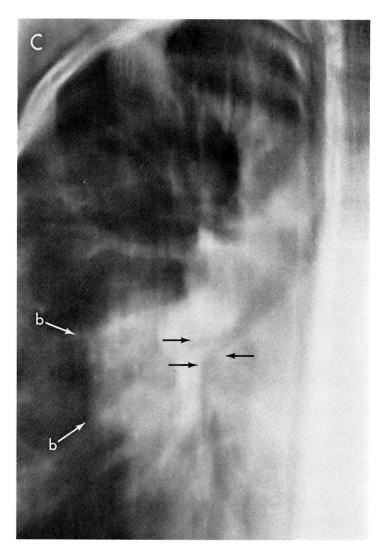

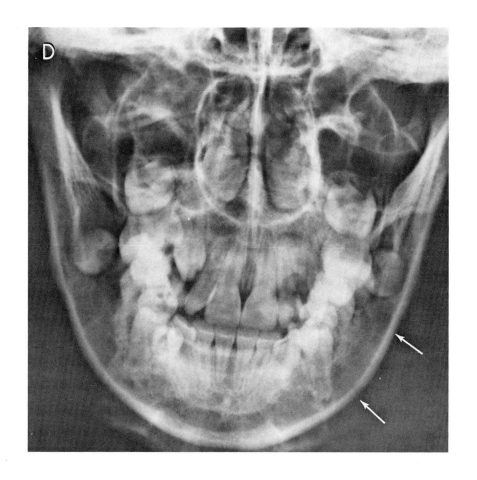

Figure 75 · Burkitt's Lymphoma / 209

PART 4

Mediastinal Tumors

General Considerations

MEDIASTINAL TUMORS present a great variety of patterns. Their variability is compounded by the fact they may arise from the tracheobronchial tree, mediastinal vessels, nerves and lymphatics plus many more potential tissues of origin within the mediastinum. Nor do they necessarily repeatedly arise from the same single site in the mediastinum. As an example, pericardial cysts may be found at any point along the entire length of the pericardium or its extensions (Figs. 101 and 102). Thymic tumors too may arise from a variety of mediastinal sites (Figs. 76–79), their only consistent characteristic being their connection with the anterior portion of the mediastinum. Because of these many manifestations of mediastinal tumors, we must limit our discussion to tumors occupying the more usual sites of origin.

The mediastinum is bounded laterally by the parietal pleura, anteriorly by the sternum and its muscles and posteriorly by the thoracic segment of the spine and its lateral appendages. Its upper limit is the thoracic inlet; its lower, the diaphragm. Divided by the heart and great vessels into the anterior and posterior portions, the mediastinal structures that occupy these two portions must be kept constantly in mind when one considers the differential diagnosis of a mediastinal tumor. Thus anteriorly one expects to find the thymus, a displaced thyroid, lymph nodes, vessels and fibroareolar tissue. Posteriorly lie the tracheal bifurcation, esophagus, descending aorta plus nerves and part of the thoracic duct. Posteriorly, too, lie the nerve tumors that arise from the spine.

Although many mediastinal tumors may be first identified in routine roentgenograms of the chest, some are never suspected until body-section studies or esophageal barium studies are obtained. The role of angiography in this group of tumors cannot be overemphasized. Less commonly employed are contrast agents, including gas and absorbable opaque solutions, which are injected interstitially into the mediastinum.

THYMOMA.—Weighing about 20 g at birth, the normal thymus enlarges slightly throughout childhood, reaching its maximum size of about 30 g at puberty. Thereafter it progressively atrophies, to disappear almost entirely in the adult.

In addition to being the progenitor of the body lymphocytes, the thymus is evidently a pivotal organ in the development of immunologic responses in man. The thymus has been blamed for many diseases to which man is host (hematologic, neuromuscular, neoplastic).

According to Robbins,[13] all tumors of the thymus are generically called "thymoma." Though unusual, their association with myasthenia gravis and their more recent identification with immunologic, blood, endocrine and neuromuscular disease has made them an extremely interesting group of tumors spanning a gamut of gross pathologic patterns which vary from sharply circumscribed and apparently well encapsulated masses to tumors that appear to be aggressive and less well delineated. Histologically thymomas usually may be classified as "small cell," "spindle cell" or "protoplasmic." In addition, the literature refers to "granulomatous" and "lymphomatous" thymomas which are often confused with Hodgkin's disease. True granulomatous thymomas have a much better prognosis than Hodgkin's disease.

Of tumors other than thyroid that arise in the upper part of the anterior mediastinum, thymic tumors are the most common. Sometimes it is extremely difficult to distinguish benign from malignant tumors. As a working rule it is well to consider all thymic tumors malignant if there is associated myasthenia gravis, so common is the relationship. In this regard it is well to recall that only 30% of patients with myasthenia gravis have an associated thymic tumor which usually proves to be of the spindle cell type.

Thymomas in general are found in the young and the old of both sexes, with the thymic lymphomas occurring more commonly in the young and the thymic carcinomas more often later in life.

The classic thymoma lies in the superior aspect of the anterior mediastinum. It is usually sharply defined, easily outlined and may or may not be rimmed by calcific plaques (Figs. 76 and 77). Some are obviously totally irregular in outline, with tumor extending through or beyond an apparently calcified capsule (Figs. 79 and 80). Despite this seeming evidence of an aggressive tumor, some, when removed, are obviously cystic and benign. Indeed, from the pleomorphic roentgen pattern alone, one cannot foretell the patient's future as these tumors often may be resectable and rarely metastasize.

Although most thymomas lie in the superior portion of the anterior mediastinum, some may lie more distally, adjoining the heart (Fig. 79). Some have even been found in the neck with but a thin thread of thymic tissue connecting them with their site of origin in the anterior mediastinum (Fig. 80). Occasionally the mediastinal component lies undiscovered or is poorly visualized, its presence overshadowed by an associated invasive pulmonary process secondary to the unsuspected primary mediastinal malignant thymoma.

As mentioned earlier, metastases to distant organs usually do not occur in thymomas. Local recurrence, or tumor implantation at the site of operation, is not uncommon.

LYMPHANGIOMAS.—Lymphangiomas are benign overgrowths of lymphatic tissue. Involving the neck and thorax, they are thought by many to be malformations rather than neoplasms. Usually they are present at birth and grow as the child grows but do not metastasize.

Lymphangiomas are of two types, the simple or capillary lymphangioma and the cavernous lymphangioma or cystic hygroma. Unlike the usual cavernous hemangiomas, cavernous lymphangiomas may become quite large, sometimes difficult to remove. They may disfigure and compress adjoining structures and thus threaten life.

In the neck, lymphangiomas tend to extend down behind the clavicle and into the mediastinum. Growth is usually self-limited and does not progress after its initial proliferation.

Radiographically, lymphangiomas usually appear as mediastinal masses with smooth margins which may extend into the neck (Figs. 82 and 84). They may change shape and size with changes in intrathoracic pressure incident to crying. Phleboliths within the mass suggest predominantly blood vessel elements which usually are benign. Often lymphangiomas remain undiscovered until adolescence or early adulthood.

THYROID TUMORS.—"Goiter" has long been the term used to describe thyroid glands that have been functionally and anatomically deranged long enough to cause hypertrophy, hyperplasia and sometimes nodularity of the gland. In such instances the thyroid is larger than normal, may progressively enlarge and remain enlarged.

Simple or colloid goiters usually are the result of iodine lack in drinking water. It is a common belief that the enlargement reflects elevated levels of thyroid-stimulating hormone (TSH) caused by a block in the output of thyroid hormone, whether acquired or familial. As a rule the enlarged simple goitrous thyroid is rather firm and gelatinous with its follicles distended by colloid.

Exophthalmic goiter, the cause of Graves' disease, is the result of acinar epithelial cell hyperplasia. Usually it is associated with an enlarged thyroid gland, the enlargement being considerably less than in colloid goiters.

Nodular or multiple colloid adenomatous goiter is still a third form of thyroid enlargement. Somewhat more common in goiter belts than elsewhere, the nodularity of the gland reflects asymmetrical focal hyperplasia, involution, hemorrhage and scarring of the glandular parenchyma. Far more common in females than in males, this type tends to develop soon after puberty. Adenomatous or nodular goiter forms the largest thyroid masses. It is this goiter that most commonly extends below the clavicles into the mediastinum to produce the so-called intrathoracic goiter (Figs. 86 and 88). Their occasional abrupt descent from the neck into the mediastinum has caused them to be known also as plunging goiters.

Of benign thyroid tumors, which may or may not arise from goiters, the most common is the adenoma. Often confused with nodular goiter (which is a regenerative rather than a neoplastic process), fibroid adenomas are true tumors, of which two forms are recognized, follicular and papillary. The follicular group includes all adenomas that produce simple acini or glandular follicles of a wide assortment. At one extreme lie the rudimentary or embryonal adenomas; at the other, the colloid adenomas; between them one finds the fetal adenomas. Thus not only is the follicular adenoma the most common adenoma, it is the one most often confused with the nodules of colloid adenomatous goiter.

The papillary adenomas include those with histologic evidence of papillary projections into glandular or cystic spaces. They run the gamut from apparently benign adenomas to adenomas with malignant anaplasia. As a group, the latter have a malignant potential that often belies their apparently benign morphology.

LEIOMYOMAS.—Leiomyomas are benign smooth muscle tumors found mainly in the gastrointestinal tract and uterus. In the chest they commonly occur as asymptomatic mediastinal masses. In the barium-filled esophagus they produce smooth, marginal, intramural masses with an intact mucosa (Figs. 92 and 93). Some may be exceedingly vascular and may arise from smooth muscle blood vessels. When leiomyomas are of this type, severe bleeding may be the presenting complaint.

These tumors have been found as primary pulmonary parenchymal lesions and endobronchial masses as well as esophageal lesions. The roentgen appearance in the esophagus may be of a smooth-edged mass protruding into either side of the chest and with intact esophageal mucosa and a smooth-margined defect in the wall. Parenchymal lesions are sharply delineated ovoid pulmonary nodules with no characteristic pattern. Endobronchial lesions may be discovered because of signs of obstruction with atelectasis and infection behind them.

Treatment is surgical removal; the prognosis is excellent.

LEIOMYOSARCOMA.—This is the malignant form of leiomyoma and occurs in the same areas. No clue except large size is useful in roentgen differentiation between the benign or malignant lesions. On occasion in the esophagus, destruction of the mucosa can be demonstrated to be quite similar to that seen in primary carcinoma. However, a large soft tissue component is usually present, suggesting the nature of the lesion.

DUPLICATION CYSTS.—Duplication cysts are congenital lesions which are remnants of the primitive foregut. As a rule they are located in the middle mediastinum near major bronchial branchings and may be found at almost any age. Occasionally they lie in a more peripheral position. As a rule they are unilocular and thin-walled and contain a mucoid fluid. Lined by epithelium, they include other elements of respiratory tissue such as cartilage, mucous glands, fibrous tissue and smooth muscle. Rarely, calcium may be present similar to the milk of calcium bile seen in abnormal gallbladders. When present, this milk of calcium may layer when the patient is in the erect position, thus furnishing a helpful diagnostic clue. Occasionally duplication cysts communicate with a bronchus.

Enteric cysts are found under 1 year of age and usually in the inferior mediastinum. They may become quite large and occasionally communicate with the esophagus or other portions of the gastrointestinal tract. The wall contains mucosa, submucosa and muscularis. A few instances of gastric mucosa with ulceration have been reported. The fluid in enteric cysts usually is mucoid. In these cysts this gastric mucosa fluid may actually contain acid.

Radiographically most duplication cysts are visible as smooth, ovoid masses that lie in the mid-mediastinum. The respiratory duplication cysts as a rule lie posterior to the trachea and major bronchial bifurcations (Figs. 94, 95 and 98). Some have been known to change in size and shape with change in position as a result of gravity, but usually this is not a helpful finding. Air and fluid levels may be seen in a few instances when communications exist with the bronchial tree.

As mentioned earlier, the esophagus must be examined routinely in all patients with mediastinal lesions. Both respiratory and enteric cysts (Figs. 99 and 100) may cause smooth defects in the wall of the barium-filled esophagus, assuming the configuration of an extrinsic pressure effect. Occasionally communications between the esophagus and the enteric duplication may be demonstrated.

PERICARDIAL CYSTS.—These cysts are probably due to developmental defects in the pericardium. As a rule they are thin-walled and fluid-filled and may have a single layer of mesothelial cells in the wall within a loose fibrous stroma. Their attachment to the pericardium may be by a thin neck or a broad base. They may be found anywhere along the pericardium and pericardial reflexions but are most common in the right cardiophrenic angle. Here they may be confused with hernias of the foramen of Morgagni or pericardial fat pads. Pericardial cysts vary in size from slight bulges of the cardiac outline to frank masses which may extend to the lateral chest wall. Calcium has rarely been reported in these cysts.

Radiographically these lesions are sharply marginated, usually smooth and apparently continuous with the cardiac outline. In the lateral projection they usually overlie the cardiac shadow and seem more dense than in the routine posteroanterior exposures (Figs. 101 and 103). Occasionally very thin-walled pericardial cysts change with changes in position, depending on gravitational forces. Occasionally kymography allows one to establish the extracardiac nature of the cyst as pulsations along the border of the cyst fail to reveal the usual characteristic pulsations of the normal cardiac border.

PRIMARY TUMORS OF THE HEART.—Primary tumors of the heart are all rare, but the most common are the *myxomas* (Figs. 109 and 110). These tumors usually arise from the interatrial septum and about 75% of the time they are on the left side in the region of the fossa ovalis. Rarely they may involve the valves. They may be sessile, pedunculated, polypoid or villous, are usually found in adults and are about equally divided between the sexes. Emboli occur occasionally. The symptoms are most commonly those of sudden onset of congestive failure, dyspnea, orthopnea, venous engorgement, with or without peripheral edema, and serous effusions. Because of the frequent location near the mitral valve, symptoms may be caused by functional stenosis of the valve.

Roentgen studies may reveal small collections of calcifications in the heart which can be distinguished from valvular deposits by location and greater excursion during the cardiac cycle. Angiocardiography is a most important diagnostic procedure when tumors are suspected and may reveal filling defects in any chamber. Occasionally filling defects in atria can be seen to move back and forth blocking valve orifices or between chambers. Perhaps coronary arteriography should be performed in all patients with suspected myxomas, as tumor vascularity has been reported in a few instances.[9]

Rhabdomyoma may occur as a solitary cardiac mass or as an invading infiltrating tumor of the myocardium. It is found most often in the left ventricle but may involve any portion of the heart, including the valve leaflets. There is a frequent association of multiple cardiac rhabdomyomas, tuberous sclerosis of the brain, adenoma sebaceum and renal fibromas. *Malignant rhabdomyosarcomas,* as well as other primary malignant cardiac tumors such as fibrosarcoma, myxosarcoma and possibly mesothelial sarcoma, have been recorded. These tumors may metastasize to pleura, lung, mediastinal lymph nodes, adrenals or brain. Radiographically the rhabdomyomas may be seen as local added masses on the cardiac outline with sharp smooth edges blending with the adjacent contours (Fig. 107). Angiocardiography or left ventriculography is useful in establishing the nature of an apparent cardiac mass and in differentiating between masses in the muscle and aneurysms of the wall. Coronary arteriography frequently allows one to distinguish pericardial from myocardial tumors and to establish the nature of a tumor in the cardiac muscle. Usually one can differentiate benign from malignant lesions by the vascular pattern.

METASTATIC CARDIAC TUMORS.—Secondary cardiac neoplasms occur more frequently than primary tumors. Invasion of the pericardium and then of the myocardium may come from local invasion by primary bronchial, esophageal, tracheal or anterior mediastinal neoplasms or from direct extension through the chest wall or diaphragm. The most frequent implants are from the bronchi and breast. Blood-borne or lymphatic extension may come from neoplasms in almost any tissue or organ and may involve the various cardiac chambers, walls or valves. We have found carcinomas of the gallbladder, kidney and colon implanted in various portions of the heart; however, only when they have caused symptoms of cardiac failure have they been discovered ante mortem. Renal carcinoma has been found extending directly into the right atrium from the renal vein and inferior vena cava. Several metastatic lesions from the thyroid have seemingly responded to ablation of the normal thyroid gland.

Local extension of lymphomas to the pericardium and then directly to the myocardium does occur infrequently. Again, there are no specific radiographic patterns, but spread may be suspected in a patient with a lymphoma who has pericardial effusion. Frequently with lymphomatous invasion, as with carcinomatous pericardial extension, the effusion may be bloody.

PARATHYROID ADENOMAS.—One to 6% of parathyroid adenomas may be found in the anterior mediastinum (Fig. 118). There is no characteristic roentgen pattern, but in the presence of hyperparathyroidism and negative results of neck exploration, selective arteriography and venography of thyroid, thyrocervical and internal mammary arteries may allow one to discover an adenoma in the mediastinum. If such is present, the vascular blush of a tumor or a normal parathyroid may be observed. Selective sampling of inferior thyroid veins and chemical analysis are now the most valuable diagnostic procedures.

TERATOMAS.—Teratomas are tumors containing tissues originating from the three germ layers: ectoderm, mesoderm, and entoderm. Therefore they may contain hair, teeth, bone, cartilage, muscle and intestinal derivatives. Any one tissue may dominate, but each should be represented to warrant the diagnosis. These tumors may be benign or malignant. The most common site of origin is the anterior mediastinum near the aortic knob and pulmonary arterial levels. They are usually sharply circumscribed and may extend into the thorax on one or both sides. Occasionally teeth or bone can be identified, especially in well-exposed tomograms of the mediastinum. If a teratoma is cystic and filled with fatty material, one can demonstrate layering with the patient in the erect position.

NEUROGENIC TUMORS.—These are relatively common in the chest, being found in the mediastinum or in the chest wall along rib margins. Very rarely are such tumors found in lung parenchyma unless they are metastatic. They may originate from peripheral nerves when in the chest wall or from sympathetic or parasympathetic trunks along the vertebrae of the thoracic spine. So-called dumbbell type lesions can be seen at neural foramina producing bone erosions. The tumors arising from peripheral nerve tissue include the neurofibromas (Fig. 122), neurilemmomas (Fig. 120) and schwannomas. All resemble one another in roentgen appearance and may produce smooth bony erosions along ribs or vertebrae with a sharply marginated soft tissue mass. The schwannomas are malignant and may metastasize to other areas.

Tumors of the sympathetic ganglions, which lie in the posterior mediastinum, are ganglioneuromas, neuroblastomas and sympathicoblastomas. The ganglioneuroma (Fig. 119) is usually the most benign of the group but can be malignant. Characteristic calcifications in paraspinal intrathoracic masses in children are quite diagnostic. Neuroblastomas and sympathicoblastomas are much more malignant, grow rapidly and have no specific roentgen patterns except their location. All may produce bony erosion or destruction, or both.

Paraganglionic cell tumors.—These are rare in the thorax. They include the so-called paragangliomas or chemodectomas and pheochromocytomas or chromaffinomas. They may be benign or malignant and seem to have no predilection for either sex. Characteristically they appear in the posterior mediastinum, are similar to the other neurogenic lesions in location and may produce similar smooth bony erosions. An unusual chemodectoma is shown (Fig. 121) appearing as a pulmonary nodule in the lung parenchyma. Usually when found like this they are metastatic.

Neurenteric cysts.—These rare mediastinal lesions are thought to represent remnants of the neurenteric canals of Kovalevski. They consist of a cystic mass in the mediastinum with a stalk extending to the spinal canal and usually a cord of tissue extending through the diaphragm to the intestinal tract. This communication may be patent or only a remaining fibrous thread. Congenital bony abnormalities of the spine are an integral part of the complex.

The roentgen findings thus consist of a smooth sharp-edged mediastinal mass with adjacent vertebral abnormalities which may be single or multiple (Fig. 123). If air and fluid are found, the communication with the intestinal tract is patent. In a few instances this communication has been demonstrated by barium in the gastrointestinal tract.

EXTRAMEDULLARY HEMOPOIESIS.—Extramedullary hemopoiesis is the development of blood-forming elements in areas outside of the normal erythropoietic tissues. This may occur when the normal areas are unable to maintain erythrocyte formation rapidly enough to keep up with the demand and may be associated with rapid red cell destruction or removal or with decrease of normal erythropoietic formation in the bone marrow. Such hemopoietic tissue may be found in the thorax and spinal canal if the normal areas of formation (liver, spleen, adrenals, heart, thymus, lungs, lymph nodes, lymphatics and occasionally retroperitoneal areas) are not able to maintain production. This abnormal formation has been described in myelofibrosis, various severe anemias, especially thalassemia, lymphomas of various kinds, carcinomatosis, hyperparathyroidism, polycythemia and erythroblastosis fetalis.

When such tissue forms in the thorax, it is usually found in the posterior mediastinum, may be unilateral or bilateral, is well demarcated in the postero-anterior projection and blends with the posterior chest wall in the lateral position (Figs. 124 and 125). Somewhat overexposed radiographs are helpful in outlining the masses. No calcifications or pulsations are demonstrable within the tissue and there is no bone erosion. A frequent associated fusiform widening of the vertebral ends of multiple ribs extending over 3–4 cm may be found. A notched appearance along the inferior rib margins distal to the widening is occasionally seen as well.[14] Biopsy or removal can be almost catastrophic because of severe bleeding, hence care must be exercised in undertaking operative procedures in suspected cases.

A related type of mass is *intrathoracic splenosis,* which may yield a similar histologic appearance or may resemble typical splenic tissue in the lung. Such lesions are found in the lower portions of the thorax, and it may be difficult to establish the intrapulmonary or pleural location of such masses. There is no typical roentgen appearance, but such lesions are invariably associated with splenic rupture. They seem to represent autotransplantation of splenic tissue into the thorax.

BIBLIOGRAPHY

1. Abrams, H. L.: *Angiography* (Boston: Little, Brown & Company, 1971).
2. Berne, A. S., *et al.*: Diagnostic carbon dioxide pneumomediastinography, New England J. Med. 267:225, 1962.
3. Boyden, A. E.: The distribution of bronchi in gross anomalies of the right upper lobe, particularly lobes subdivided by the azygos vein and those containing pre-epiarterial bronchi, Radiology 58:797, 1952.

4. Fleischner, F. G.: Mediastinal lymphadenopathy in bronchial carcinoma, Radiology 58:48, 1952.
5. Fraser, R. G., and Pare, J. A. P.: *Diagnosis of Diseases of the Chest* (Philadelphia: W. B. Saunders Company).
6. Greenspan, R. H.: Pulmonary angiography in lesions of the chest, Radiol. Clin. North America 1:315, 1963.
7. Herlitzka, A. J., and Gale, J. W.: Tumors and cysts of the mediastinum, Arch. Surg. 78:697, 1958.
8. Leigh, T. F.: Mass lesions of the mediastinum, Radiol. Clin. North America 1:377, 1963.
9. Marshall, W. H., *et al.:* Tumor vascularity in left atrial myxoma demonstrated by selective coronary arteriography, Radiology 93:815, 1969.
10. McCort, J. J., and Robbins, L. L.: Lymph node metastases in carcinoma of the lung, Radiology 57:339, 1951.
11. Michelson, E., and Salik, J. C.: The vascular pattern of the lung as seen on routine and tomographic studies, Radiology 73:511, 1959.
12. Neuhauser, E. B. D., and Harris, G. B. C.: Roentgenographic features of neurenteric cysts, 79:235, 1958.
13. Robbins, S. L.: *Pathology* (3rd ed.; Philadelphia: W. B. Saunders Company, 1967).
14. Ross, P. L.: Roentgen findings in extramedullary hematopoiesis, Am. J. Roentgenol. 106:604, 1969.
15. Shanks, S. C., and Kerley, P. (ed.): *A Textbook of X-ray Diagnosis* (3rd ed.; Philadelphia: W. B. Saunders Company, 1962), Vol. II.
16. Schinz, H. R., *et al.*: *Roentgen Diagnostics* (1st Am. ed.; edited by J. T. Case) (New York: Grune & Stratton, Inc., 1953).
17. Simon, G.: *Principles of Chest X-ray Diagnosis* (New York: Appleton-Century-Crofts, Inc., 1971).
18. Steinberg, I., and Finby, N.: Great vessel involvement in lung cancer: Angiocardiographic report on 250 consecutive proved cases, Am. J. Roentgenol. 81:807, 1959.
19. Leigh, T. H., and Weems, S.: Roentgen aspects of mediastinal lesions, Seminars Roentgenol. 4:59, 1969.

Figure 76.—Thymoma.

A, posteroanterior radiograph: Delineating a large mass with a peripheral rim of eggshell calcification in the left hemithorax. The lesion seems to arise in the region of the anterior mediastinum. No pulmonary pseudopods extend beyond the rim of the lesion. The rim of calcification along the medial margin separates the mass from the cardiac shadow.

B, lateral view: Demonstrating the anterior position of the mass with its calcified rim (**arrows**). An air space is demonstrable between the mass and the sternum (**a**). Normal vessels can be seen through the mass. The density is

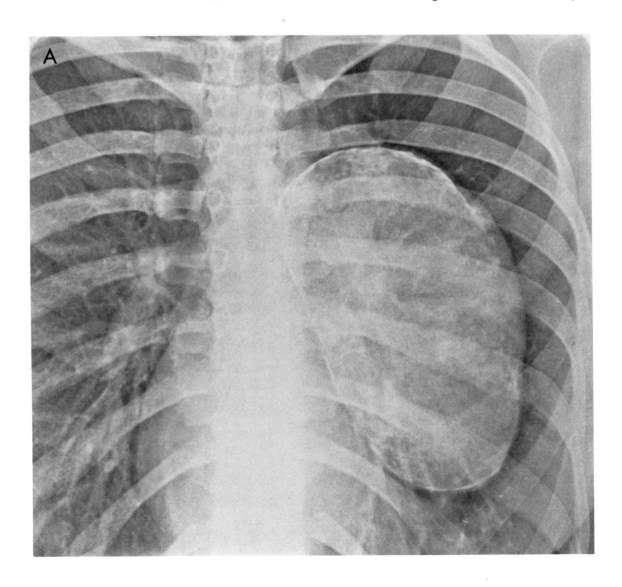

somewhat less than one expects for a mass of this size, suggesting the presence of substantial amounts of fat. The fluoroscopic examination revealed pulsations synchronous with the cardiac pulsations; these were believed to be transmitted.

A 28-year-old teacher required an annual physical examination, including a chest radiograph. She had no chest symptoms. As a result of the radiographic observations thoracotomy was done, where the mass was easily removed from the anterior mediastinum. Pathologic diagnosis was thymoma, which appeared to be malignant microscopically. Five years later there was a small recurrence in the left base. This, too, was removed easily. When last seen 10 years after the initial removal, the patient was well.

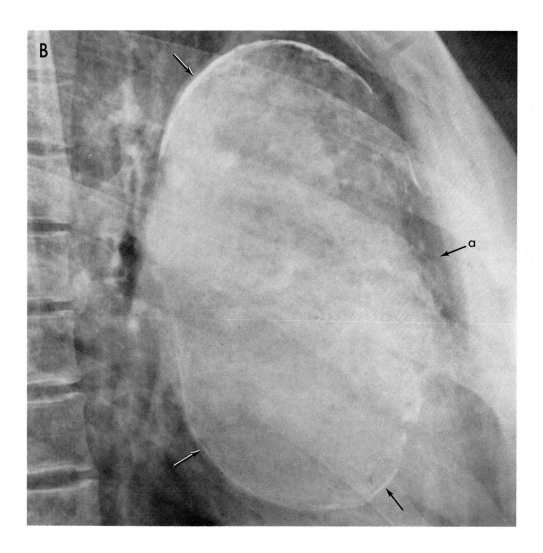

Figure 76 · Thymoma / 223

Figure 77.—Thymoma.

A, a somewhat lordotic posteroanterior view: Revealing a multilobulated mass extending down from the region of the top of the ascending aorta to the midportion of the right atrium (**arrows**). An eggshell rim of calcification is present in the inferior portion of this mass (**a**). All of the vascular markings are prominent.

B, enlargement of the lobulated mass in **A.**

C, lateral body-section radiograph through the anterior mediastinum: Revealing the eggshell calcifications in several portions of the lobulated mass

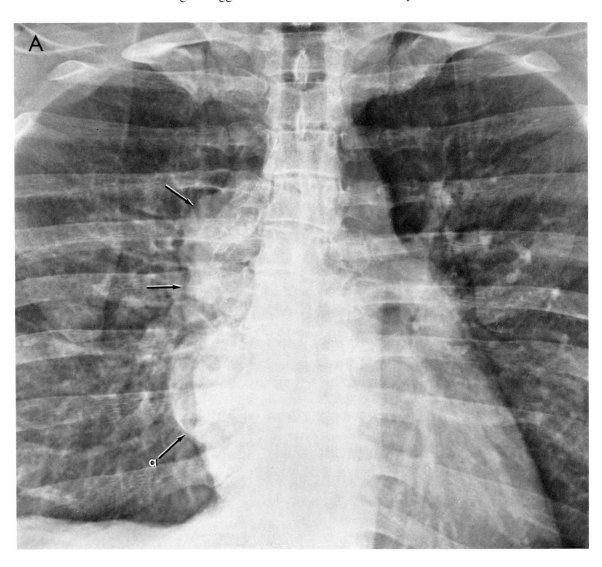

(**arrows**) with more speckled calcifications in the superior portions (**a**). The eggshell calcification in masses of this nature in this location is fairly characteristic of thymic lesions which may be benign or malignant.

At thoracotomy a thymic lesion was shelled out easily. Pathologic study revealed a thymic neoplasm of moderate differentiation. The patient was well three years after removal.

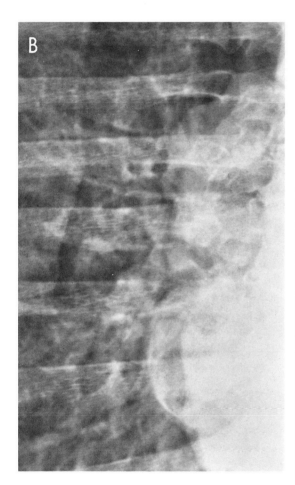

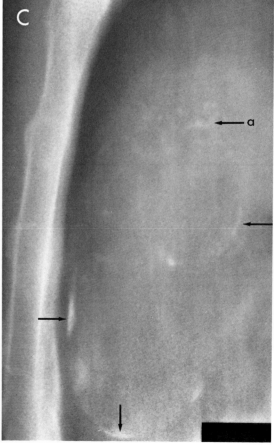

Figure 77 · Thymoma / 225

Figure 78.—Thymoma.

A, posteroanterior radiograph: Revealing a smooth-edged mass (**arrow**) adjacent to the left cardiac border.

B, close-up of mass in **A**: Through this mass (**arrow**) one can see the pulmonary hilar vessels (**a**) and the aortic arch (**b**). The inferior portion (**c**) blends with the cardiac outline, indicating the anterior position of the mass. Several small unrelated calcifications are present in the left upper lobe.

C, more heavily exposed radiograph of the area in **B**: Showing to better advantage the nature of the shadow which is superimposed on the aortic margins (**b**) and the pulmonary hilar vessels (**a**). In the lateral projection one could not determine the precise location of the mass; it was suggested that it lay in the anterior portion of the mediastinum.

A thin 26-year-old woman was examined because of symptoms of myasthenia gravis. Thoracotomy revealed a thymoma which contained a large amount of fat, probably the cause of our inability to define the mass in the lateral projection.

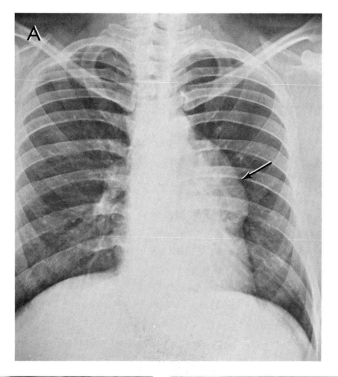

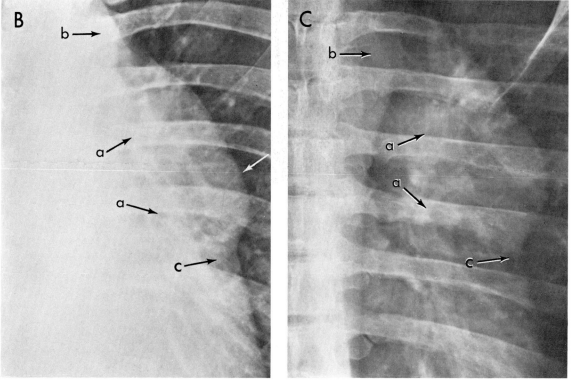

Figure 78 · Thymoma / 227

Figure 79.—Thymoma.

A, posteroanterior radiograph: Showing a peculiar left cardiac border resembling the classic outline of a ventricular aneurysm (**a**). The density of the abnormal shadow at the apex of the heart (**a**) is exactly that of the heart, of which it seems to be a part. A second curved density, continuous with the outer margin of the apical shadow (**b**), extends to the area of the aortic knob which it crosses and ends at its superior margin.

B, lateral radiograph: Demonstrating a dense, ovoid, sharp-edged mass overlying the cardiac shadow. In this projection it is apparent that the density of the mass is indeed added to the cardiac shadow and is not a portion of the heart.

Fluoroscopic studies were of no aid in differentiating the edges of the cardiac margin. Venous angiocardiography confirmed that the mass was extracardiac.

A 20-year-old girl wanted to play on a company softball team, and as part of her physical examination her chest was examined radiographically. The abnormality was discovered at this time. At thoracotomy a soft mass was found overlying the pericardium. A thin tongue of tissue extended into the anterior mediastinum. Grossly and microscopically the tumor resembled adult thymic tissue and was believed to be a thymoma.

She remained asymptomatic for 5 years, when a similar mass was found to the right of the mediastinum. This was also excised; like the earlier tumor, this had the histologic appearance of adult thymic tissue. The patient remained asymptomatic, and 10 years after the original resection was healthy.

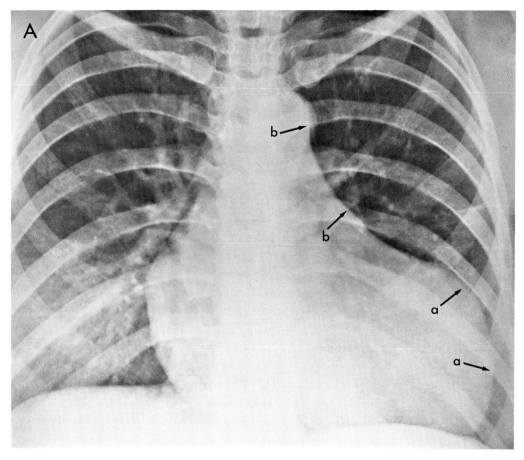

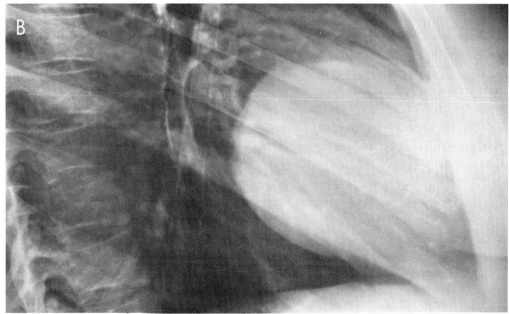

Figure 79 · Thymoma / 229

Figure 80.—Thymoma.

A, posteroanterior radiograph: Revealing a large mass with smooth undulating margins blending with the entire right cardiac border (**arrows**). The density is similar to that of the adjacent heart. Undistorted pulmonary vessels are seen through the mass (**a**).

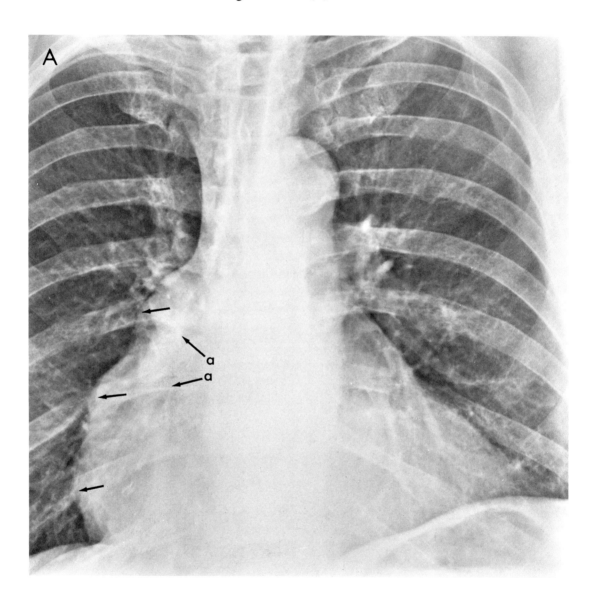

B, lateral projection: Showing the mass superimposed on the cardiac shadow (**arrows**) extending upward toward the mediastinum. Its proximal edges blend with the heart superiorly. Major pulmonary vessels appear to be normal; the esophagus is not displaced.

A 57-year-old man was examined because of weakness, easy fatigability and some weight loss. Thoracotomy revealed a lobulated soft mass with a thin isthmus of tissue extending to the anterior mediastinum. This was easily peeled from the pericardium. Pathologic diagnosis was thymoma.

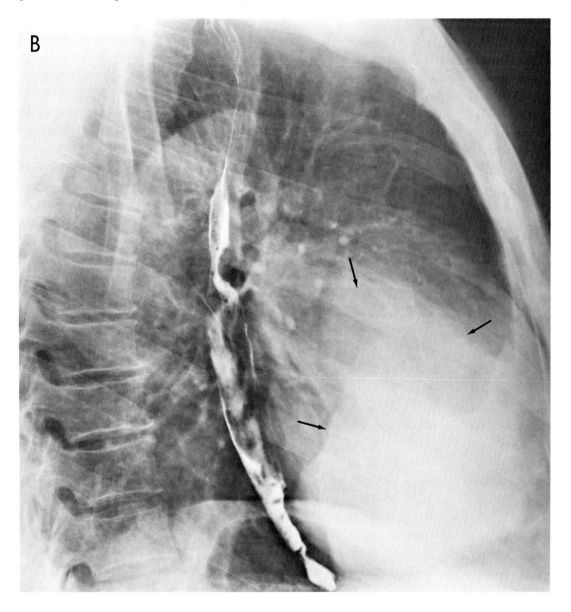

Figure 80 · Thymoma / 231

Figure 81.—Thymic cyst.

A, posteroanterior radiograph: Revealing widening of the superior mediastinum (**arrows**) beginning above the arch of the aorta. The margins are sharp on the left side and somewhat less well defined on the right.

B, lateral projection: Demonstrating loss of the outline of the proximal aortic arch and an overlying soft tissue mass (**x**) which extends to the thoracic inlet (**arrows**). On fluoroscopy the mass did not move during swallowing and the esophagus was not displaced.

A 65-year-old man complained of increasing weakness and fatigue. No chest symptoms were elicited. Thoracotomy revealed a cystic lesion arising in the anterior mediastinum. The pathologic diagnosis was thymic cyst.

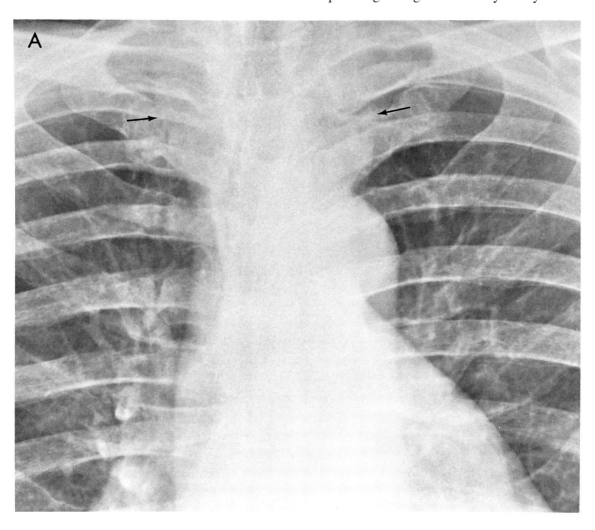

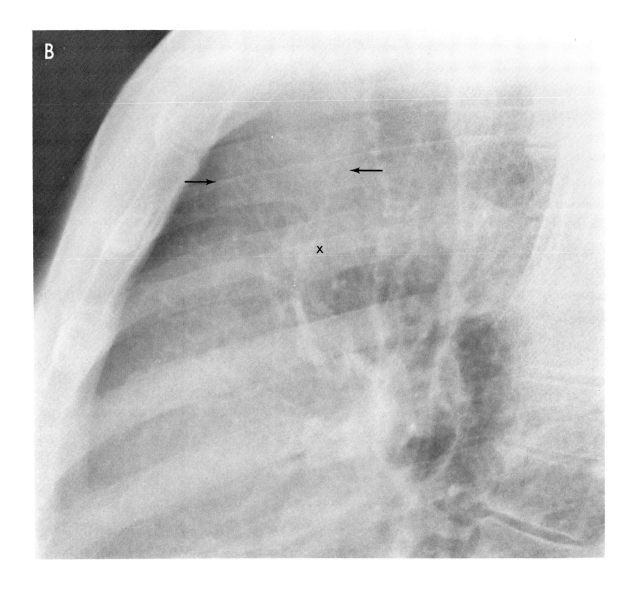

Figure 81 · Thymic Cyst / 233

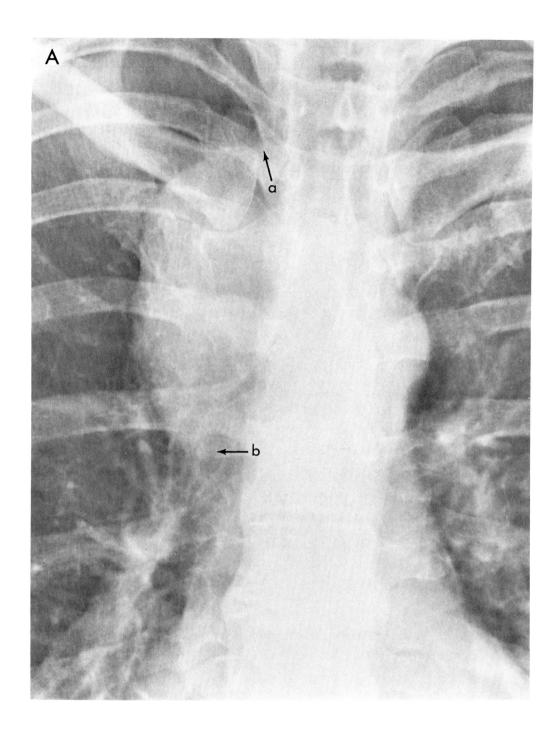

Figure 82.—Lymphangioma.

A, enlargement of the posteroanterior projection (**B**): Demonstrating a smooth-margined lesion to the right of the mediastinum with somewhat convex upper border (**a**) and a lower border that blends with the vascular structures in the hilus (**b**). The mass is unilateral; the left side of the mediastinum, hilar vessels and cardiac outline are normal.

B, routine posteroanterior radiograph.

C, lateral projection: Showing the anterior mediastinal mass (**arrows**) displacing the trachea slightly posteriorly. The ascending aortic outline is lost in the shadow of the mass (**x**). The hilar vessels are normal.

A 38-year-old man entered the hospital for inguinal hernia repair. No chest symptoms were elicited; the general physical examination disclosed no abnormalities. Thoracotomy revealed a thin-walled cystic anterior mediastinal lesion, proved on histologic study to be a lymphangioma.

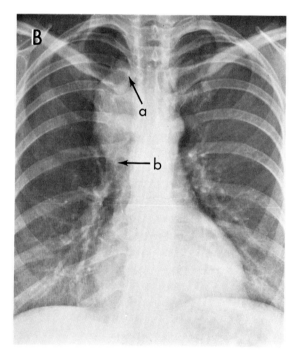
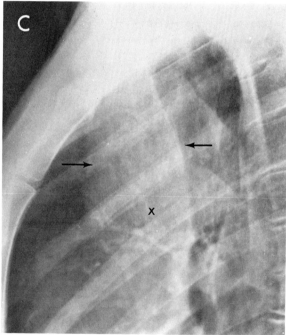

Figure 82 · Lymphangioma / 235

Figure 83.—Cystic lymphangioma.

A, posteroanterior radiograph: Revealing a smooth, sharp-edged, kidney-shaped mass adjacent to the right pulmonary artery. The vessels can be seen through the mass (**a**). Small pleural plaques are present on each diaphragmatic leaf (**b**).

B, lateral radiograph: Showing the lesion superimposed on the hilar vascular shadows (**arrows**). The tracheal bifurcation (**c**) is clearly seen through the mass without distortion of the bifurcation or the adjacent vessels.

C, close-up of the lesion seen in **A:** Pulmonary vessels are visible at **a.**

D, close-up of the lesion seen in **B:** the tracheal bifurcation (**c**) and lesion (**arrows**) are more clearly depicted here.

A 50-year-old shipyard worker had handled asbestos for many years. The abnormality was discovered on a routine survey of the chest. The prolonged asbestos exposure made one suspect a neoplasm. Thoracotomy revealed a thin-walled, cystic lesion. Pathologic diagnosis was cystic lymphangioma.

Figure 83, courtesy of Dr. Walter Miller, City Health Center, Seattle, Wash.

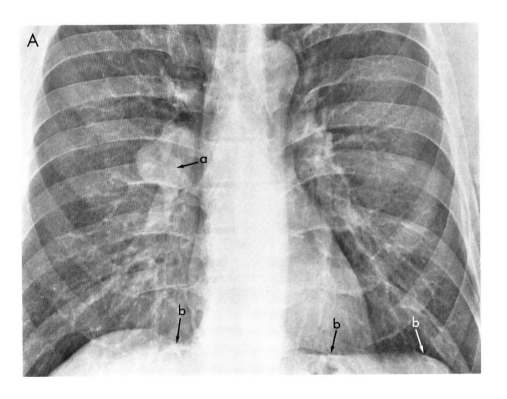

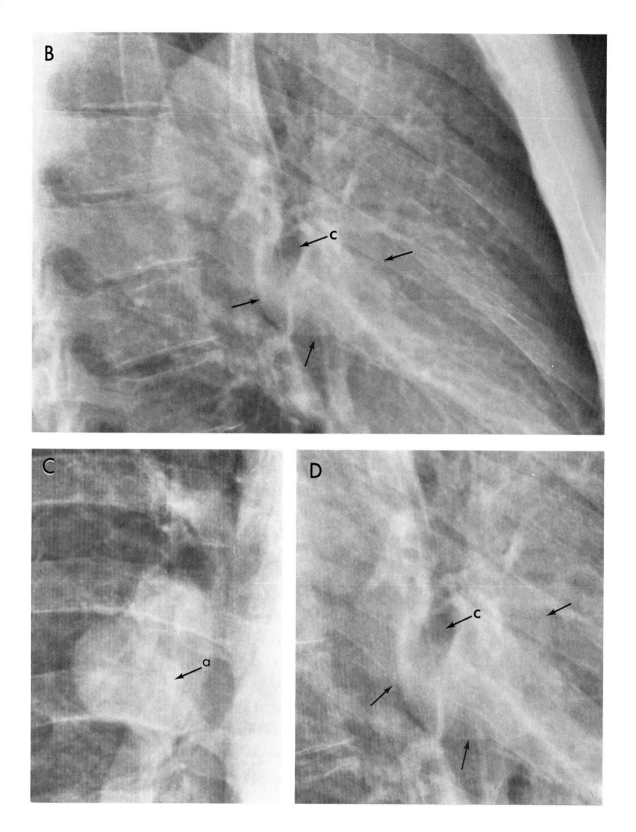

Figure 83 · Cystic Lymphangioma / 237

Figure 84.—Lymphangioma.

A, posteroanterior radiograph: Showing a mass with undulating margins beginning at the left thoracic inlet and extending down and blending with the cardiac shadow inferiorly (**a**). Within the mass are several ringlike calcified nodules resembling phleboliths (**arrows**). The density of the mass is similar to that of the cardiac shadow. The lower trachea (**b**) is displaced slightly to the right, but the lumen does not seem to be compromised.

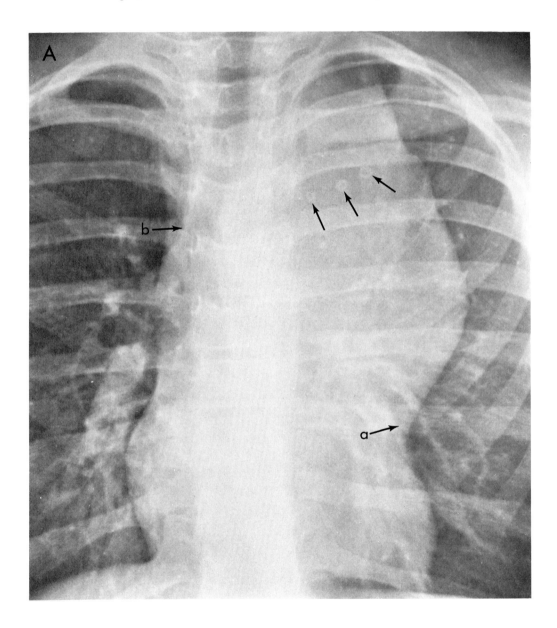

B, lateral projection: Demonstrating the sharp outline of the posterior margin of the mass (**arrows**). Anteriorly the mass fades into the mediastinum (**x**). No significant vascular distortion is seen in either projection.

An 8-year-old boy had a soft tissue mass in the neck discovered by his parents several days before this roentgen examination. On close questioning the parents were unable to remember any abnormality prior to this time. On physical examination the mass was somewhat nodular and wormy in texture. No change in size could be detected on physical examination or under the fluoroscope with changes in intrathoracic pressure. Thoracotomy revealed a large mass which was soft and extremely vascular. Histologically the lesion proved to be a lymphangioma.

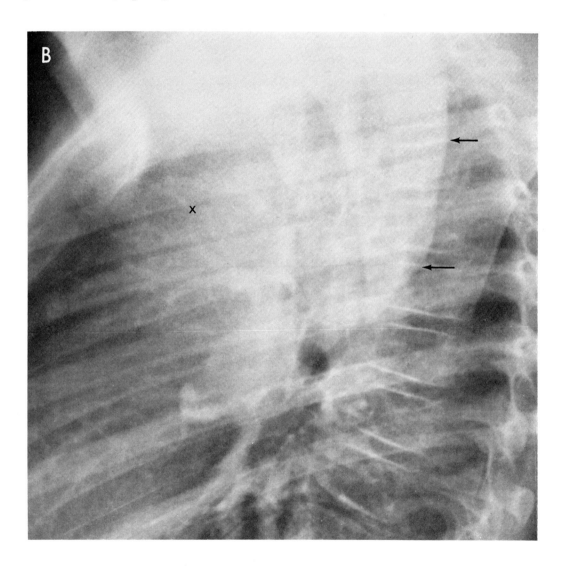

Figure 84 · Lymphangioma / 239

Figure 85.—Huge substernal extension of the thyroid gland.

A, posteroanterior radiograph: Revealing a huge undulating, sharply marginated anterior mediastinal mass extending into each hemithorax with the upper margins lost in the soft tissues of the thoracic inlet. The trachea and esophagus (**arrows**) are displaced slightly to the right. There is a narrowing of the left main stem bronchus (**a**).

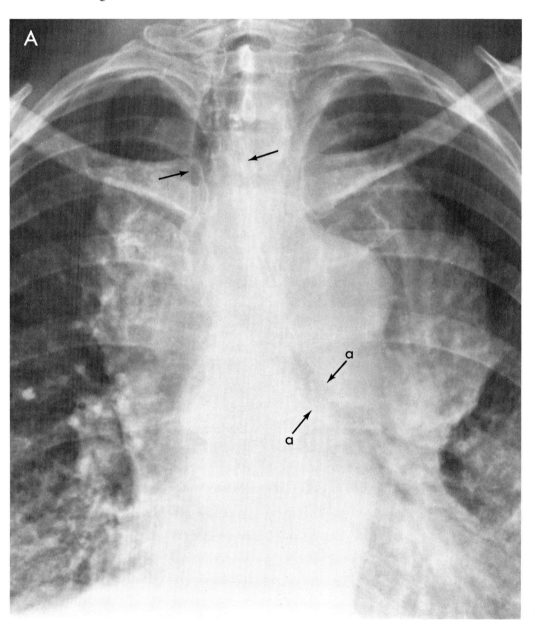

B, lateral view: Showing the esophagus and trachea displaced posteriorly by the huge anterior mediastinal mass (**arrows**). Just below the thoracic inlet the trachea seems somewhat narrowed from front to back (**b**). It is more apparent in this lateral projection that the mass may extend into the neck or from the neck into the mediastinum. The sternum is intact.

Fluoroscopically, considerable upward motion of the mass was observed with swallowing.

Operation revealed the enormous substernal thyroid which on pathologic study was found to be a colloid goiter.

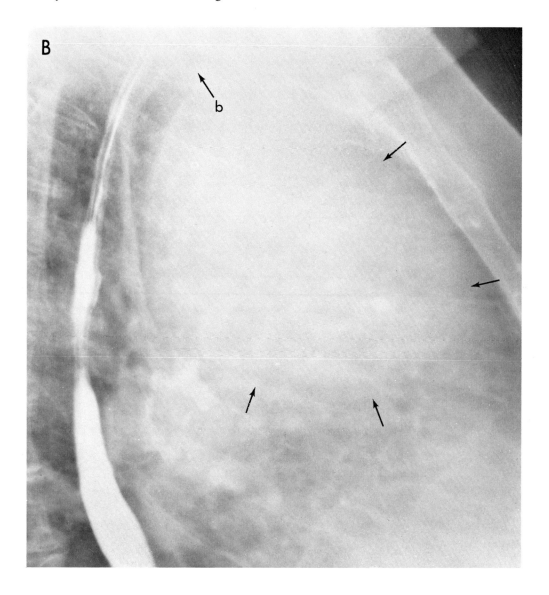

Figure 85 · Substernal Extension of Thyroid / 241

Figure 86.—Intrathoracic thyroid gland.

A, posteroanterior radiograph: Showing a sharply circumscribed nodular mass adjacent to the mediastinum and extending into the right hemithorax. The fluoroscopist thought it moved upward with swallowing. In spite of its convex upper margin, the mass was thought to be the thyroid gland. No significant tracheal narrowing or esophageal displacement is present.

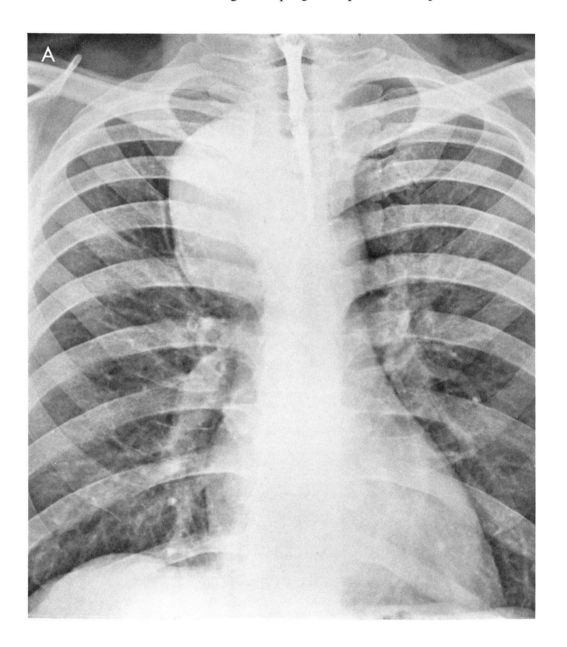

B, lateral projection: Revealing a somewhat vague soft tissue mass (**arrows**) in the superior mediastinum which does not interfere with the air-filled tracheal outline. The esophagus is not displaced.

Radioactive ^{131}I uptake study revealed some uptake of the radioactive material in the region of the mediastinal mass.

A 38-year-old woman was studied as part of a yearly physical examination. No pulmonary symptoms were elicited during routine history-taking. Results of the general physical examination were essentially normal, as were the routine laboratory studies. Pathologic study of the removed mass revealed thyroid tissue which was essentially normal in appearance. No malignant cells were identified.

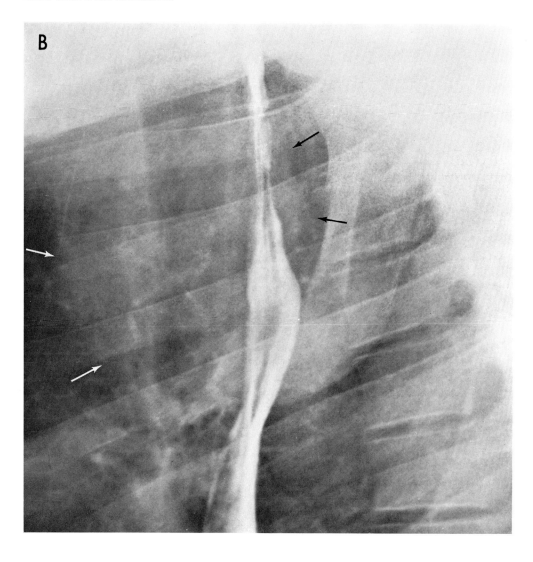

Figure 86 · Intrathoracic Thyroid / 243

Figure 87.—Intrathoracic thyroid gland.

A, posteroanterior radiograph: Revealing a smooth, lobulated soft tissue mass in the superior mediastinum on the right. Some lateral esophageal displacement (**arrows**) but no tracheal displacement or narrowing is apparent. On fluoroscopy the mass moved with swallowing.

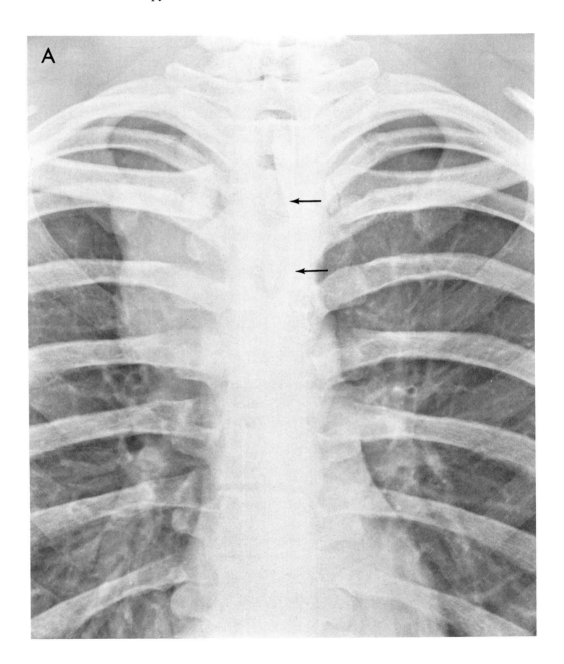

B, the lateral view: Showing the posterior margin of the mass overlying the trachea (**arrows**). The latter is not displaced, but the esophagus does seem to be a little farther back than normal.

A 40-year-old woman consulted her physician because of swallowing difficulties. At operation an intrathoracic thyroid was found.

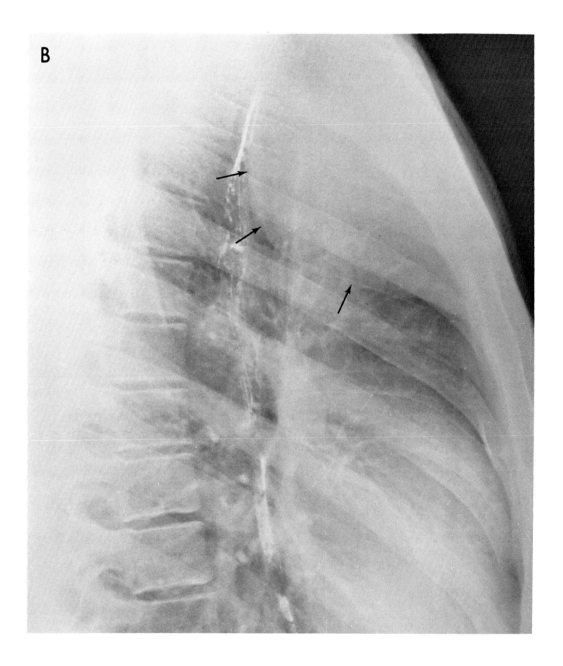

Figure 87 · Intrathoracic Thyroid / 245

Figure 88.—Intrathoracic thyroid gland.

A, close-up of the initial posteroanterior radiograph: Revealing a sharp-edged mass (**arrows**) adjacent to or overlying the aortic knob (**x**). The upper margins of the mass are indistinct and blend into the surrounding soft tissues. Because one of the patient's physicians suspected that this might be an aortic aneurysm, angiocardiography was performed which showed the mass to be extravascular.

B, enlargement of a posteroanterior chest study made 18 years after **A:** Showing increase in size of the mass, which now contains calcifications (**arrows**). The aorta (**x**) is still clearly seen through the mass. It too is more dense and contains some calcification in its wall. At this time the routine chest study revealed cardiac enlargement, vascular congestion and bilateral pleural fluid indicative of congestive heart failure.

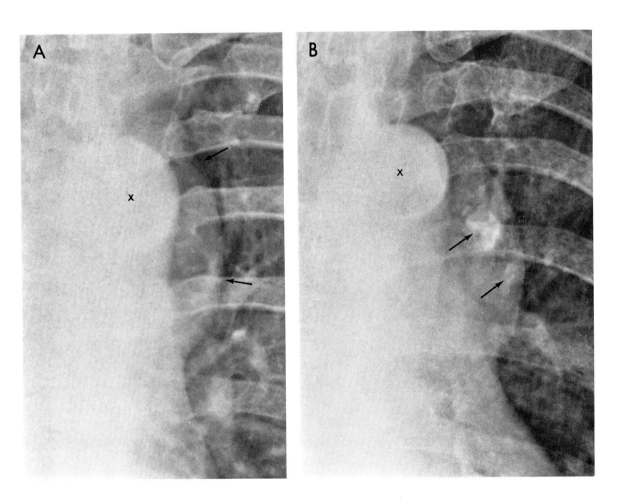

C, close-up of a lateral projection: Demonstrating the anterior location of the mass (**arrows**) and irregular calcifications within it. It is difficult to separate the mass from the base of the aorta in this projection. Calcified paratracheal nodes are present (**a**).

A 74-year-old woman complained of dyspnea and ankle edema. She was thought to be in congestive failure. In a review of her history it was learned that a mediastinal mass had been found 18 years previously (**A**). She had refused treatment at that time.

A thyroid scan revealed marked uptake of ^{131}I at the time of the second examination, when the patient was in cardiac failure. Treatment with antithyroid drugs reduced the hyperthyroidism. Biopsy of the mass revealed thyroid tissue. The patient refused operative removal.

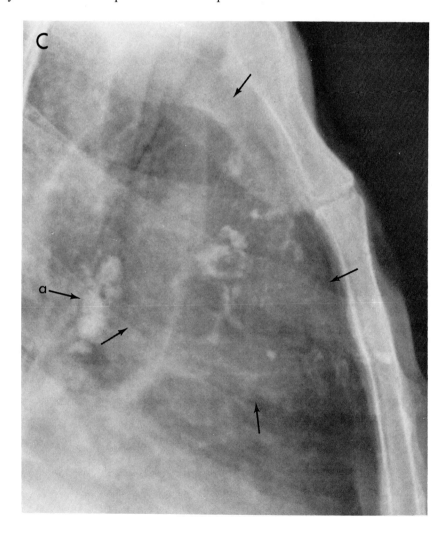

Figure 88 · Intrathoracic Thyroid / 247

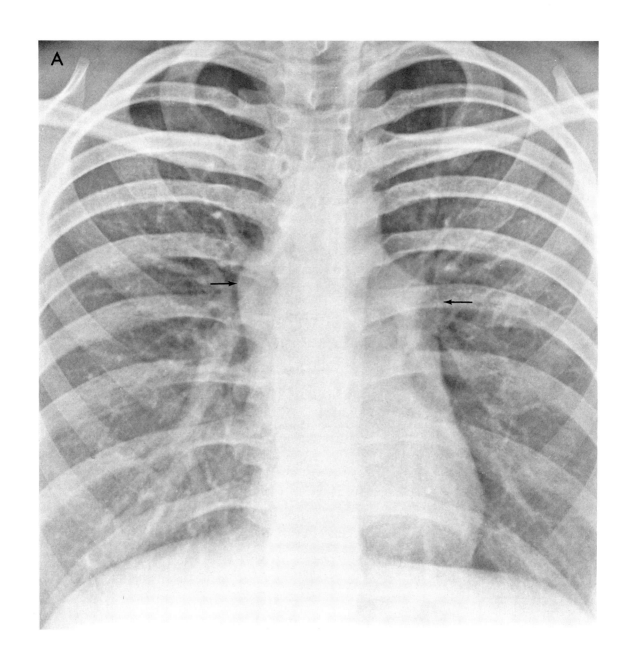

Figure 89.—Vascular teratoma.

A, posteroanterior radiograph: Revealing widening of the mediastinum (**arrows**) at the level of the pulmonary vessels. One loses the normal origin and contour of the pulmonary arteries and veins in each hilar region. The mass is smooth on the right side and somewhat tented on the left.

B, close-up of widened mediastinum seen in **A.**

(*Continued.*)

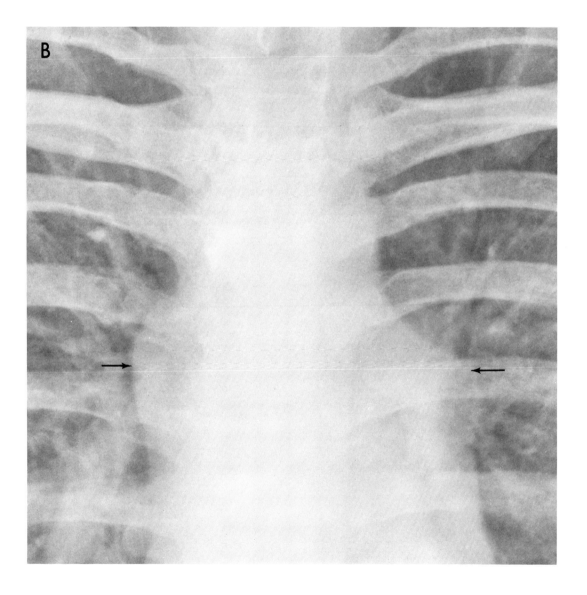

Figure 89 · Vascular Teratoma / 249

Figure 89 (cont.).—Vascular teratoma.

C, lateral view: Demonstrating absence of the normal retrosternal air space and the outlines of the ascending and proximal transverse aorta. A well-defined mass cannot be identified. Such changes are indicative of an anterior mediastinal abnormality. The smooth character of the mass seen in the posteroanterior view (**A** and **B**), plus the fact that it is ill-defined in the lateral projection suggest an infiltrative process.

D, close-up of a lateral body-section study: Confirming the findings in **C.** No substernal air space is visible, nor can a discrete mass be seen. The ill-defined shadow blends with the upper pulmonary vessels.

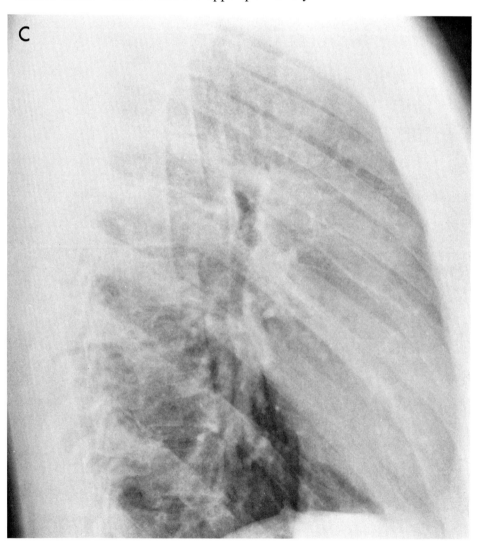

A 19-year-old student nurse required a chest examination at the conclusion of an assigned period on an infectious disease nursing service. A chest radiograph made at the beginning of her training was normal. Thoracotomy revealed an extremely vascular lesion arising in the region of the thymus. With difficulty the lesion could be peeled from adjacent structures. The pathological diagnosis was vascular teratoma.

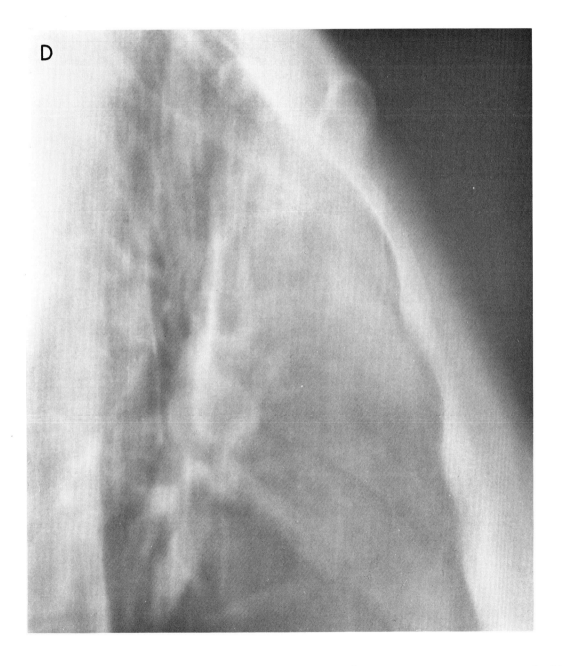

Figure 89 · Vascular Teratoma / 251

Figure 90.—Foramen of Morgagni hernia.

A, posteroanterior radiograph: Delineating the sharply demarcated superior border of a large mass (**arrow**) extending into the right inferior hemithorax and blending with the right cardiac border and medial portion of the diaphragm. The lateral margin gradually fades into the adjacent lung.

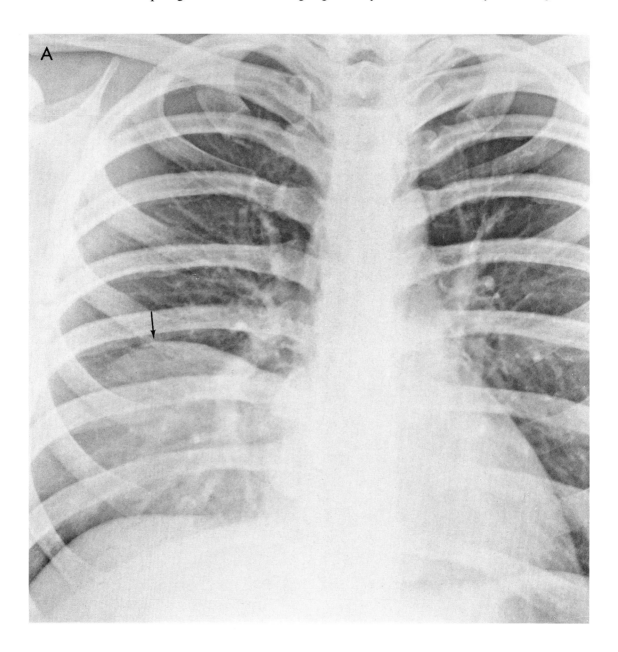

B, lateral projection: Demonstrating the anterior position of the mass, which is peeling pleura from the anterior chest wall (**a**). The inferior portion blends with the diaphragm anteriorly (**x**), suggesting the subdiaphragmatic origin of the mass. No bowel gas is visible.

The patient was a 40-year-old asymptomatic man who had a routine study while he was in jail. At thoracotomy a hernia was found, originating in the foramen of Morgagni. The hernial contents were almost completely omental in origin.

Figure 90, courtesy of Dr. Walter Miller, City Health Center, Seattle, Wash.

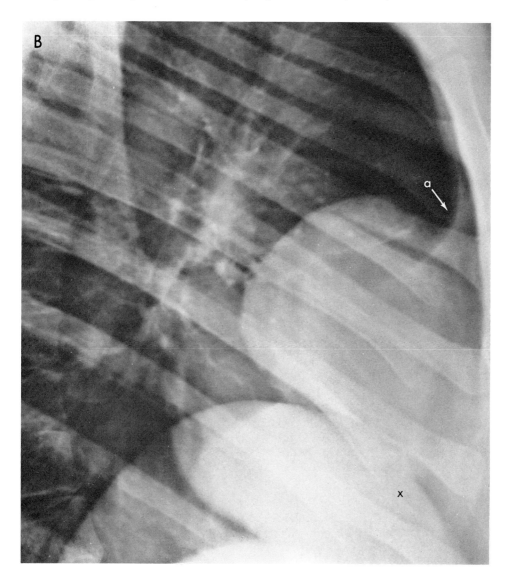

Figure 90 · Hernia of Foramen of Morgagni / 253

Figure 91.—Hernia of the foramen of Bochdalek.

A, posteroanterior radiograph, barium study: Demonstrating a faintly outlined rounded shadow behind the heart at the level of the esophageal hiatus (**arrows**). The barium-filled esophagus is not displaced.

B, lateral projection: Showing a smooth-edged soft tissue mass adjacent to the spine (**arrows**). No bony change is evident. Herniation in the foramen of Bochdalek was suspected.

C, magnification of the mass in **B.**

A 58-year-old man was studied because of vague abdominal pain. The posterior mass was discovered on routine chest study. Operation revealed a hernia of the foramen of Bochdalek containing omentum but no bowel loops.

Figure 91, courtesy of Dr. H. S. Neal, Media, Pa.

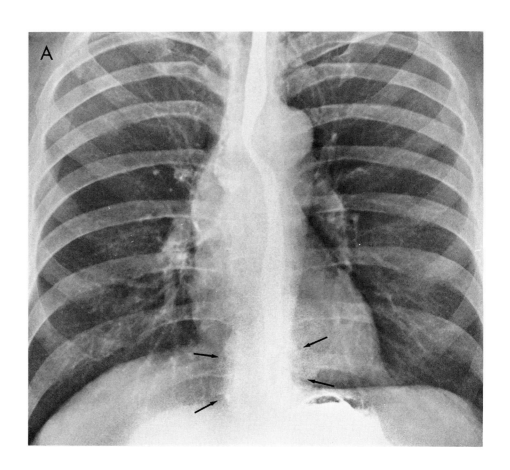

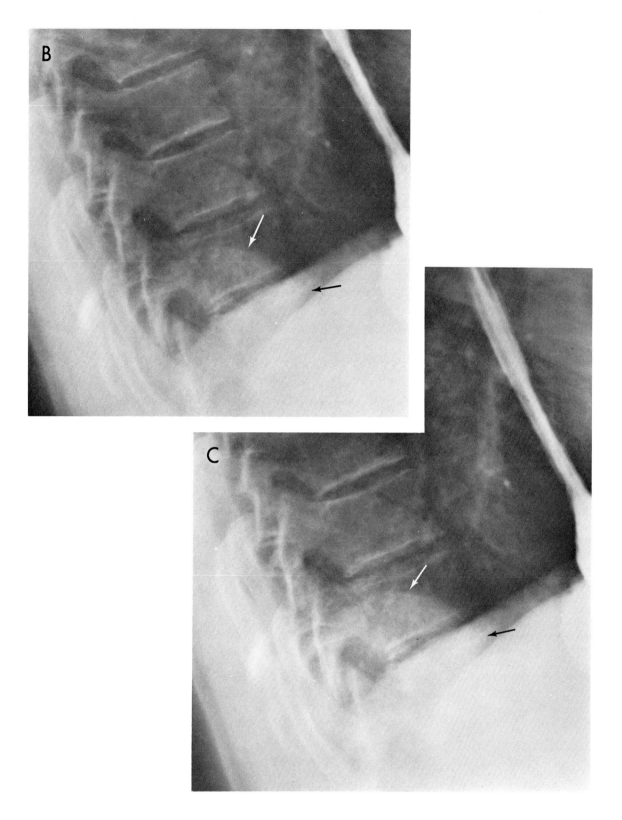

Figure 91 · Hernia of Foramen of Bochdalek / 255

Figure 92.—Leiomyoma of the esophagus.

A, posteroanterior radiograph: Revealing a smooth-bordered elliptical mass in the right hemithorax above the pulmonary artery and obscuring its outline (**arrow**).

B, close-up posteroanterior view of the barium-filled esophagus: Showing distortion due to an intramural mass (**arrows**) which extends to the right of the midline (**x**). The beaking and sharp margins seen in the esophagus are rather characteristic of intramural lesions.

C, close-up lateral view of the mass (**x**), which lies partially between the esophagus and trachea and which is displacing the esophagus posteriorly and the trachea anteriorly.

A 32-year-old man was seen for his annual physical examination while in the Navy. The shadow was detected at this time. At operation the mass was easily shelled out of the esophagus and proved to be a benign leiomyoma.

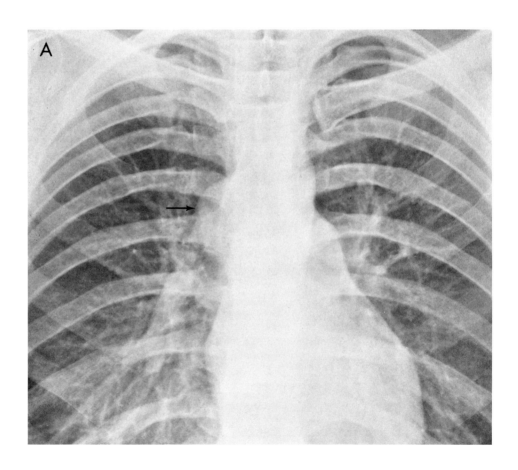

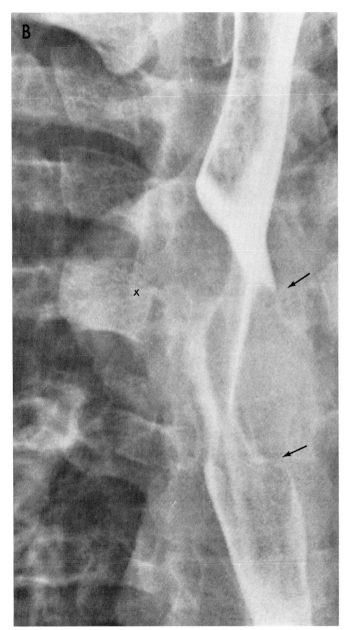

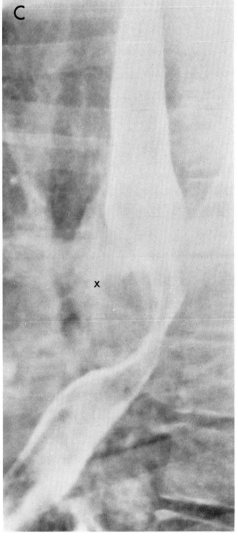

Figure 92 · Leiomyoma of Esophagus / 257

Figure 93.—Leiomyoma of the distal esophagus.

A, posteroanterior projection: Demonstrating a sharply marginated mass seen through the cardiac shadow extending to both sides of the midline (**arrows**). On fluoroscopy the mass seemed to pulsate. As with all masses adjacent to major vessels or the heart, one could not determine whether these pulsations were transmitted or expansile.

B, close-up view of the barium-filled esophagus: Revealing a sharply outlined impression of the mass on the esophageal column with mucosa which is displaced but seems intact (**a**). The upper edge of the rounded mass is sharp and slightly beaked (**b**). The findings are characteristic of an intramural lesion of the esophageal wall.

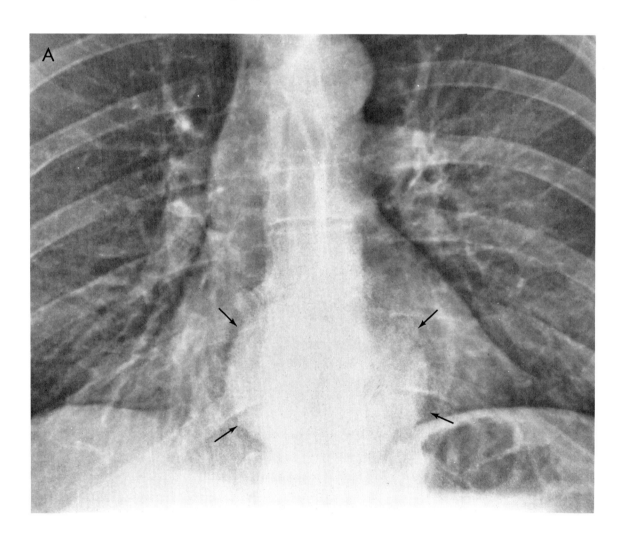

C, close-up view of the esophagus taken immediately after **B: a** and **b,** as in **B.**

A 45-year-old man was referred for a gastrointestinal examination because of epigastric discomfort which was relieved when he took food and alkali. The chest examination was incidental to the intestinal study. At thoracotomy the mass easily was shelled out of the esophageal wall. Pathologic diagnosis was leiomyoma.

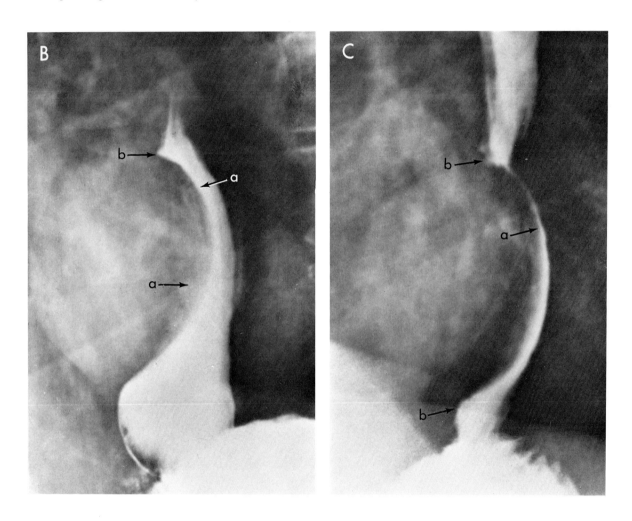

Figure 93 · Leiomyoma of Esophagus / 259

Figure 94.—Respiratory duplication.

A, posteroanterior projection: Revealing a mass the size of a golf ball occupying a portion of the mediastinum. Its right lateral border (**arrow**) is round and smooth. There is abrupt esophageal displacement to the left (**a**).

B, lateral view: Showing the mass (**arrows**) posterior to the normal-appearing major pulmonary vessels and just below and behind the tracheal bifurcation. The esophagus is not deviated backward or forward.

C, close-up of a contrast study: Intravenous angiogram delineating the superior vena cava (**b**) and right atrium (**c**) as well as barium in the esophagus (**a**) and indicating the central location of the mass (**x**) which does not involve any adjacent vascular structures.

A 23-year-old man had a survey chest radiograph made while applying for a new job. The abnormality caused no symptoms. Prior to thoracotomy it was suspected that this lesion was a leiomyoma. However, a thin-walled cystic lesion was found which proved to be a respiratory duplication.

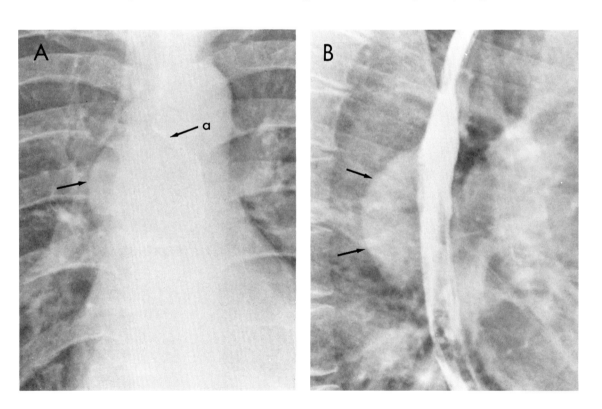

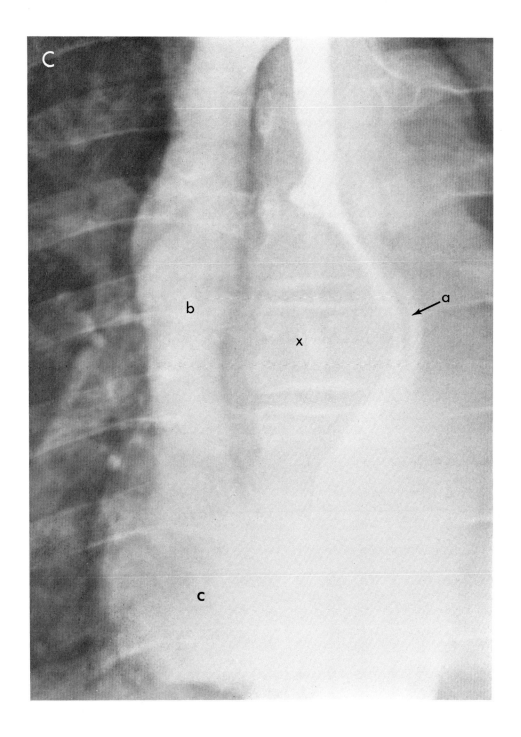

Figure 94 · Respiratory Duplication / 261

Figure 95.—Respiratory duplication.

A, close-up view of a posteroanterior radiograph: Illustrating a sharp-edged, semilunar shadow (**arrow**) along the right mediastinal border through which the edge of the superior vena cava (**a**) and upper pulmonary vessels are clearly visible. The lower edge crosses the junction of the superior vena cava and right atrium (**b**). The fact that the vena cava and hilar vessels can be seen through the mass indicates that the mass lies at a different level in the mediastinum. The trachea and esophagus are not displaced.

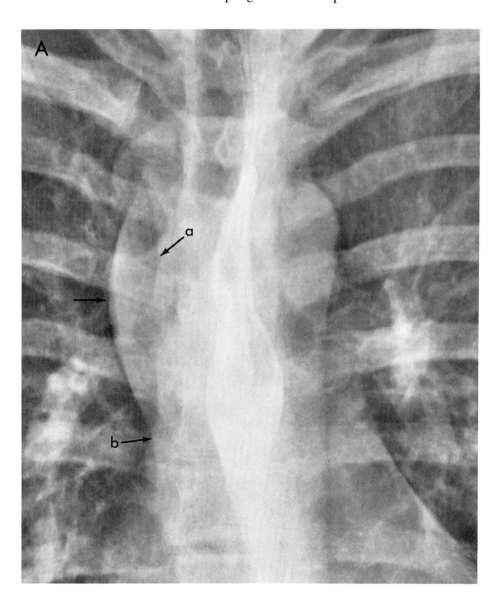

B, close-up view of a lateral projection: Delineating the elongated, ovoid character of the mass (**arrows**) superimposed on the normal esophagus. The tracheal bifurcation and pulmonary vessels are normal.

A 24-year-old Navy seaman reported for his annual physical examination, at which time the abnormality was discovered. Thoracotomy revealed a thin-walled cyst which pathologic analysis showed to be a respiratory duplication.

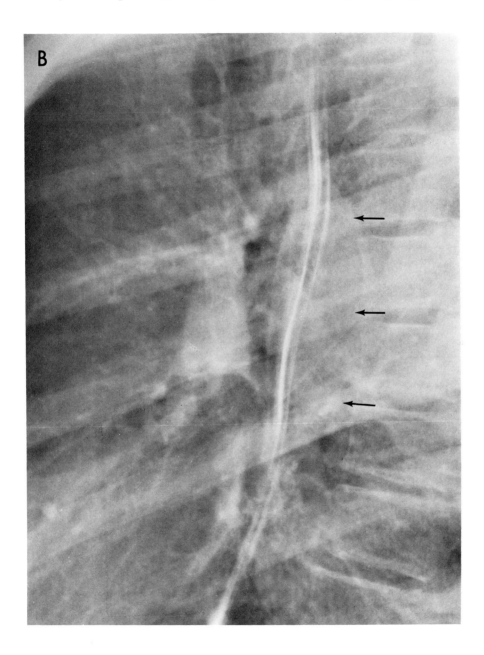

Figure 95 · Respiratory Duplication / 263

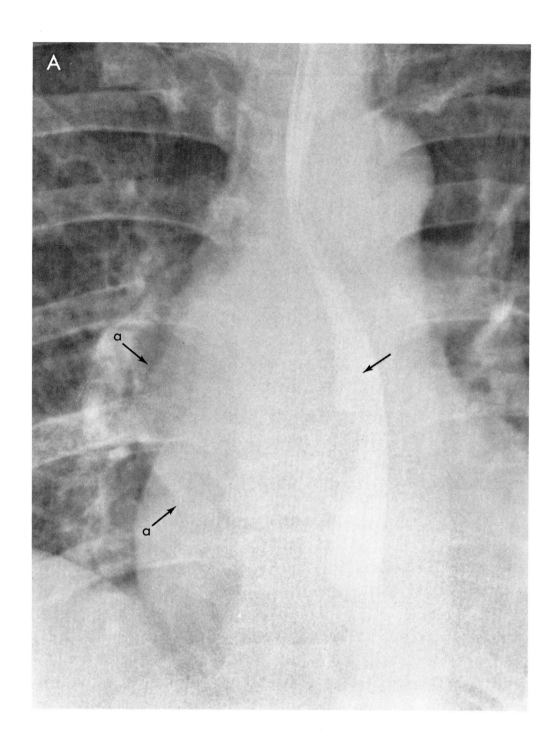

Figure 96.—Respiratory duplication cyst.

A, close-up of a posteroanterior radiograph: Showing a large, rather sharply marginated mass (**a**) in the midportion of the mediastinum that causes lateral displacement of the esophagus (**arrow**). No motion was evident with swallowing.

B, lateral projection: The major pulmonary vessels are ill-defined. The mass (**a**) extends posterior to the esophagus but does not displace it.

(*Continued.*)

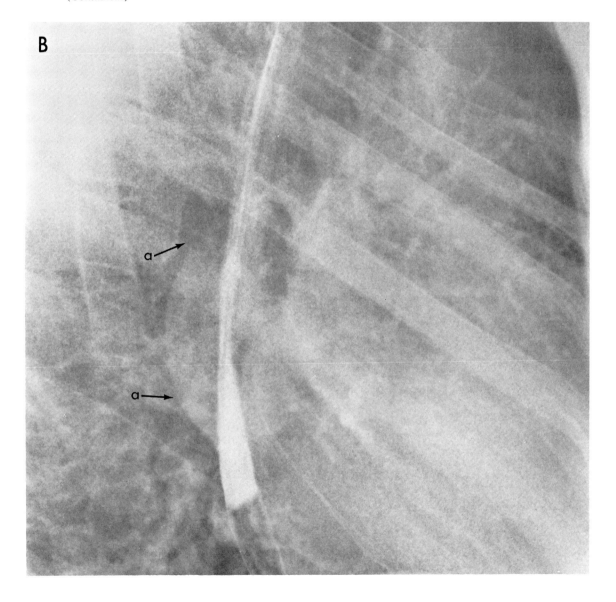

Figure 96 · Respiratory Duplication Cyst / 265

C, close-up of anteroposterior body-section radiograph: Revealing the sharply outlined mass (**a**) elevating the left main stem bronchus (**b**). There is slight narrowing of the lumen of the left main stem bronchus (**c**).

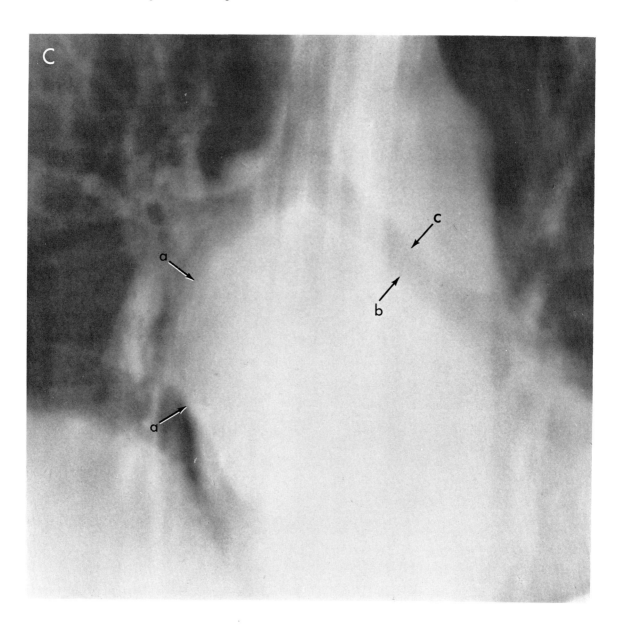

D, close-up of lateral body-section radiograph: Showing the mass (**a**) displacing the left main stem bronchus (**b**) posteriorly.

A 48-year-old man saw his physician because of an intermittent wheeze which seemed unrelated to anything specific. On physical examination the wheeze was detected, but no other positive findings were elicited. Bronchoscopy showed smooth extrinsic pressure on the midportion of the left main stem bronchus. Thoracotomy revealed a thin-walled cystic lesion in the mediastinum. The pathologic interpretation was a respiratory duplication cyst.

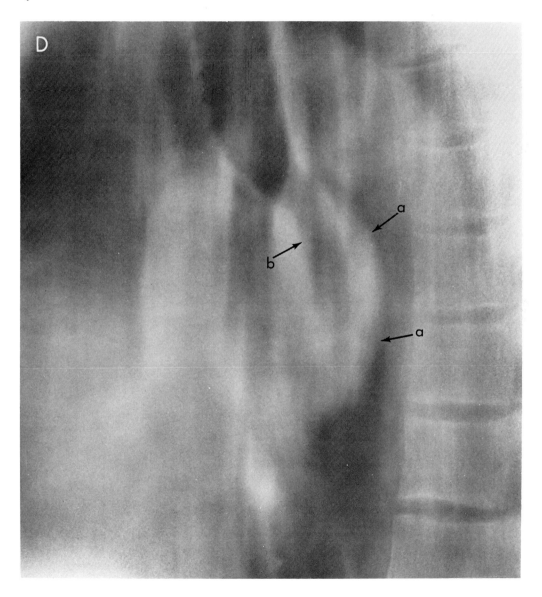

Figure 96 · Respiratory Duplication Cyst / 267

Figure 97.—Respiratory duplication cyst.

A, close-up of a posteroanterior radiograph: Demonstrating a smooth-edged ovoid mass inferior to the aortic knob (**arrows**). The upper and lower margins of the mass are clearly visible through the aorta. The adjacent pulmonary artery (**a**) and cardiac shadow are also visible through the mass, indicating the posterior position of the abnormality. The esophagus is normal.

B, close-up of an oblique projection with barium in the normal esophagus: Revealing the posterior location of the mass (**arrows**). It appears to be intrapulmonary. No bony changes are present.

Aortography delineated a normal-appearing thoracic aorta and body-section studies disclosed no bony erosions.

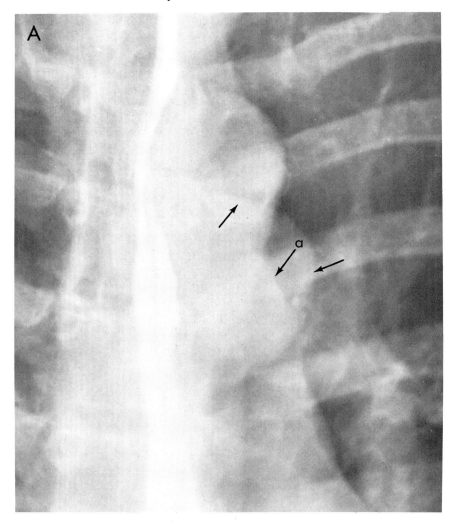

A 40-year-old woman saw her physician for a routine physical examination, at which time the mass was discovered. Thoracotomy revealed the cystic nature of the lesion.

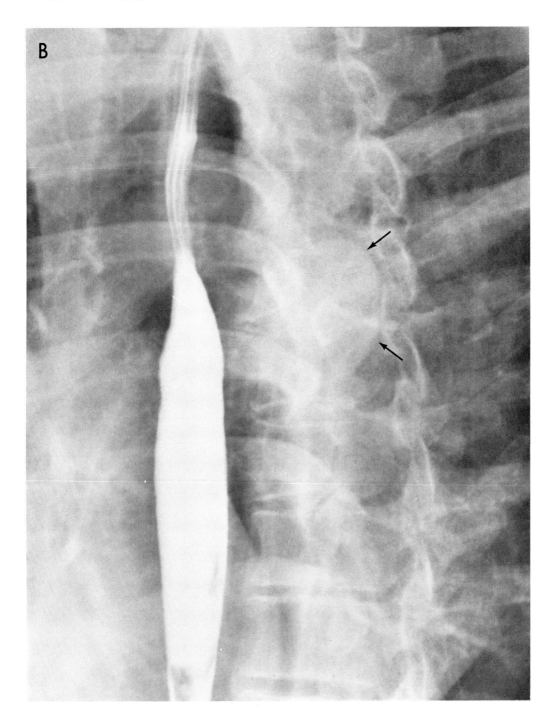

Figure 97 · Respiratory Duplication Cyst / 269

Figure 98.—Mediastinal bronchogenic cyst.

A, posteroanterior radiograph: Revealing a lobulated mass (**arrow**) in the right hemithorax adjacent to the mediastinum. Speckled calcification is detectable at the inferior margin of the mass (**a**). The outline of the pulmonary vessels near the right hilus is lost.

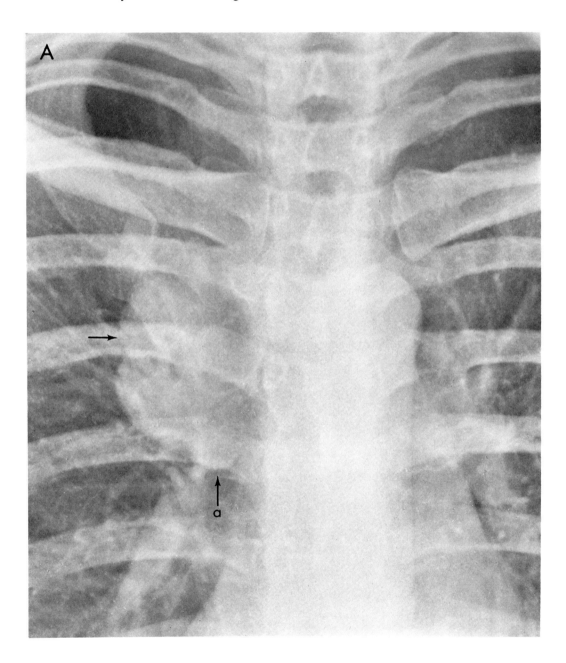

B, lateral radiograph: Demonstrating the anterior location of the mass. There is no distortion of the trachea (**b**) or the pulmonary vessels (**arrows**). Speckled calcification (**a**) is seen in the inferior portion of the mass.

(Continued.)

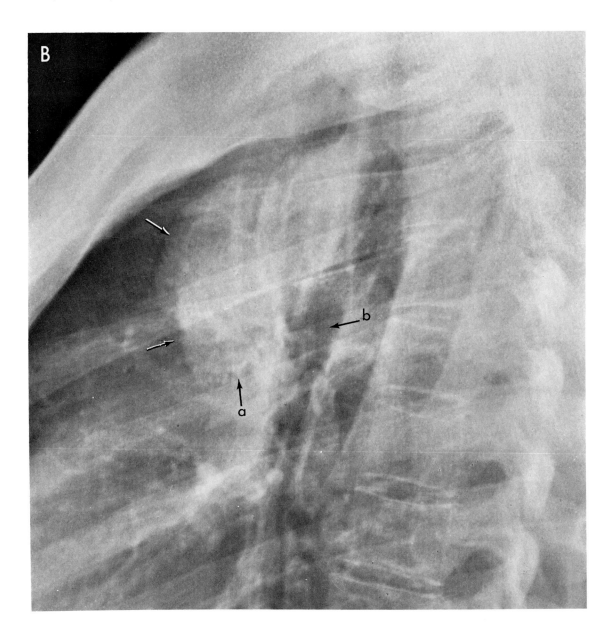

Figure 98 · Mediastinal Bronchogenic Cyst / 271

Figure 98 (cont.).—Mediastinal bronchogenic cyst.

C, two months later, posteroanterior view: Showing an increase in the size of the mass (**arrow**), which now is more lobulated. The calcium within it is much more apparent and has increased in amount. A layered level of calcium (**b**) is clearly seen in the inferior portion of the mass, and speckled calcifications are scattered throughout the remaining portions.

D, lateral projection: Confirming the increase in size of the mass (**arrows**) and its calcification (**b**).

E, body-section radiograph: Demonstrating movement of the dependent calcification (**b** in **C** and **D**) to other portions of the mass when the patient is placed in the supine position. This change indicates that the lesion is cystic. The margins of the mass are sharp, without pulmonary or mediastinal extensions.

An asymptomatic 26-year-old man was found to have an abnormality during a routine chest survey. On removal of the mass, pathologic study demonstrated a bronchogenic cyst containing calcium.

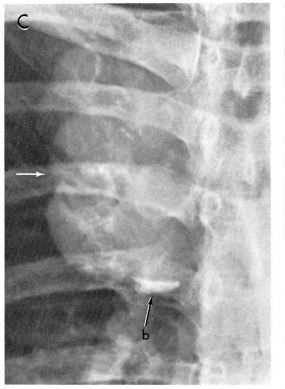
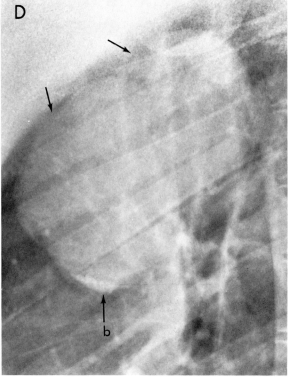

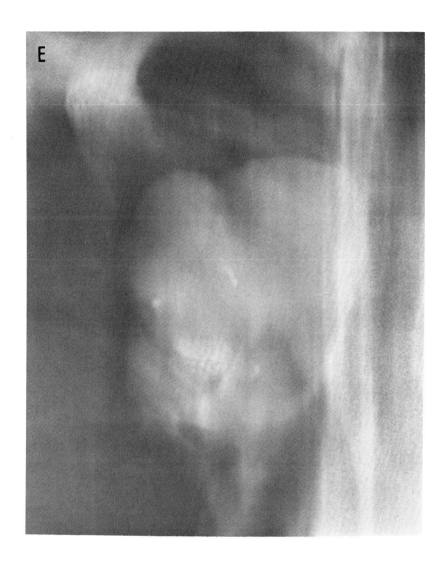

E

Figure 98 · Mediastinal Bronchogenic Cyst / 273

Figure 99.—Bronchogenic cyst arising from the trachea.

Posteroanterior radiograph: Revealing a smooth-edged egg-shaped mass with a concave inferior medial border (**arrow**) blending with the cardiac border. A small spotted calcification overlies the inferior portion of the mass (**a**). The superior medial margin is lost in the mediastinum. The trachea is deviated to the left (**b**).

A 24-year-old man had a routine chest survey, in which the mass was detected. Thoracotomy disclosed a thin-walled cyst adherent to the trachea, which was filled with clear yellowish fluid. Pathologic study of the wall revealed bronchial epithelium characteristic of a respiratory duplication.

Figure 99, courtesy of Dr. Walter Miller, City Health Center, Seattle, Wash.

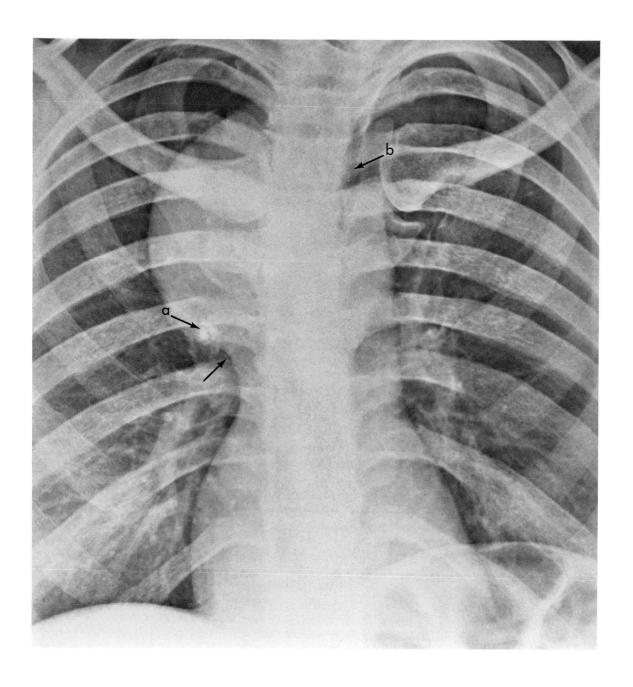

Figure 99 · Bronchogenic Cyst from Trachea / 275

Figure 100.—Enteric duplication cyst.

A, posteroanterior radiograph: Revealing a round, smoothly marginated soft tissue mass (**arrows**) near the esophageal hiatus. This causes deviation of the distal esophagus (**a**), but the esophageal mucosa appears to be intact. There are multiple rib anomalies on the left.

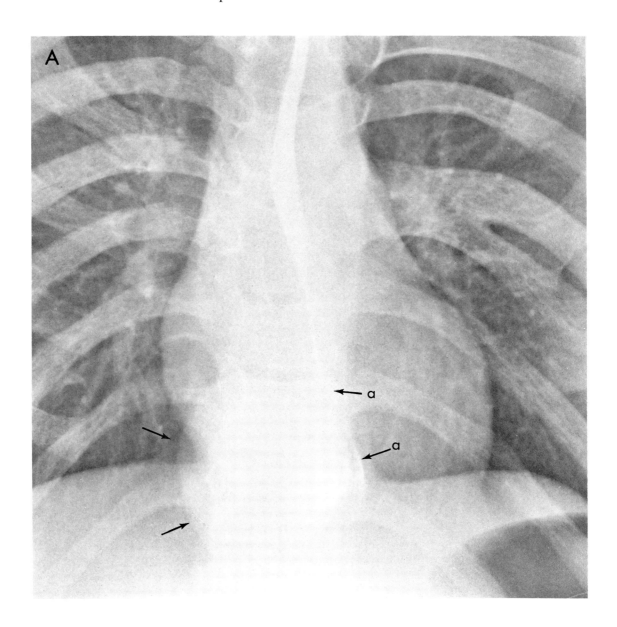

B, lateral radiograph: Showing the rounded margins of the soft tissue mass (**arrows**) near the esophageal hiatus. Additional barium studies revealed no communication with the gastrointestinal tract.

A 13-year-old girl was studied because of epigastric pain. The mass was removed through the abdomen and pathologic study indicated a gastric duplication.

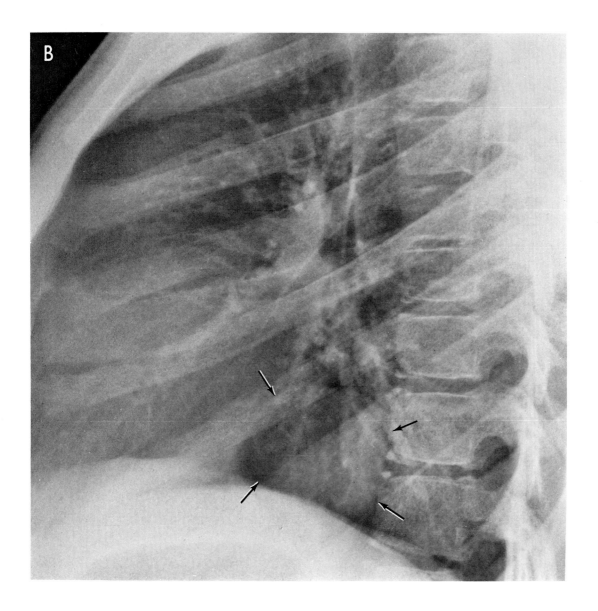

Figure 100 · Enteric Duplication Cyst / 277

Figure 101.—Pericardial cyst.

A, posteroanterior radiograph: Revealing a smooth, sharp-edged mass adjacent to the right cardiac shadow (**arrow**), obliterating the normal cardiophrenic angle. Pulmonary markings are visible through the mass, which seems slightly less dense than the cardiac shadow. The upper margin blends with the cardiac contour.

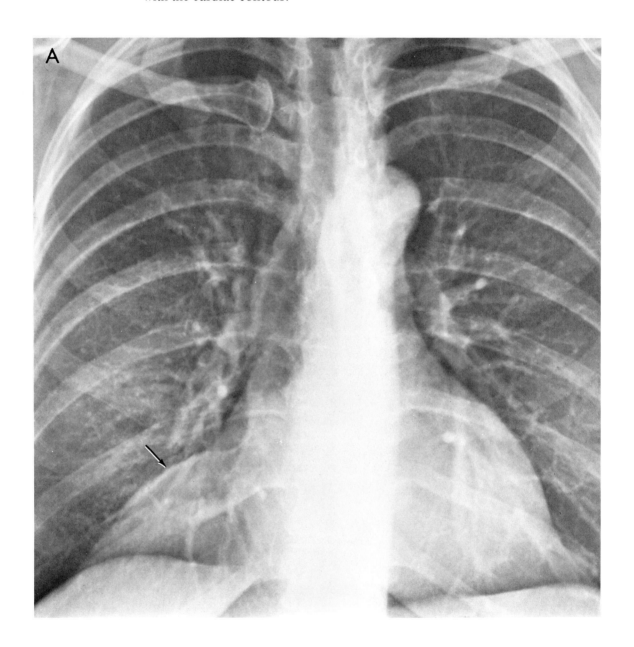

B, lateral projection: The mass (**arrows**) obviously overlies the heart. The location is a helpful clue to diagnosis.

A 41-year-old woman had no chest complaints but described minor right upper quadrant discomfort. Thoracotomy revealed a typical thin-walled cystic lesion of the pericardium filled with clear yellow fluid.

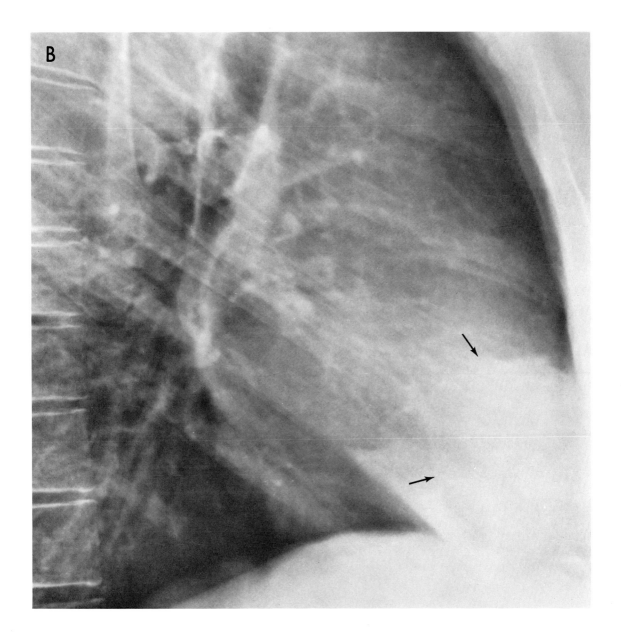

Figure 101 · Pericardial Cyst / 279

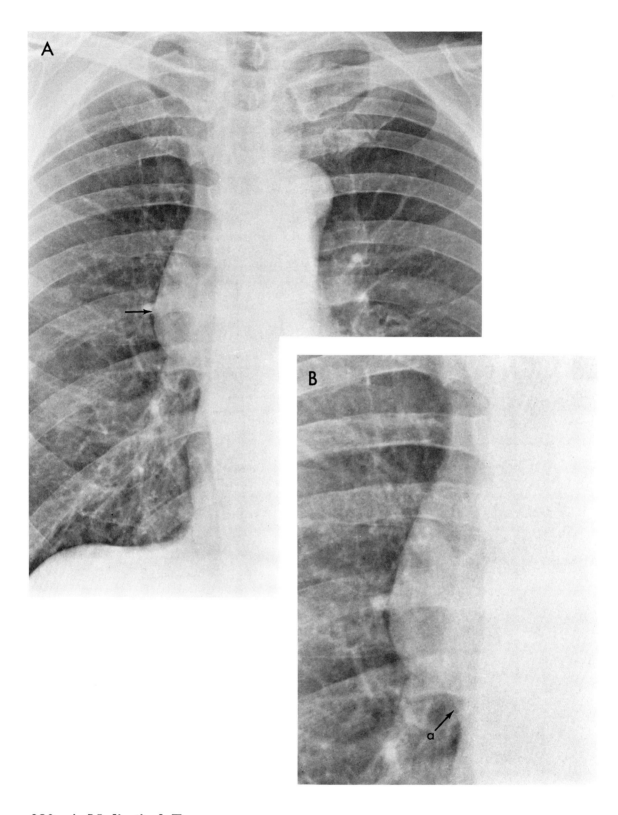

Figure 102.—Pericardial cyst.

A, posteroanterior radiograph: Showing a smoothly contoured, tear-drop-shaped mass adjacent to the mediastinum on the right side (**arrow**).

B, close-up of the lesion in **A:** Revealing the right pulmonary vessels visible through the mass; they do not appear to be distorted. The inferior margin of the mass (**a**) is continuous with the edge of the cardiac shadow.

C, close-up of an oblique projection: Showing the intimate relationship of the mass (**arrows**) and the ascending aorta.

A 45-year-old man entered the hospital for an elective operative procedure, at which time the chest study was made. Thoracotomy revealed a thin-walled cystic lesion which was filled with pericardial fluid and extended from the adjacent pericardium.

Figure 102, courtesy of Dr. Philip Gilbert, Cooper Hospital, Camden, N. J.

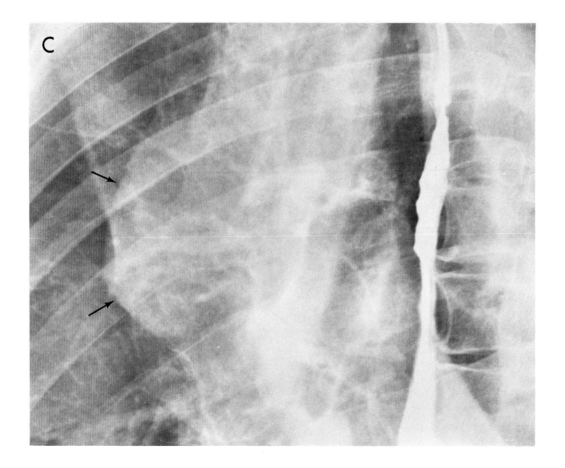

Figure 102 · Pericardial Cyst / 281

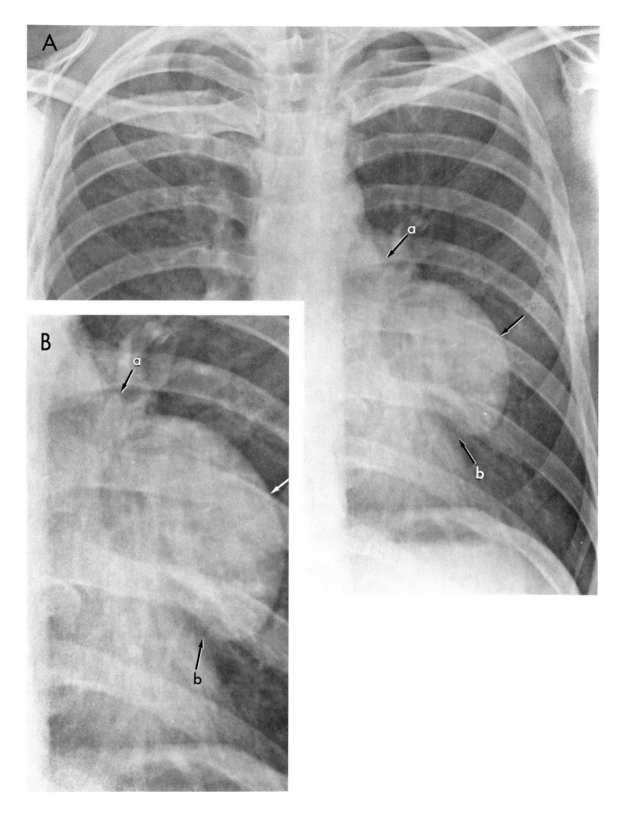

Figure 103.—Pericardial cyst.

A, posteroanterior radiograph: Showing a smooth-edged ovoid mass (**arrow**) blending with the left cardiac border. The upper margin is continuous with the pericardial reflection (**a**). A notch between the mass and the cardiac edge is seen inferiorly (**b**).

B, close-up of the lesion in **A.**

C, lateral projection: Confirming the ovoid character of the mass, which overlies the cardiac shadow (**arrows**). No calcification is visible.

A 30-year-old Army officer was up for his promotional physical examination when the lesion was discovered. At thoracotomy a typical thin-walled, fluid-filled pericardial cyst was found.

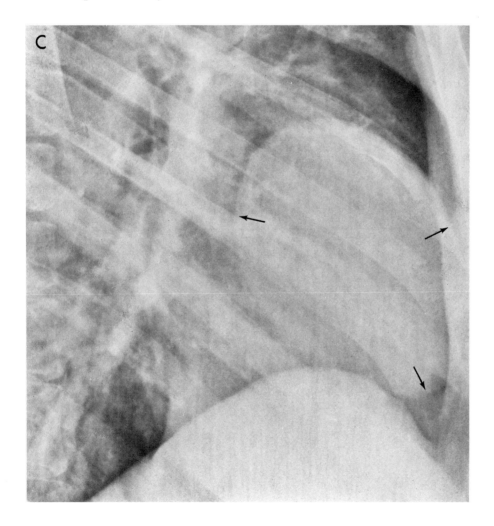

Figure 103 · Pericardial Cyst / 283

Figure 104.—Aortic aneurysm.

Posteroanterior projection: Illustrating a large, sharply defined mass containing multiple linear layers of calcification intimately associated with the aortic arch. The pulmonary hilar vessels on the left are obscured by the mass, which is of a density similar to that of the cardiac shadow. At least one draining pulmonary vessel from the upper lobe is displaced downward and bowed (**arrow**).

A 70-year-old man had intermittent chest pain and a 4+ serologic reaction. The aneurysm remained unchanged for years, but finally ruptured.

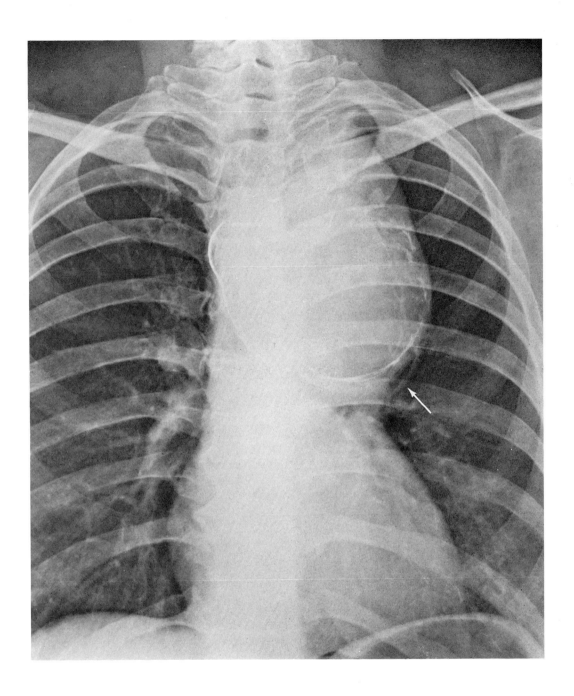

Figure 104 · Aortic Aneurysm / 285

Figure 105.—Aortic aneurysm.

A, close-up of a posteroanterior radiograph: Revealing a sharply outlined mass (**x**) adjacent to the aortic knob and seemingly separate from it (**a**).

B, lateral projection: Showing a sharply edged, somewhat wavy lesion overlying the proximal portion of the arch of the aorta (**arrows**).

C, body-section radiograph: Demonstrating a smooth, sharply marginated mass (**x**) which seems separate from the aorta (**a**). At this point, it was considered unnecessary to obtain an aortogram and thoracotomy was carried out.

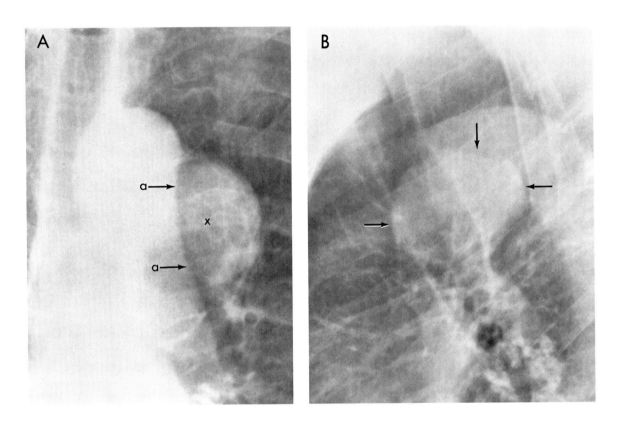

A 75-year-old man with no chest symptoms presented himself to his physician with hoarseness due to left vocal cord paralysis. Thoracotomy revealed a thin-walled, narrow-necked aortic aneurysm arising from the under surface of the proximal aortic arch and thought to be arteriosclerotic in nature.

Comment: In view of the relative safety of contrast substances, one is justified in opacifying vascular structures when masses are found immediately adjacent to mediastinal vascular structures.

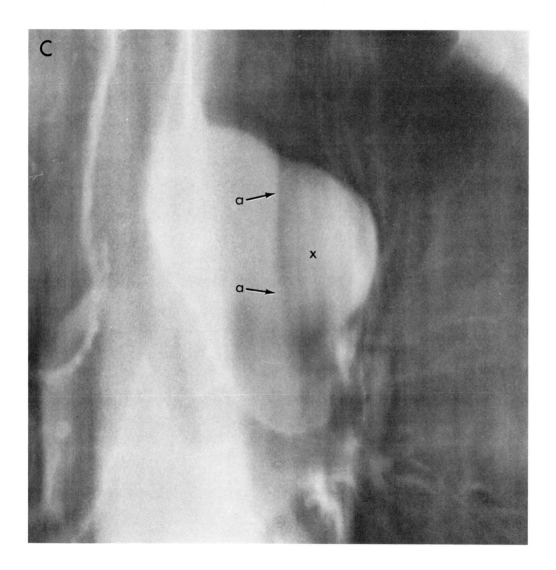

Figure 105 · Aortic Aneurysm / 287

Figure 106.—Aortic aneurysm.

Posteroanterior radiograph: Revealing a large, smoothly marginated mass in the left hemithorax (**x**). The normal aortic knob shadow is lost in the mass and its interwoven, matted, fine metallic wire. The nest of wire extends across the midline and into the region of the ascending aorta (**arrow**).

This is an ancient radiograph taken about six months after the diffuse silver wiring had been interlaced into the thoracic aneurysm. In spite of the wiring, lateral extension has continued, as shown by the soft tissue mass beyond the wire (**x**).

Figure 106, courtesy of Dr. Walter Miller, City Health Service, Seattle, Wash.

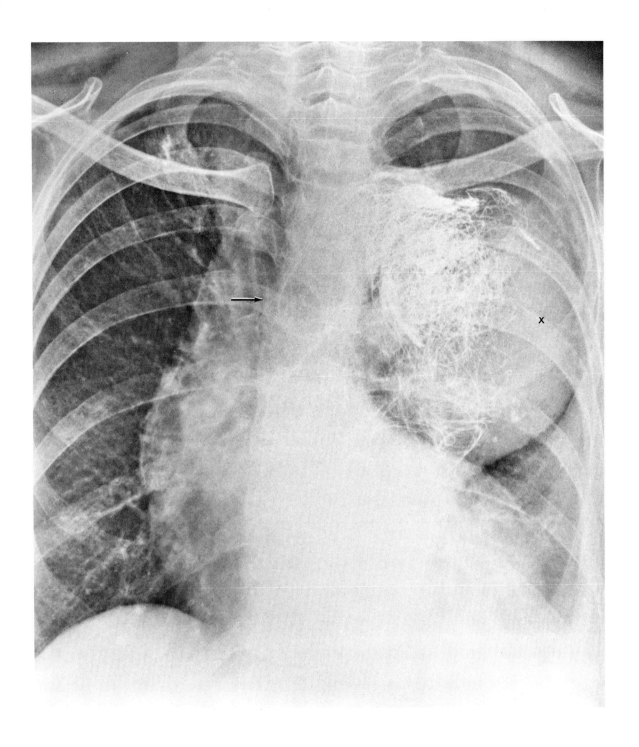

Figure 106 · Aortic Aneurysm / 289

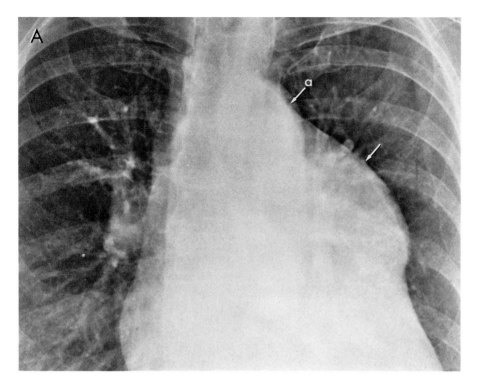

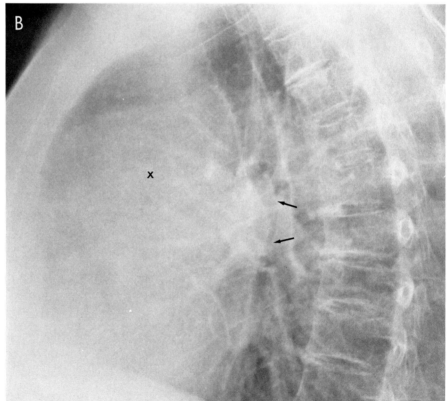

Figure 107.—Rhabdomyosarcoma of the heart.

A, posteroanterior radiograph: Revealing a mass with a sharply marginated lateral border overlying the pulmonary vessels and seemingly part of the cardiac outline on the left (**arrow**). This shadow extends across the aortic knob (**a**) but cannot be separated from the heart. The sharp outline of the aortic knob indicates that the mass lies anterior to the aortic arch.

B, lateral projection: Showing opacification of the supracardiac area anteriorly (**x**). The mass blends with the proximal portion of the aortic arch but also is indistinguishable from the cardiac border. The pulmonary hilar vessels appear to be normal (**arrows**).

C, retrograde aortogram: Defining very sharp outlines of the walls of the aorta. There are stretching, elongation and tortuosity of the left coronary artery (**arrows**). No tumor stain is evident. In spite of the absence of tumor stain, the abnormal coronary vessels indicate the mass to be a part of the cardiac muscle wall and not of extracardiac origin.

This 68-year-old woman had nonspecific chest pain and a peculiar cardiac arrhythmia when first seen. Thoracotomy revealed a primary rhabdomyosarcoma of the heart.

Figure 107, courtesy of Dr. Paul A. Riemenschneider, Cottage Hospital, Santa Barbara, Calif.

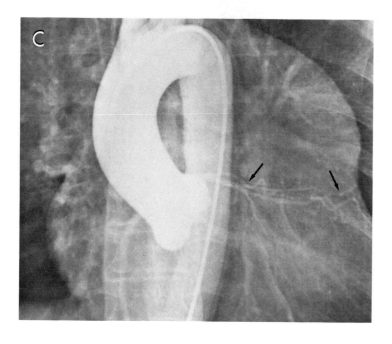

Figure 107 · Cardiac Rhabdomyosarcoma / 291

Figure 108.—Cardiac osteosarcoma.

A, initial posteroanterior radiograph: Revealing a densely calcified mass in the region of the pulmonary outflow tract of the right ventricle (**arrows**). A faint calcification is also visible along the right cardiac margin just within the border (**a**).

B, lateral projection: Showing the mass lying anterior to the pulmonary vessels but still seemingly within the cardiac shadow. A layer of calcification is clearly evident along the posterior cardiac margin (**arrows**).

(Continued.)

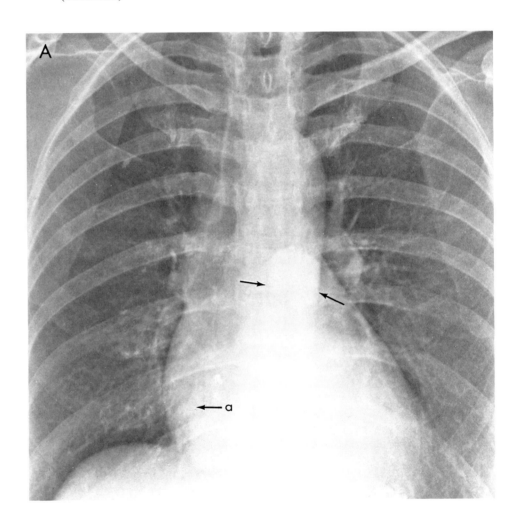

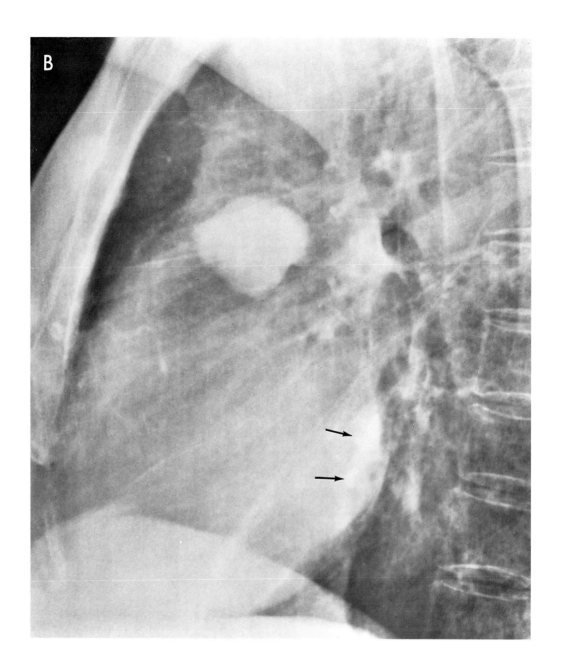

Figure 108 · Cardiac Osteosarcoma / 293

Figure 108 (cont.).—Cardiac osteosarcoma.

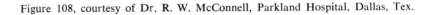

C, posteroanterior view three years after thoracotomy and partial removal of the original main calcified mass: Indicating that masses have recurred and increased in size. An effusion is present in the right pleural space.

D, close-up of a lateral projection: Revealing the extensive nature of the calcification.

A 53-year-old woman was seen initially with a history of recent progressive dyspnea and left-sided chest pain. On physical examination a systolic murmur was noted along the left sternal border as well as a split cardiac second sound. The electrocardiogram showed right axis deviation with right ventricular hypertrophy. Results of laboratory studies were within normal limits. At thoracotomy the main calcified mass was removed from the right ventricle. Pathologic diagnosis was primary cardiac osteosarcoma.

Figure 108, courtesy of Dr. R. W. McConnell, Parkland Hospital, Dallas, Tex.

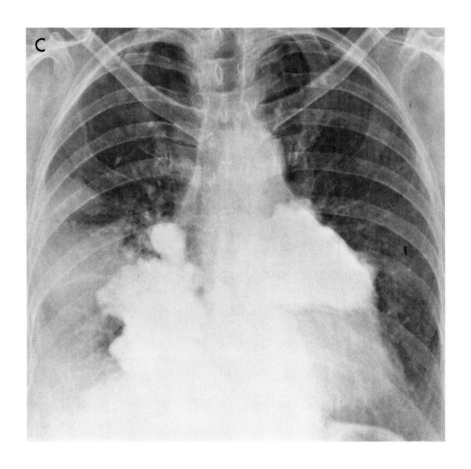

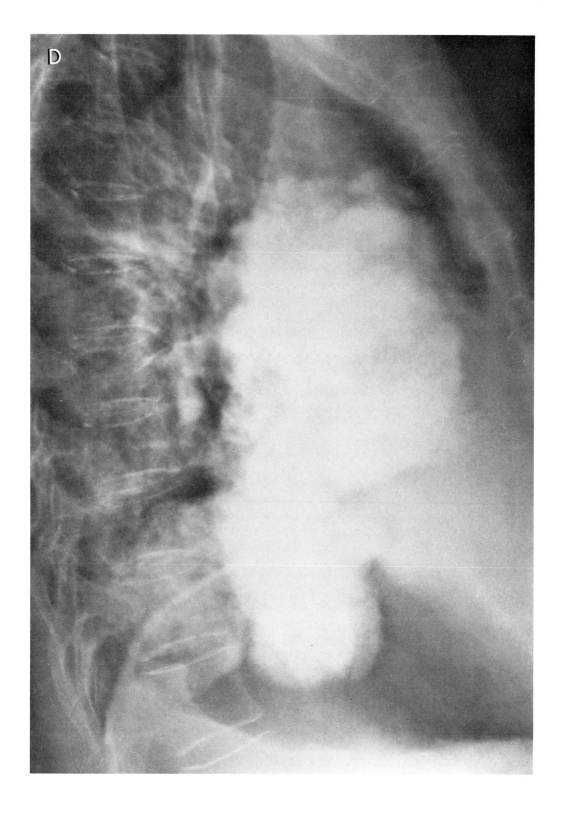

Figure 108 · Cardiac Osteosarcoma / 295

Figure 109.—Bilateral atrial myxoma.

A, initial posteroanterior radiograph: Revealing no abnormalities. At this time the patient complained of intermittent fever, night sweats and fatigue. She also was anemic and had a peculiar cardiac murmur.

B, lateral exposure: Also showing no abnormalities.

C, posteroanterior exposure five years after **A** and **B:** Showing increase in size of the heart shadow and several calcifications within the right cardiac border (**a**). The pulmonary vasculature is unchanged and within normal limits. At this time the patient's original symptoms of fever, night sweats, fatigue, anemia and heart murmur had recurred. The cardiac murmur, however, had changed in character. During the five year interval she was variously thought to have acute rheumatic fever, subacute bacterial endocarditis, rheumatic heart disease with mitral regurgitation and stenosis.

(Continued.)

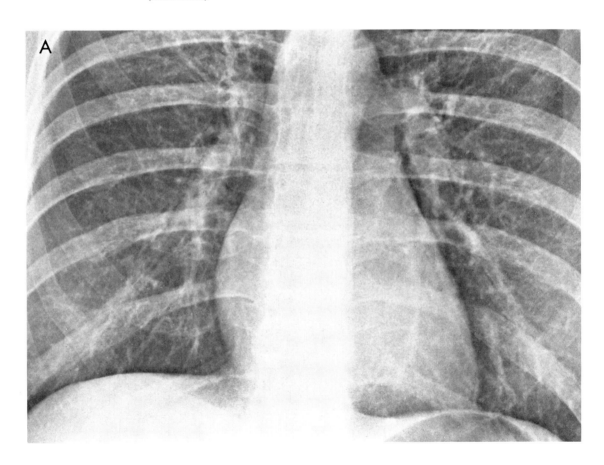

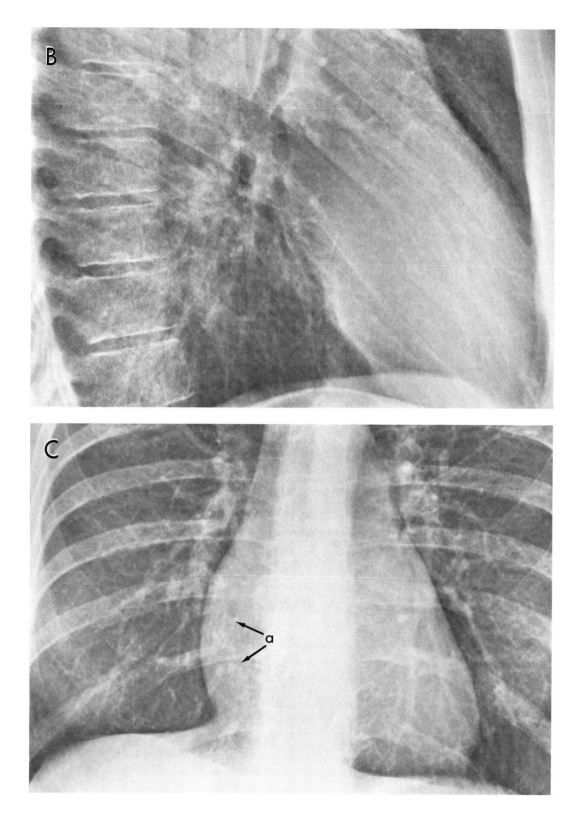

Figure 109 · Bilateral Atrial Myxoma / 297

Figure 109 (cont.).—Bilateral atrial myxoma.

D, posteroanterior exposure six months later: Demonstrating further increase in heart size and more clearly evident calcifications within the right heart border (**a**). Again, the pulmonary vasculature is normal.

E, lateral radiograph when **D** was obtained: Showing the increased heart size and a slight posterior impression on the esophagus (**b**). The calcifications (**a**) lie anteriorly and must be within the right atrium. Again, the pulmonary vasculature is normal.

(Continued.)

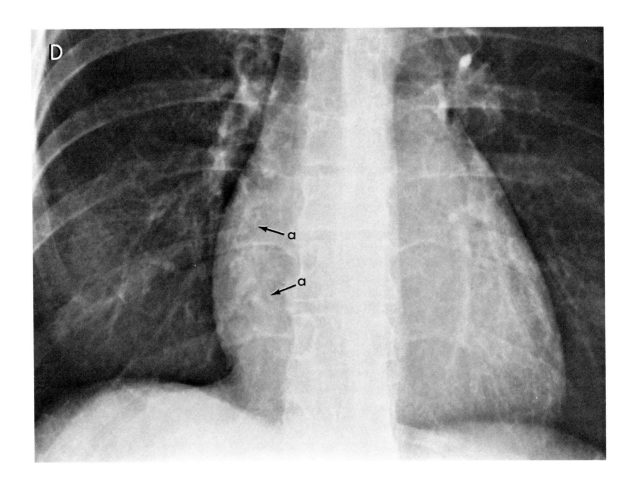

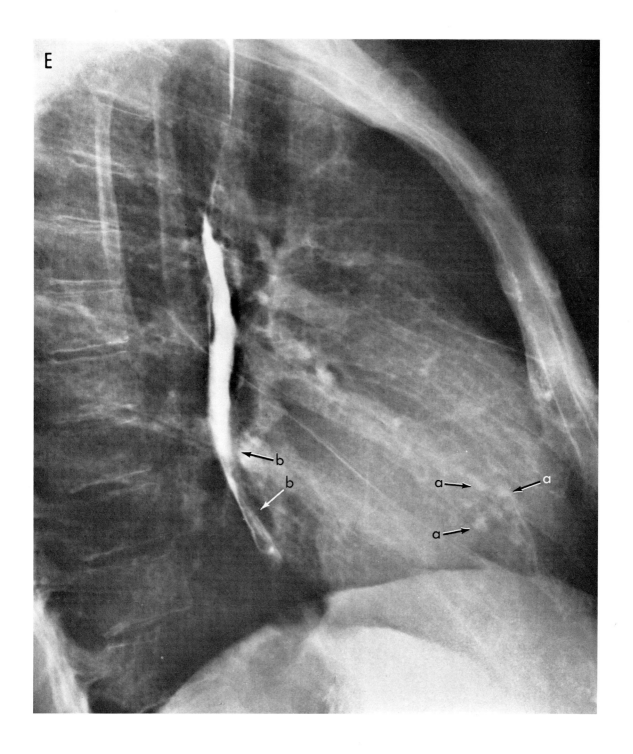

Figure 109 · Bilateral Atrial Myxoma / 299

Figure 109 (cont.).—Bilateral atrial myxoma.

F, anteroposterior projection during venous angiocardiography through a catheter in the right proximal atrium (**c**): Showing a large ovoid negative defect within the opaque column (**arrows**) in the more dependent portion of the atrium. Contrast material is visible in the normal-appearing right ventricle and pulmonary artery (**d**).

G, radiograph in the same sequence but several seconds after **F:** Delineating herniation of a portion of the filling defect through the tricuspid valve and lying partially in both right-sided chambers (**arrows**).

H, lateral projection during venous angiocardiography: Showing a huge multilobulated filling defect (**arrows**) in both the right atrium and ventricle.

(*Continued.*)

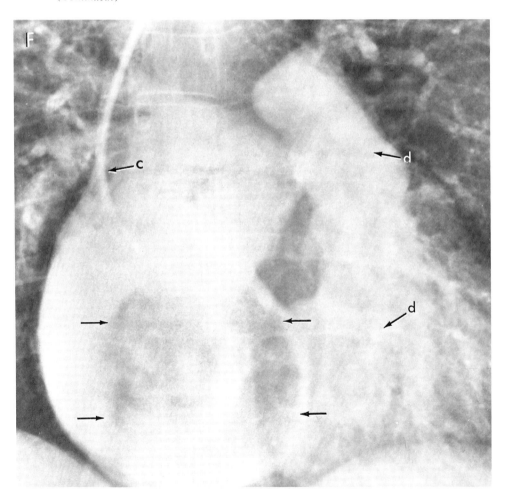

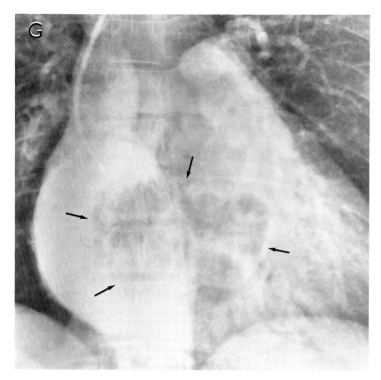

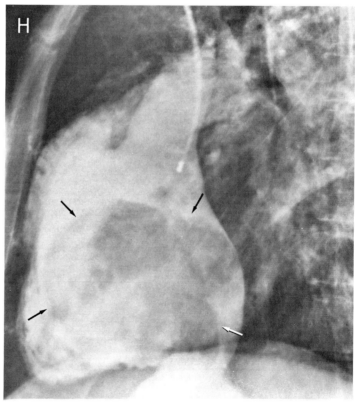

Figure 109 · Bilateral Atrial Myxoma / 301

Figure 109 (cont.).—Bilateral atrial myxoma.

I, lateral projection during filling of the left side of the heart: Revealing a smaller negative shadow across the area of the mitral valve (**arrows**) partially in the left atrium and ventricle. This, too, was seen to move from atrium to ventricle.

J, radiograph of the specimen removed from the right atrium: Showing the multilobulated character of the right-sided mass and the surprisingly dense character of the calcification within it.

On hospitalization this 37-year-old woman had a two week history of nonproductive cough, fever, ankle swelling and palpitations. Blood pressure was 105/65, pulse 108, respirations 16. There were some splinter hemorrhages of the nails of the right index and ring fingers. The neck veins were slightly distended. An apical systolic murmur radiating to the left axilla was present with a diastolic rumble. The liver was palpable.

The lesions were excised and a patch put on the atrial septum. The patient did fairly well for a while, but died two years later with extensive recurrent tumor in the cardiac chambers, at which time further attempted removal was unsuccessful. Pathologic study each time revealed similar material believed to represent atrial myxoma.

Figure 109, courtesy of Dr. Melvin Figley, University of Washington, School of Medicine, Seattle.

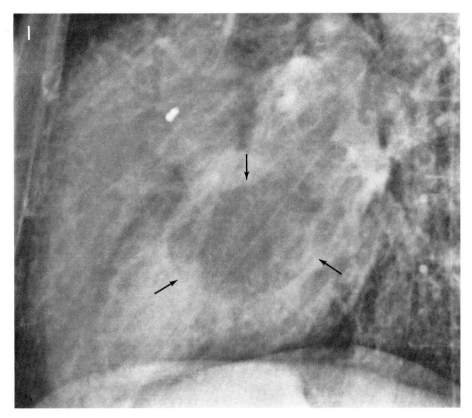

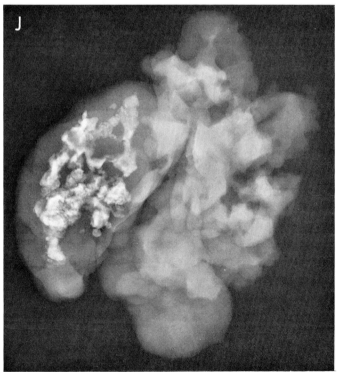

Figure 109 · Bilateral Atrial Myxoma / 303

Figure 110.—Fibromyxosarcoma of the pulmonary valve.

A, posteroanterior radiograph: Normal findings, with normal-appearing pulmonary artery and veins.

B, posteroanterior view three years later: Revealing marked decrease in the size of the vessels to the left lower lobe (a), several of which are now but

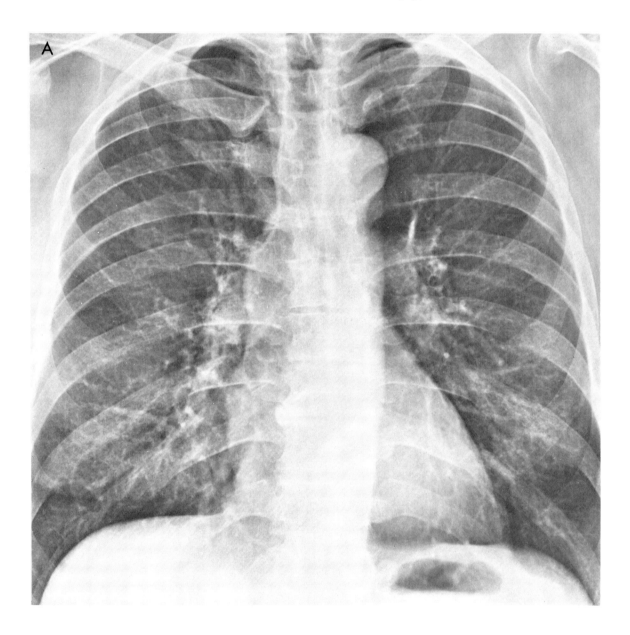

thin linear streaks (**b**). On the right, the entire pulmonary artery and all its branches also have diminished in size (**c**). The more peripheral vessels are reduced to strands. The only normal-appearing residual vascularity is in the left upper lobe.

(*Continued.*)

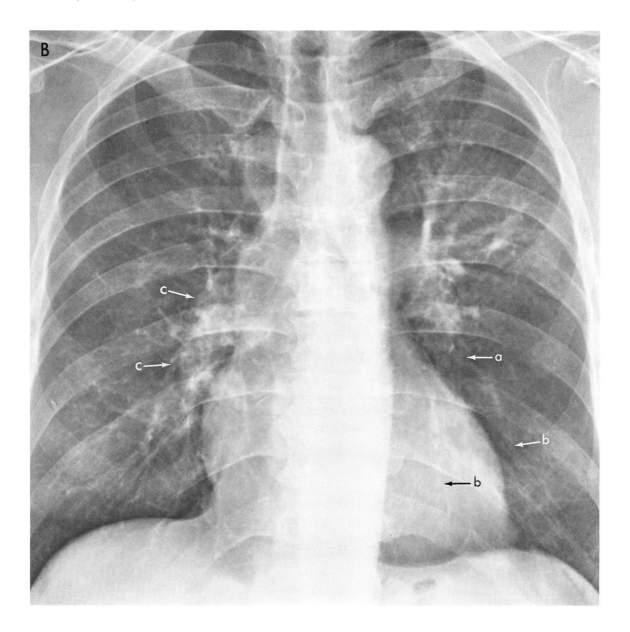

Figure 110 · Fibromyxosarcoma / 305

Figure 110 (cont.).—Fibromyxosarcoma of the pulmonary valve.

C, radiograph from a pulmonary angiogram series four months after **B:** Demonstrating absence of vascular filling to the left lower lobe (**x**), an irregular filling defect in the left pulmonary artery (**d**) and multiple round filling defects in the right pulmonary artery (**e**) obstructing most of the arterial branches. Note the vascular void in most of the right lung. Some contrast agent fills a single vessel to the right upper lobe, but even this is compromised by tumor deposits (**arrows**).

A 53-year-old man was seen because of sudden onset of left anterior chest pain, productive cough and blood-streaked sputum. On physical examination, a cardiac murmur, not present previously, also was detected. **B** was made at this time. Clinical diagnosis was pulmonary embolism and the patient was treated with anticoagulants. Four months later he complained of severe dyspnea, weakness and faintness but no chest pain. Shortly after hospitalization he had an episode of cyanosis and hypotension and the electrocardiogram showed some T-wave changes and ST depression. He improved somewhat but remained cyanotic without oxygen delivered nasally. There was no venous distention or leg pain. Cardiac murmur was still present and quite harsh. At this time pulmonary angiography (**C**) was done, followed by surgery.

A large myxomatous mass was found, apparently arising from the region of the pulmonary valve and involving the pulmonary outflow tract of the right ventricle, extending to the pulmonary bifurcation. Attempts at removal failed because the heart would not maintain normal rhythm. The patient died on the operating table. At autopsy a pleomorphic tumor was found apparently arising from the sinus of the pulmonary valve and situated in the main pulmonary artery. Old areas of infarction were observed in both lungs. This was thought to represent a fibromyxosarcoma arising from the pulmonary valve region.

Figure 110, courtesy of Dr. Melvin Figley, University of Washington, School of Medicine, Seattle.

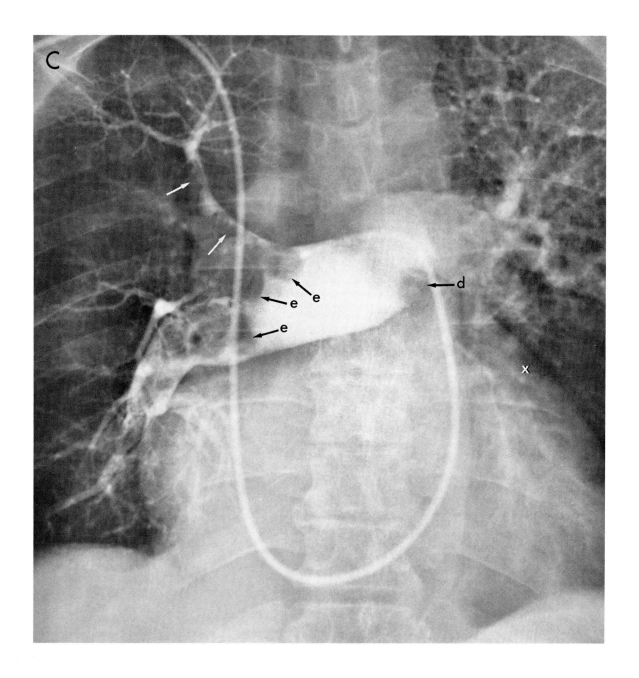

Figure 110 · Fibromyxosarcoma / 307

Figure 111.—Subclavian artery aneurysm.

A somewhat overexposed posteroanterior radiograph: Showing a smooth-edged homogeneous mass similar in density to the cardiac shadow with no visible calcification and no demonstrable bony erosion. Its marked convexity plus the acute angles formed by the mass laterally and medially (**arrow**) indicate the extrapleural nature of the lesion.

A 22-year-old man had a history of a knife injury two years prior to this roentgen study. At this time he had some minor discomfort over the right shoulder. This study dates back to the time before angiography was a commonly accepted procedure. Operation revealed a huge thin-walled subclavian artery aneurysm.

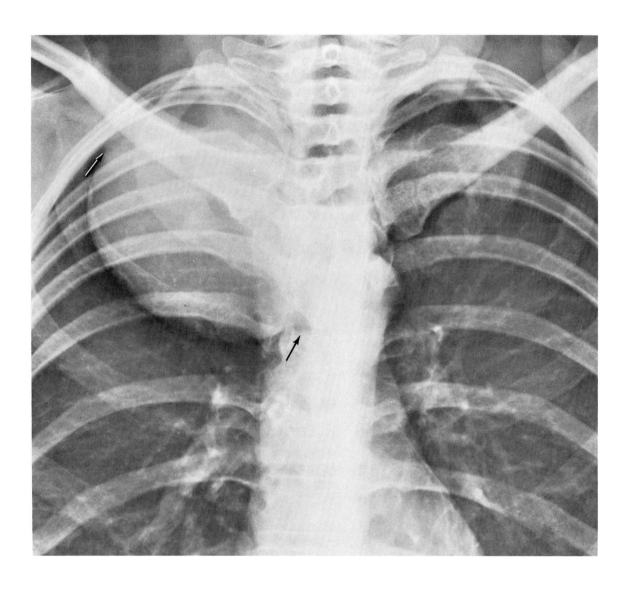

Figure 111 · Subclavian Artery Aneurysm / 309

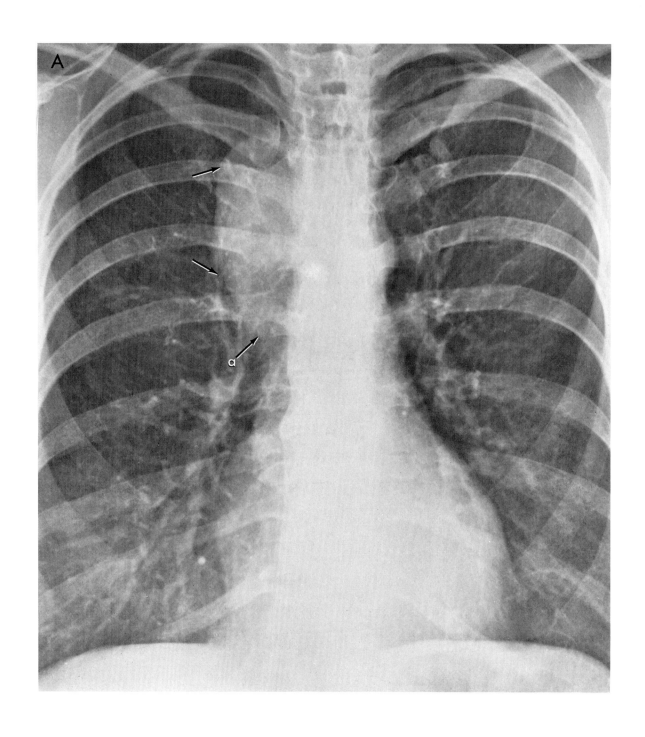

Figure 112.—Pulmonary vein aneurysm.

A, posteroanterior projection: Revealing a sharply demarcated mass in the region of the superior pulmonary vascular shadows on the right, with extension to the mediastinum (**arrows**). No major pulmonary vessel shadows can be seen through the mass, whose inferior portions seem to occupy the space where one would expect to find normal blood vessels (**a**). The density is slightly less than the cardiac and aortic shadows.

B, close-up of the mass in **A.**

No mass was visible in lateral projections, hence these are not included.

This study was part of a routine physical examination of a 28-year-old hospital employe. Thoracotomy revealed a thin-walled aneurysm in one of the large draining pulmonary veins.

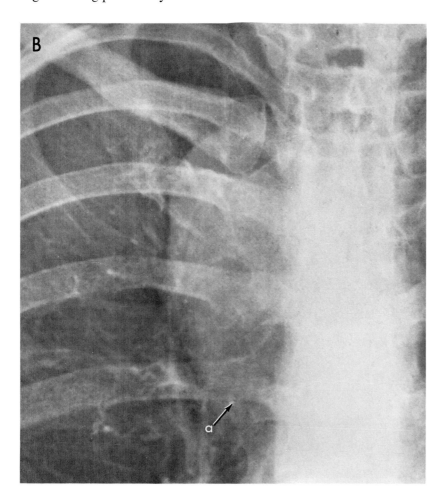

Figure 112 · Pulmonary Vein Aneurysm / 311

Figure 113.—Pulmonary artery aneurysm.

A, close-up of a posteroanterior radiograph: Demonstrating a sharply marginated abnormal shadow (**x**) intimately related to the vascular structures and lying just below the aortic arch in the left side. It is separate from the descending aorta (**arrow**). Just lateral to the mass one can see clearly the branches of the left pulmonary artery which are normal in size, shape and location (**a**).

B, lateral projection: Revealing a faint, rather ill-defined density (**arrows**). The branching pulmonary arteries appear to be normal. The trachea and major bifurcation are also normal.

(*Continued.*)

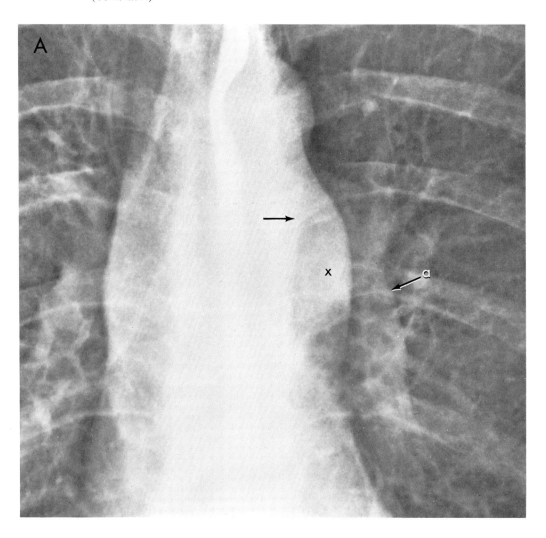

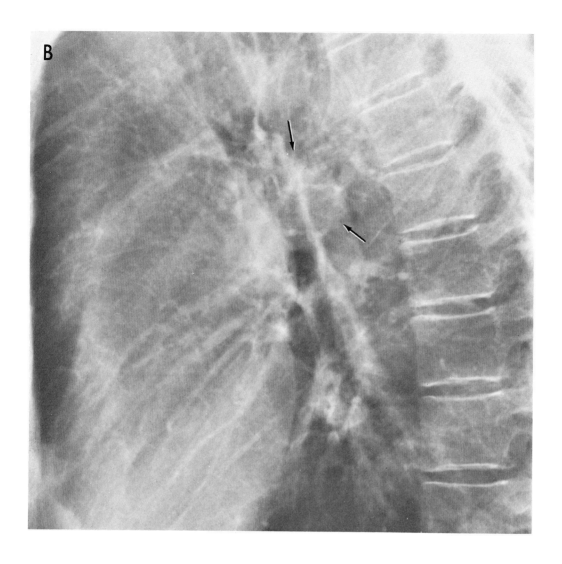

Figure 113 · Pulmonary Artery Aneurysm / 313

Figure 113 (cont.).—Pulmonary artery aneurysm.

C, body-section radiograph through the mass: Delineating its slightly lobulated appearance seemingly continuous with the left pulmonary artery (**arrows**).

D, pulmonary angiogram: Demonstrating marked dilatation of the main pulmonary artery with an obvious aneurysmal appearance (**x**) accounting for the entire shadow seen in the left hilar region.

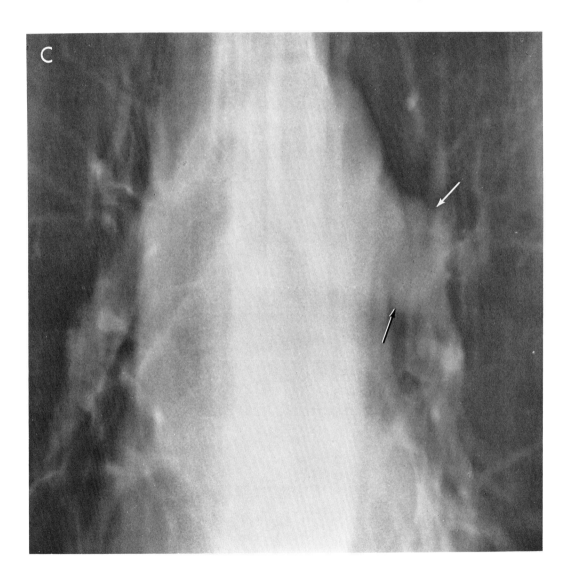

A 41-year-old teacher, on changing her position from one school to another, required a physical examination and chest radiograph. Results of the physical examination and routine laboratory studies, as well as an electrocardiogram and more extensive blood studies, were within normal limits. No treatment was deemed necessary, and when last seen five years after the diagnosis, the patient continued to be asymptomatic and chest radiographs were unchanged in appearance from those presented here.

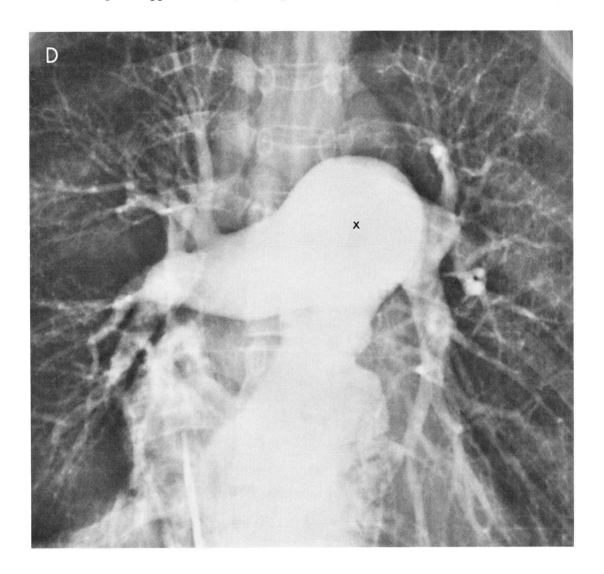

Figure 113 · Pulmonary Artery Aneurysm / 315

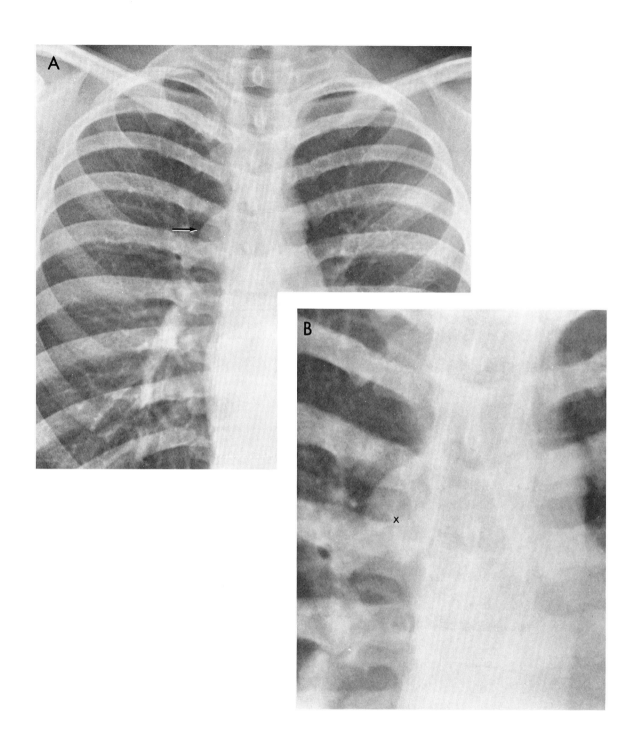

Figure 114.—Prominent azygos vein.

A, posteroanterior radiograph: Revealing a sharp-edged shadow (**arrow**) opposite the aortic knob extending to the right of the mediastinum and occupying the position of the azygos vein but seeming much larger than it should be. Adjacent pulmonary arteries and veins in the hilus are normal in contour and position.

B, close-up of the apparent tumor (**x**) in **A.**

C, interosseous venogram. Showing filling of the shadow (**x**) which represents a normal azygos vein.

A 24-year-old medical student had a survey chest radiograph just prior to graduation, at which time the suspected abnormality was discovered.

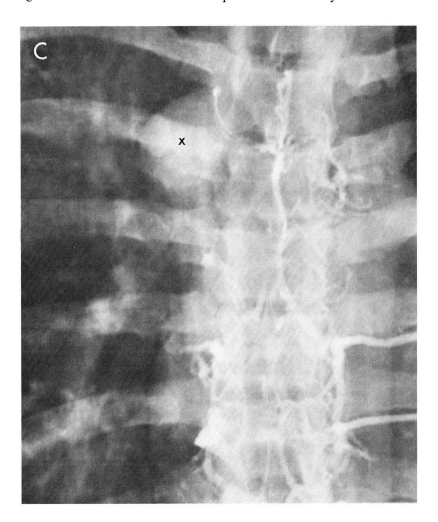

Figure 114 · Prominent Azygos Vein / 317

Figure 115.—Lymphoid hyperplasia.

A, a posteroanterior exposure: Revealing an egg-shaped paratracheal mass (**x**) on the right causing slight deviation of the trachea to the left and lateral displacement of several upper lobe vessels (**arrows**).

B, lateral body-section radiograph: Emphasizing the multilobulated character of the smooth mass and its intimate tracheal relationship (**arrows**). An unimpeded airway (**y**) is preserved.

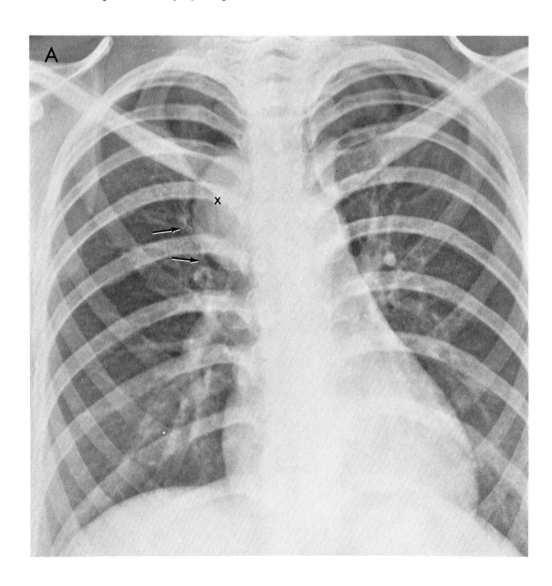

A 24-year-old woman had complained of dyspnea and chest pain for six months prior to this study. Six years previously a diagnosis of a mediastinal tumor had been made on the basis of a survey chest radiograph, but she had refused to have an operation. As on earlier studies, again no other abnormalities were found and laboratory studies were not helpful. This time the patient agreed to a thoracotomy, and pathologic study after removal of the mass revealed lymphoid hyperplasia.

Figure 115, courtesy of Dr. R. Shell, Ann Arbor, Mich.

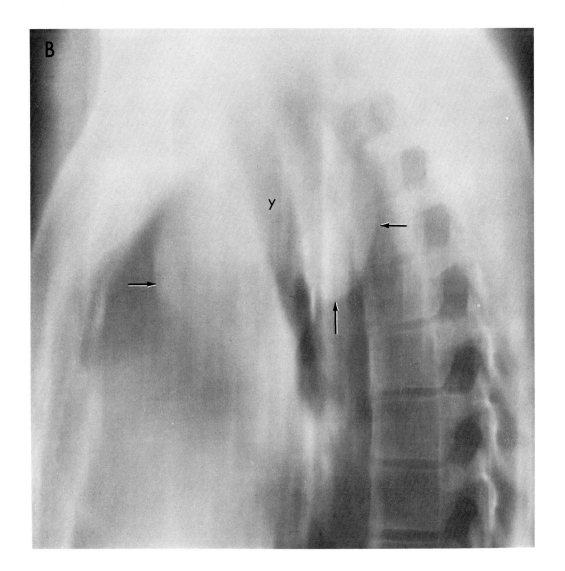

Figure 115 · Lymphoid Hyperplasia / 319

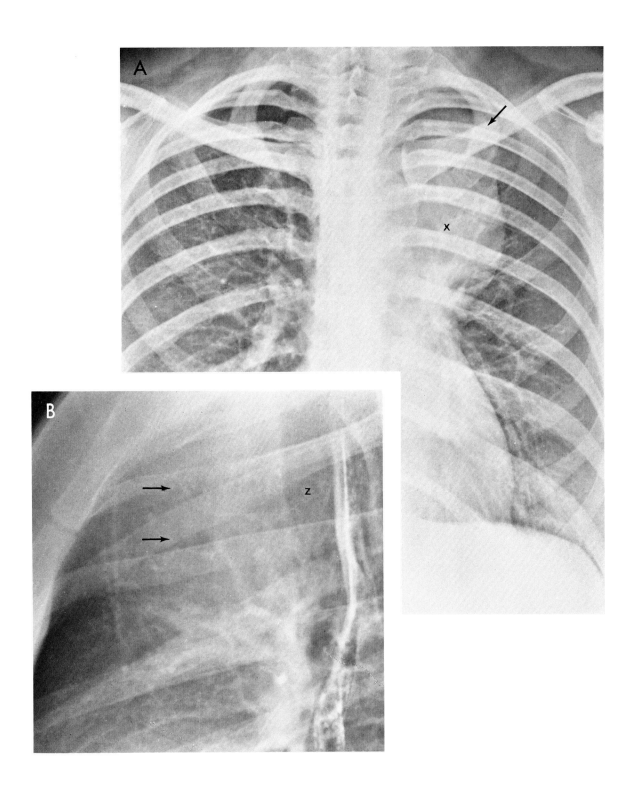

Figure 116.—Lipoma of the left upper lobe.

A, posteroanterior radiograph: Revealing a mass (**x**) with a smooth left lateral margin which gradually fades as it approaches the apex of the lung (**arrow**).

B, lateral projection: In which only a vague indication of a mass is visible (**arrows**). The tracheal outline (**z**) is smooth, regular and not displaced. The barium-filled esophagus is also normal. The ill-defined appearance in the lateral projection and the fading off of the superior margins suggest the fatty nature of the lesion.

C, close-up of the lesion in **A:** Disclosing the sternum (**a**) and aorta (**b**) through the mass. Note the normal hilar vessels (**y**). Some clear lung is visible in the apex of the left lung.

An asymptomatic 20-year-old student, on entering college, had a chest radiograph, at which time the shadow was detected. Operative intervention revealed the fatty nature of the lesion, which proved to be a benign lipoma.

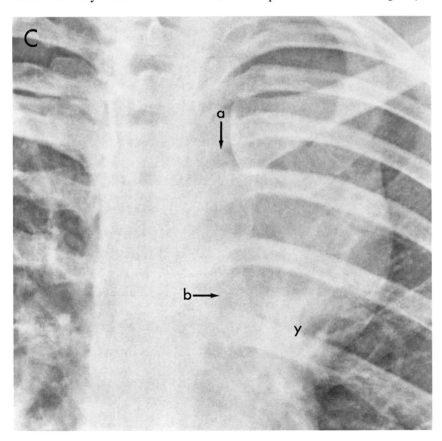

Figure 116 · Lipoma of Left Upper Lobe / 321

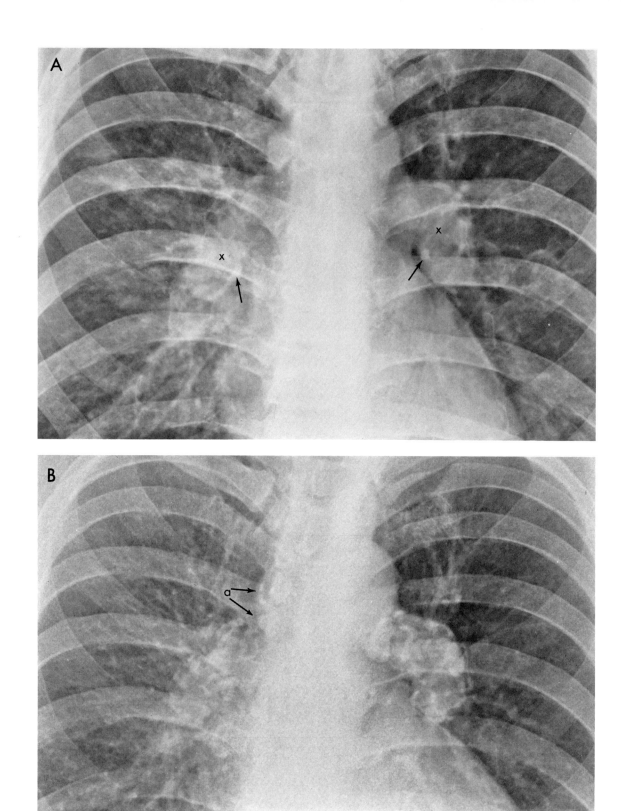

Figure 117.—Sarcoid.

A, posteroanterior radiograph: Showing bilateral hilar enlargements (**x**). The shadows are obviously extravascular: they contain fine calcific deposits (**arrows**). Small nodules lie in both lungs.

B, posteroanterior radiograph 15 years later: Revealing marked calcifications in both hili and obvious calcification in the paratracheal nodes at (**a**). The pulmonary parenchymal nodules have diminished in size.

C, lateral projection: Demonstrating the hilar and paratracheal nodes (**a**) and a group of anterior mediastinal nodes (**b**). An unexpected cluster of calcified nodes is present in the region of the diaphragm and in the immediate subxiphoid area (**c**).

A 42-year-old company executive was asymptomatic when he reported for his annual physical examination. Lung biopsy at this time revealed sarcoid.

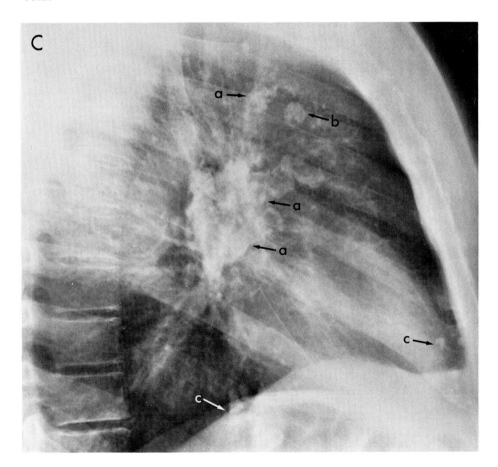

Figure 117 · Sarcoid / 323

Figure 118.—Mediastinal parathyroid adenoma.

A, posteroanterior radiograph: Demonstrating a sharply outlined mass in the right hemithorax (**x**). This blends with the ascending aorta and the right cardiac border.

B, oblique projection: Showing the sharply outlined ovoid mass (**arrows**) blending with the aorta and the right cardiac margin. The position and shape of the mass suggest a tumor of thymic origin, a paracardial or duplication cyst.

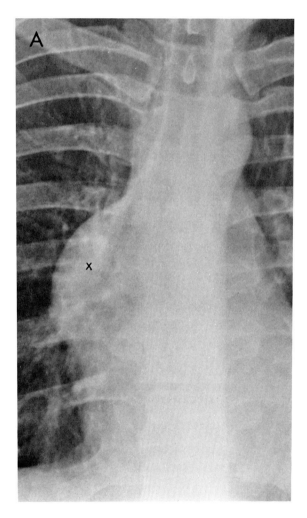 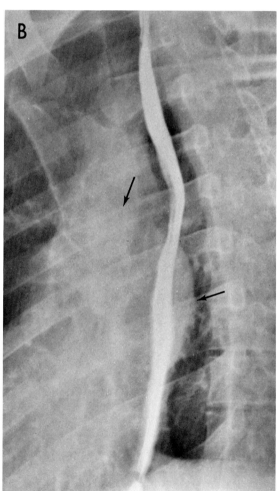

C, lateral view: Revealing a very ill-defined soft tissue shadow (**y**) superimposed on the region of the ascending aorta and possibly extending into the anterior mediastinum. The space anterior to the cardiac shadow is quite clear (**arrow**).

In this 30-year-old asymptomatic man, the chest mass was discovered on a survey examination of the chest. At the time of hospitalization the results of laboratory studies were within normal limits and the patient had no abnormal physical findings. At thoracotomy a cystic mass covered with mediastinal pleura and closely related to the ascending aorta and right cardiac border was identified. This was peeled readily from the adjacent structures and from the anterior mediastinum. The initial pathologic impression was of a cystic thymoma with somewhat peculiar cells. Review at the Penrose Cancer Seminar resulted in an opinion that this most likely represented a parathyroid adenoma.

Six years later a mass recurred in this region and in the region of the parathyroids, suggesting that this was indeed a parathyroid adenoma.

Figure 118, courtesy of Dr. David J. Stevenson, Lutheran Hospital and Medical Center, Denver, Colo.

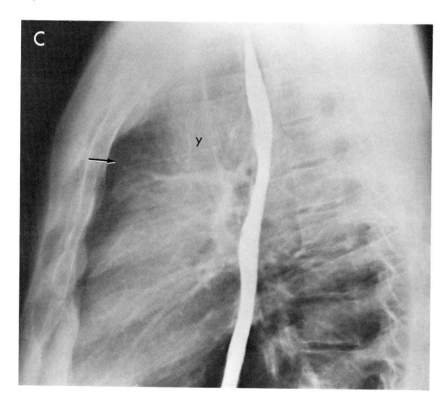

Figure 118 · Mediastinal Parathyroid Adenoma / 325

Figure 119.—Ganglioneuroma.

A, posteroanterior exposure: Revealing an elliptical, sharply outlined paraspinal mass visible through the cardiac shadow (**arrows**). The silhouette of the mass seen through the cardiac outline indicates its posterior nature. Diffuse speckled calcification is evident throughout the mass. Underlying and adjacent bony structures are normal.

B, close-up of the lesion in **A:** Showing the speckled calcific debris to better advantage (**arrows**). In a young patient the most likely diagnosis of a mass in the paraspinal area with this peculiar calcification would be a neurogenic tumor, probably a ganglioneuroma.

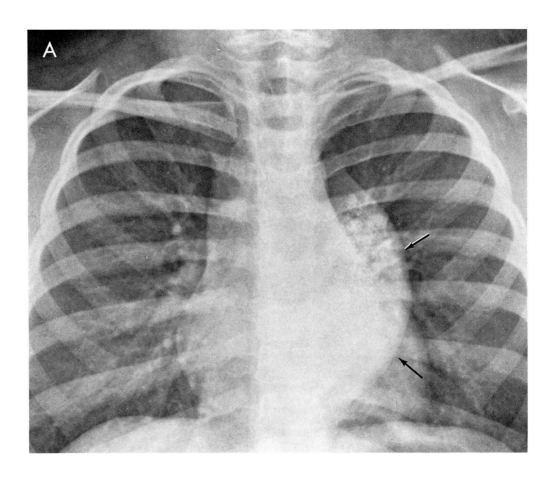

A 3-year-old girl was studied as part of a continuing examination following removal of an adrenal neuroblastoma. The paraspinal mass (**A**) was discovered approximately one year after removal of the primary lesion and following radiation therapy directed to the operative field. Further pathologic analysis and removal of a portion of this mass resulted in a diagnosis of ganglioneuroma. At this time there was speculation about the role of the radiation therapy in the conversion of the neuroblastoma to the more adult ganglioneuroma.

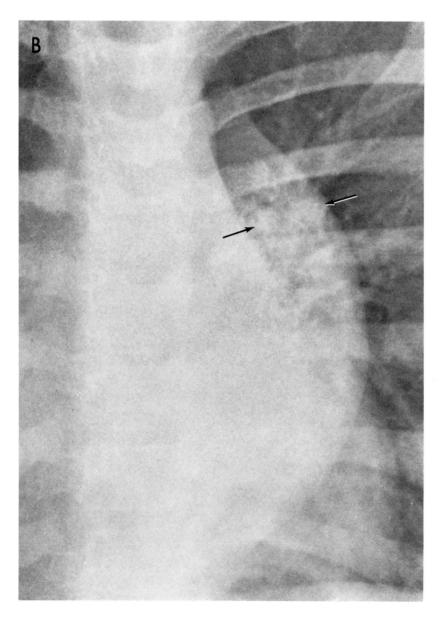

Figure 119 · Ganglioneuroma / 327

Figure 120.—Neurilemmoma.

Posteroanterior radiograph: Showing a smooth-edged mass over the right upper lobe and extending to the thoracic inlet. Its acute-angled margins (**arrows**) at the chest wall and mediastinum plus the convex outline indicate its extrapleural nature. Smooth vertebral and costal bony erosions are present (**a**).

A 30-year-old man complained of a heavy sensation in the right side of his chest. No other symptoms or positive physical findings were elicited. Laboratory studies were not contributory. At operation a neurilemmoma (pathologic diagnosis) was removed.

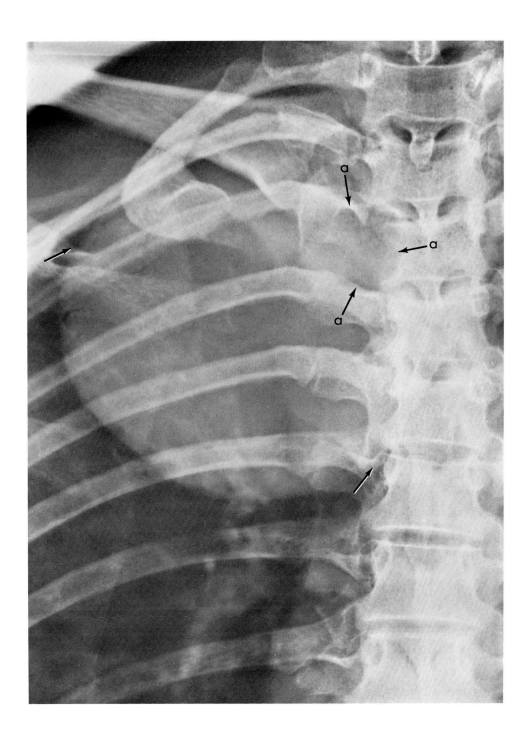

Figure 120 · Neurilemmoma / 329

Figure 121.—Paraganglioma.

A, posteroanterior radiograph: Revealing a mass (**x**) with elevation of the paraspinal soft tissues to the left of the spine (**arrows**), indicating the extrapleural nature of the lesion. Pulmonary vessels are seen clearly through the mass.

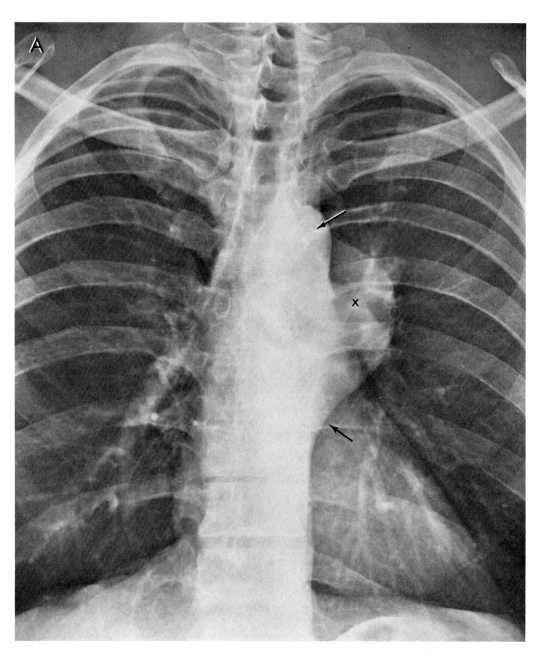

B, body-section radiograph: Demonstrating vertebral erosion (**arrows**) and elevation of the paraspinal soft tissues (**a**), confirming the extrapleural location of the lesion.

A 38-year-old man was examined because of pain in the midthoracic area. No neurologic changes were found, and results of physical examination and laboratory studies were normal. At operation a solid mass was found which proved on pathologic examination to be a paraganglioma.

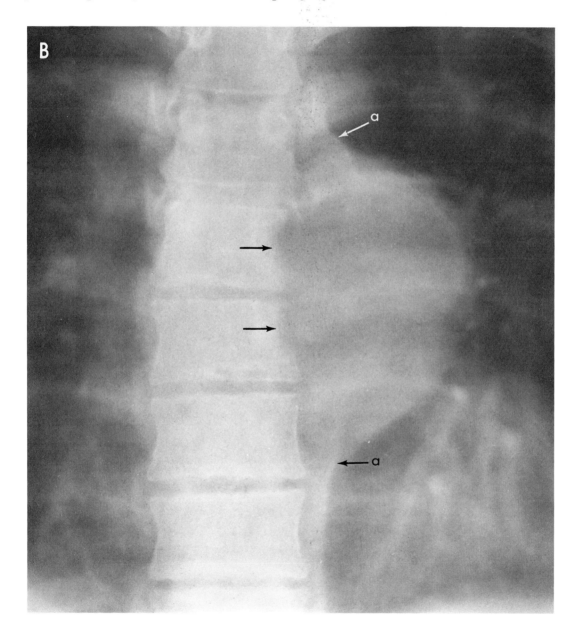

Figure 121 · Paraganglioma / 331

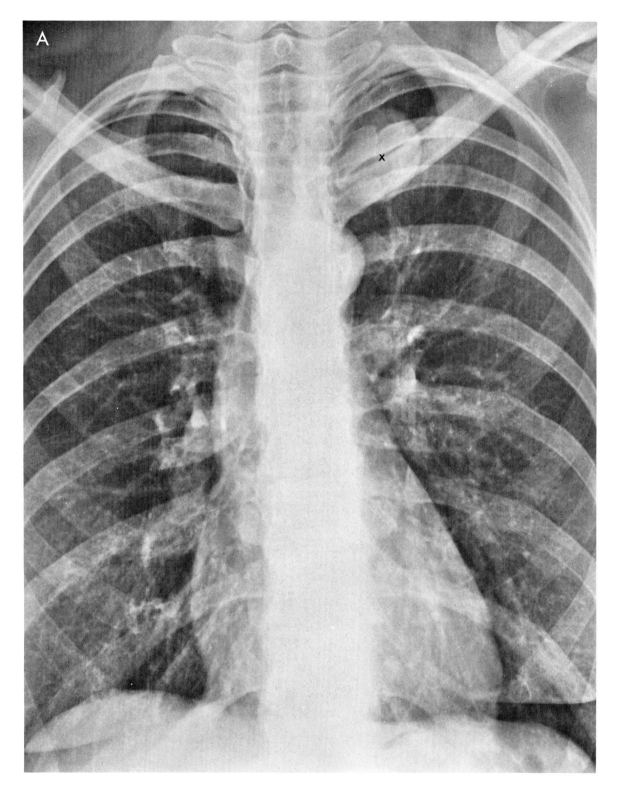

Figure 122.—Neurofibroma.

A, posteroanterior radiograph: Revealing a smooth-edged mass (**x**) overlying the left upper lobe adjacent to the mediastinum. No vascular distortion or bony change is visible.

B, a grid anteroposterior exposure: Demonstrating bony erosion of the vertebra (**arrow**) and proximal rib (**a**), suggesting the neurogenic origin of the mass.

(Continued.)

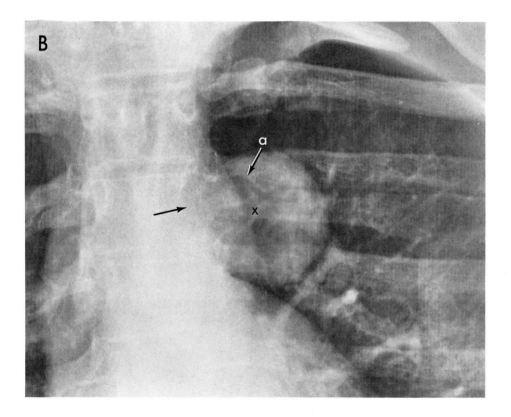

Figure 122 · Neurofibroma / 333

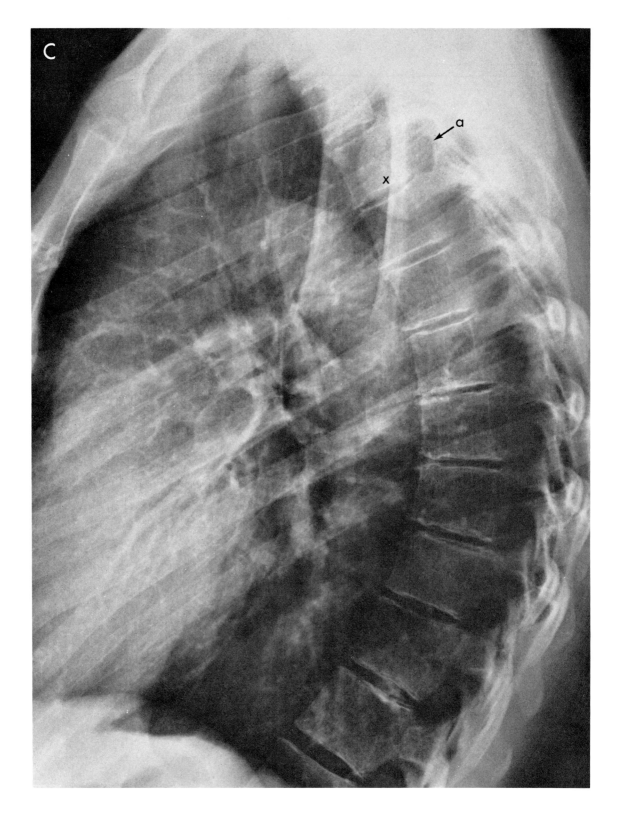

C, lateral projection: Showing the posterior location of the lesion (**x**) adjacent to the spine. One of the intervertebral foramina (**a**) is larger than those above and below.

D, close-up of **C:** Delineating smooth enlargement of the neural foramen (**a**) with its dense white border suggesting the slowly growing nature of the lesion.

A 40-year-old man was studied because of an abnormality detected on a minifilm survey by the city health clinic. On surgical removal of the lesion, pathologic study revealed a neurofibroma.

Figure 122, courtesy of Dr. Walter Miller, City Health Center, Seattle, Wash.

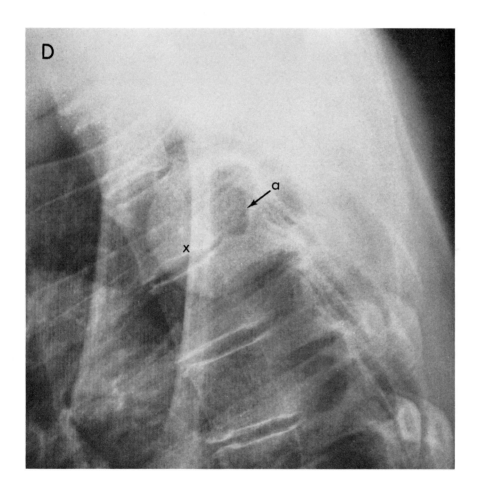

Figure 122 · Neurofibroma / 335

Figure 123.—Neurenteric cyst.

A, posteroanterior radiograph: Revealing a dense soft tissue mass (**x**) in the left superior mediastinum.

B, close-up of the mass in A: Demonstrating a thin rim of calcium in the wall (**arrows**).

(*Continued.*)

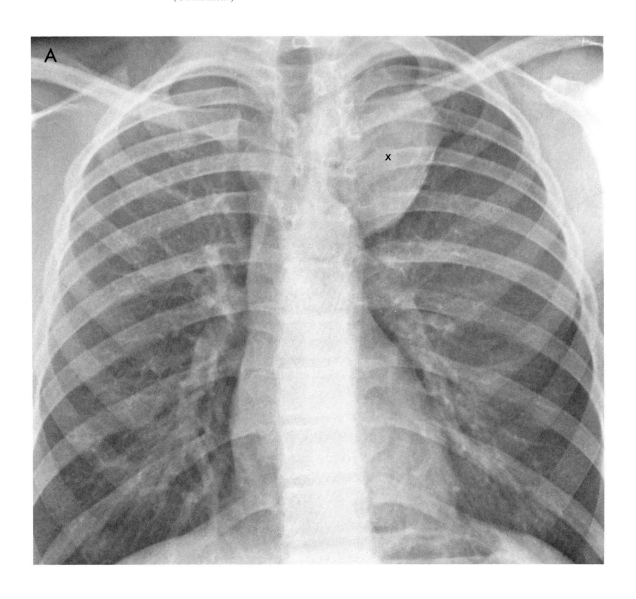

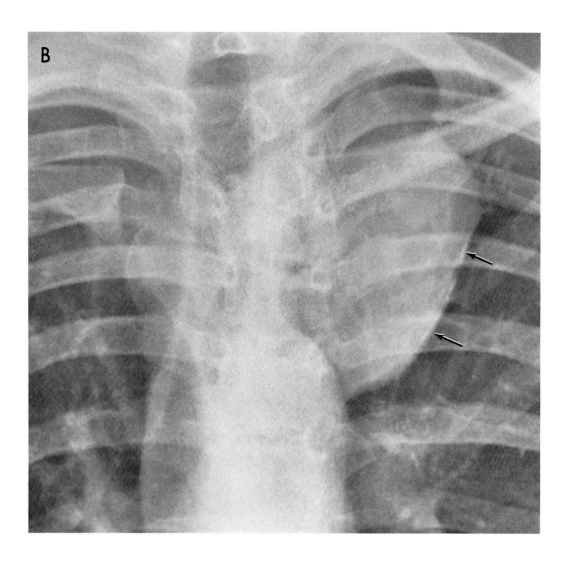

Figure 123 · Neurenteric Cyst / 337

C, anteroposterior radiograph exposed to illustrate the spine: Indicating a hemivertebra (**a**) and several defects in the neural arch (**b**).

D, lateral exposure: Demonstrating the posterior location of the mass adjacent to the thoracic segment of the spine (**arrows**). Enlargements of the intervertebral foramina are not delineated in this view.

In this 20-year-old asymptomatic man the mass was discovered on a routine survey of the chest. Operation revealed a neurenteric cyst.

Comment: Neurenteric cysts are thought to originate from unobliterated remnants of the accessory neurenteric canals of Kovalevski. The mediastinal cystic lesion is often connected to the spinal canal by a patent or fibrous stalk. Congenital anomalies of the spine are consistently associated, often in the form of hemivertebrae or cleft vertebrae. Occasionally a patent, or closed, connection between the cyst and alimentary tract, usually the upper small intestine, persists. Rarely, this communication can be demonstrated by opaque contrast medium filling the communicating tube and a portion of the cyst. When such an opening is present, air may be seen initially in the cystic lesion.

Figure 123, courtesy of Dr. T. F. Leigh, Atlanta, Ga.

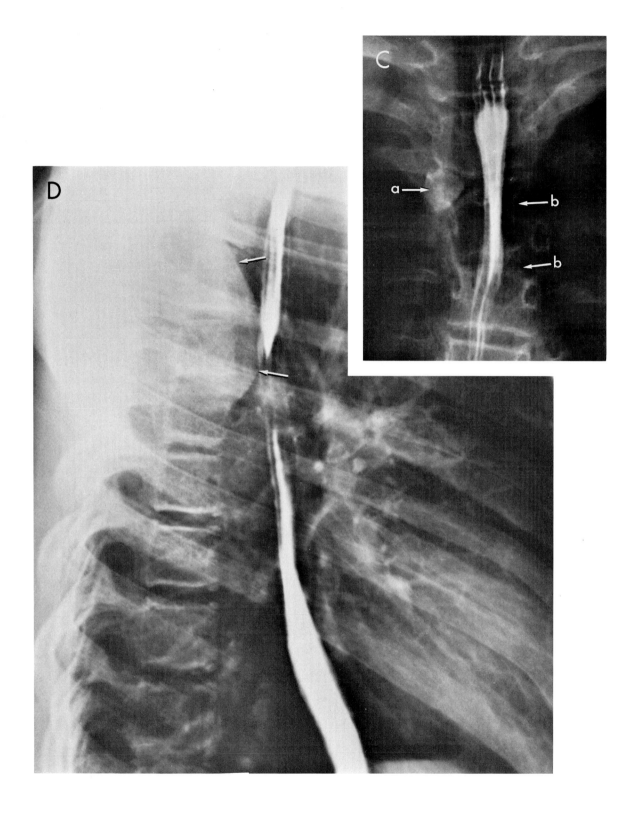

Figure 123 · Neurenteric Cyst / 339

Figure 124.—Extramedullary hemopoiesis.

A, posteroanterior radiograph: Revealing a smooth soft tissue mass seen through the cardiac shadow (**arrows**) which is separate from the aortic margins. No distortion, displacement or destruction of adjacent tissues is apparent. There is fusiform widening of the dorsal aspects of multiple ribs (**x**).

B, lateral projection: Showing the ill-defined mass (**arrows**), barely perceptible as it overlies the spine.

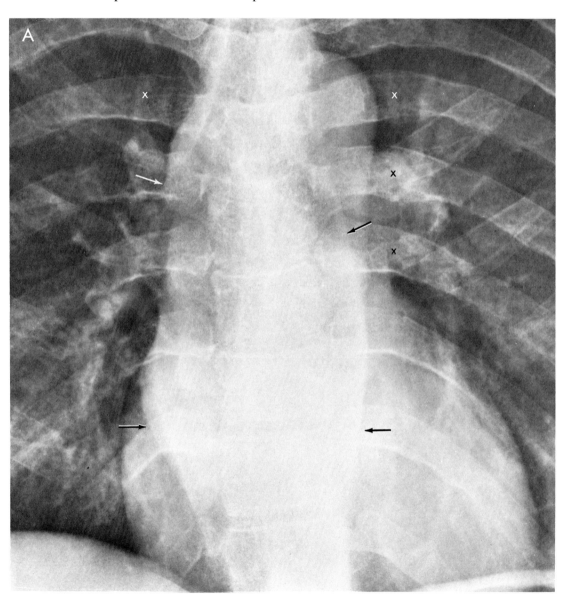

A 33-year-old woman had a history of hemolytic anemia and leg weakness. As part of her study, a chest radiograph was obtained and the abnormality discovered. Biopsy confirmed the diagnosis.

Comment: The association of the lobulated paraspinous mass without bone erosion and the fusiform dilatation of the dorsal aspects of the ribs in a patient with anemia should lead one to the diagnosis of extramedullary hemopoiesis.

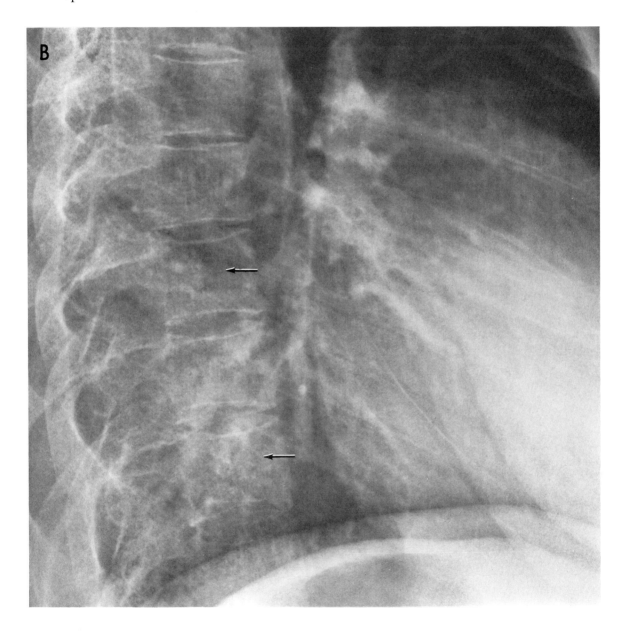

Figure 124 · Extramedullary Hemopoiesis / 341

Figure 125.—Extramedullary hemopoiesis.

A, posteroanterior radiograph: Revealing a smooth-marginated paraspinal mass extending into each hemithorax and clearly visible through the cardiac and aortic shadows (**arrows**). There is some fusiform widening of the dorsal aspects of several ribs (**x**).

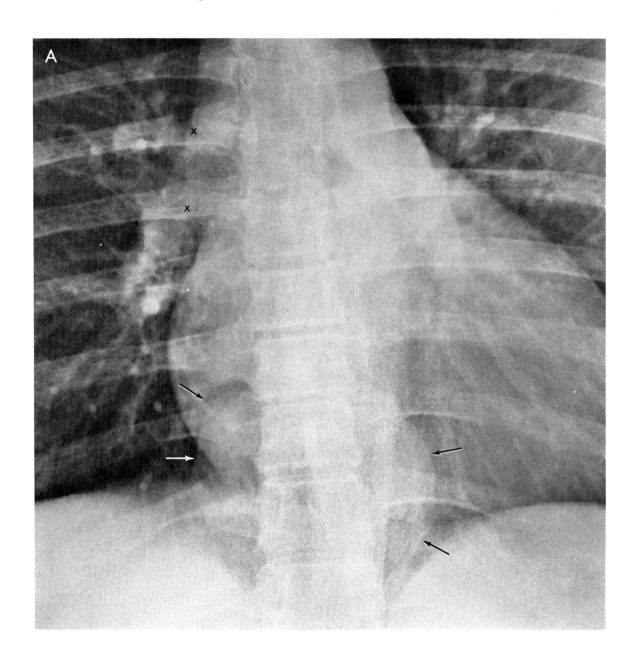

B, lateral projection: Showing an ill-defined mass overlying the lower dorsal spine (**arrows**), without bone erosion. No calcifications are visible within the mass.

A 24-year-old man with hereditary spherocytosis was examined because of increasing fatigue and weakness. The spleen was large. The abnormality was discovered on the chest roentgen studies. Biopsy was followed by considerable bleeding.

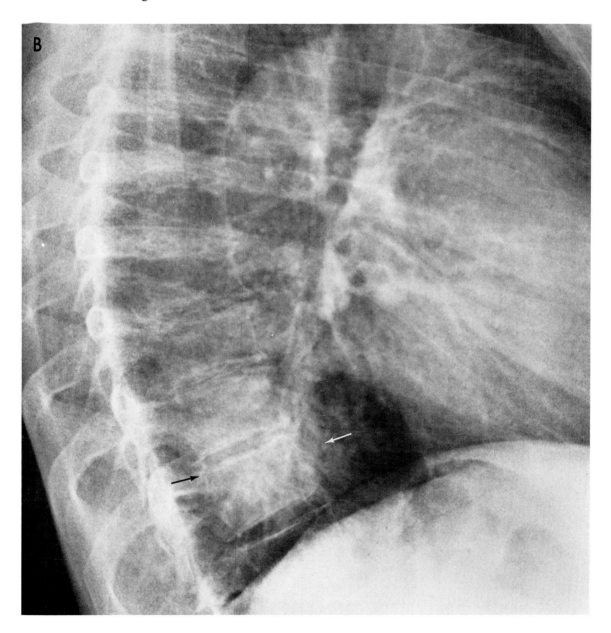

Figure 125 · Extramedullary Hemopoiesis / 343

PART 5

Parenchymal Tumors

General Characteristics

THE POSSIBILITY of a large number of different neoplasms arising in the thorax is obvious from the multiple types of tissues present as well as the complicated embryologic development of the thoracic contents. The most common tumors are illustrated here along with a few uncommon ones. There may be a few isolated, most unusual types of tumors that we have been unable to locate, but an end to the search for unusual neoplasms had to be declared in order to finish this volume.

As with all body areas there is a limit to the way an abnormality may present itself in the thorax. The manner of presentation and the effect on local related structures usually allow one to arrive at a logical conclusion. Unusual tumors may not present themselves in typical fashion or act in an expected manner, suggesting to the careful observer that he may be dealing with an uncommon lesion. Rare abnormalities are not discussed in detail, but a few descriptions are given that may be helpful.

HAMARTOMA.—Hamartomas are tumorlike malformations containing only an abnormal mixture of the normal constituents of the organ in which they are found. These malformations may consist of a change in the quantity, arrangement, degree of differentiation or any combination of these. They are found in the periphery of the lung and are usually incidentally discovered in a chest roentgenogram as a solitary pulmonary nodule (Figs. 126–128). They are spherical or ovoid and have smooth, sharply demarcated margins. When calcification is visible it is of the "popcorn" variety in the center of a solitary nodule (Figs. 126 and 128). As a rule these tumors grow slowly and very rarely may enlarge enough to produce obstructive bronchial symptoms. Rapid growth has been reported in a few instances, but this is a rare occurrence. Removal is the treatment of choice when nodules do not contain characteristic calcification.

BRONCHIAL ADENOMAS.—Bronchial adenomas constitute 6–10% of primary neoplasms of the lung and occur with about equal frequency in the two sexes. Average age is between 35 and 40, with 80% occurring before the age of 50. There are two major types: about 15% are carcinoid, and the remainder cylindromatous. The tumors are quite vascular, with hemoptysis the most common presenting complaint and occurring in about 60% of patients with adenoma. Pain and wheezing are quite frequent. Metastases are rare, but local spread and invasion are usual and there is a great tendency to local recurrence. The position in major bronchi or the trachea many times makes complete local removal difficult. About 90% can be seen on bronchoscopy. They are somewhat more common on the right side than on the left, and there is a much larger lesion beneath the surface than is immediately apparent.

The roentgen patterns may be those of obstruction with localized emphysema early; later there are infection and collapse behind the occluding tumor (Figs. 129 and 130). Frequently, on body-section radiography rounded masses may be demonstrated in the trachea or bronchi.

Treatment is removal whenever possible. Repeated coring out of tumor through the bronchoscope has been successfully carried out over a period of years in many patients when the mass could not be removed for one reason or another. Radiation therapy has not been very helpful.

ALVEOLAR CELL CARCINOMA.—Alveolar cell carcinoma, bronchiolar carcinoma, pulmonary adenomyomatosis, diffuse bronchiolar carcinoma and multiple alveolar carcinomas seem to be distinct from bronchogenic carcinoma of the lung, although apparent confusion exists as to the cells of origin. Whether they are derived from alveolar epithelium, basal cells of terminal bronchioles or are of mesenchymal origin is still undecided. The histologic similarity to a viral disease in sheep, *jagziekte,* is well known. Although the tumor may be unicentric in origin, the frequent diffuse pattern suggests the probability of a multifocal origin. Its relatively benign histologic appearance, failure of wide metastatic spread and bilateral involvement in 80% of the patients separate it from the more common bronchogenic or squamous cell tumor. In experimental animals a similar disease can be induced by a variety of etiologic agents. The clinical presentation is nonspecific, but frequently hemoptysis is an initial complaint. Classically, large amounts of gelatinous sputum are usually remembered as a prominent clinical feature, but probably this only occurs in a small number of patients with the disease. The incidence is appreciably higher in women than in men.

The roentgen changes vary widely, from a diffuse alveolar lesion producing no antemortem visible shadow to all variations of diffuse nodular pulmonary disease involving small lung areas to the entire visible pulmonary parenchyma (Figs. 131 and 132).

In some patients solitary or multiple discrete pulmonary nodules may be found. When this type of lesion is present, the margins are ill-defined and fluffy, with pseudopods extending into adjacent lung, and thus radiographically may be indistinguishable from other types of lung cancer. Nodular lesions with diffuse coalescent areas may be found in the same patient. Diffuse fine pulmonary nodules resembling pneumoconioses can be seen throughout both lungs. Cavitation is uncommon but does occur. Metastases may be to any organ, but they occur 50% of the time or less. The varied ubiquitous patterns should raise the suspicion of alveolar cell carcinoma in a patient with prolonged extensive roentgen evidence of pulmonary changes and few clinical findings.

The only successful treatment at present is surgical removal of small nodular lesions. No effective method is available for treating the diffuse disease. Radiation therapy has been of little benefit.

VASCULAR MALFORMATIONS.—Vascular tumors, arteriovenous fistulas, hemangioma and telangiectasis are lesions of uncertain cellular origin but have large, dilated, tortuous vascular channels with communications between arterial and venous channels. Some may be present at birth, but many are not discovered until adult life. Most seem to remain static after discovery, especially in patients with extensive involvement of both lungs, precluding removal.

Presenting complaints may be cyanosis, clubbing of fingers, hemoptysis, extracardiac bruit and dyspnea. Frequently associated are polycythemia and peripheral arterial desaturation; however, cardiac output is usually normal. Complications are cerebral thrombosis and massive pulmonary hemorrhage. They may be discovered incidentally in the chest roentgenogram. Characteristically the shadows are sharp-edged, single or multiple in a lobe, lung or both sides of the chest. Usually a large vessel can be seen entering or leaving the nodule or nodules (Figs. 135 and 136). Angiocardiography is diagnostic and essential because of the frequent multiplicity of the lesions and to aid in planning possible removal.

BRONCHOPULMONARY SEQUESTRATION.—Bronchopulmonary sequestration is a segment of lung completely or partially separated from adjacent normal lung. There are intra- and extralobar types, which usually cannot be differentiated by radiographic study. There usually is no communication with the normal bronchial tree, and the blood supply is via a large artery originating directly from the aorta below the diaphragm. The lesion is usually in the right lower lobe, although the extralobar type is more common in the left lower lobe and may have multiple vessels arising from the aorta.

Pathologically, these masses are usually composed of firm fibrotic lung; they may be cystic and filled with a mucoid material. Often abscesses and pus are found within them.

The roentgen appearance in a child or young adult is that of a parenchymal mass, the margins of which are reasonably sharp (Fig. 137). If suspected, aortography and selective cannulation of the aberrant vessels will establish the diagnosis. Surgical removal is the treatment of choice.

LIPOID PNEUMONIA.—This occasionally is found in the form of a solid pulmonary mass and offers a problem of differentiation in chest radiographs. Very often these masses are found in survey radiographs of the chest in asymptomatic individuals. If the possibility of lipoid deposits in the lung is considered, a history of some type of exposure to oil can be elicited. Frequently this is obtained after removal of the mass, but even if suspected, lung biopsy or removal of the offending segment or lobe may be the treatment of choice. Most often the chronic use of oily nosedrops or of mineral oil as a laxative has been the major factor, but on occasion the oily mediums used for bronchography or inhalation of fine mists of machine oil may cause lipoid pneumonia. The right middle lobe and the lower lobes are most often affected, but in debilitated patients the upper lobes may be involved. When the roentgen appearance is diffuse there is no great problem, but quite frequently these pneumonias are discovered as ill-defined, rough-margined nodules which cannot be differentiated from a carcinoma (Fig. 138).

Conglomerate masses of silicosis.—Certain inflammatory masses are easily confused with neoplasms. One of the most difficult lesions to differentiate is the conglomerate mass of silicosis. Such masses are most often seen in the upper lobes but may be found in any portion of the lung. They develop in lung tissue which is diffusely involved with nodular silicosis and secondarily infected (Fig. 129). The masses may vary from 5–6 mm up to 5–10 cm in diameter. Pathologically these are dense areas of scar tissue which seem to form in silicotic lung parenchyma in response to some kind of infection. Most often the offending organism is the tubercle bacillus, although various other bacteria also have been implicated. The patients have a history of industrial exposure to silica, but they may present any symptoms of carcinoma of the lung, including cough, pain, wheezing and hemoptysis.

In the radiographic examination these masses have sharp irregular margins with multiple pseudopods emanating from the edges. Clear areas of adjacent lung are usually present. It may be difficult or impossible to differentiate these masses from bronchogenic neoplasms if they are solitary. A useful clue in differentiation is a tendency for the conglomerate mass to be flat in one plane rather than spherical, as are the bronchogenic cancers (Fig. 139). Unfortunately one cannot always determine this flatness. On some occasions conglomerate masses will evacuate and air–fluid levels then appear within them (Fig. 140). At this stage it may be quite difficult to differentiate between squamous cell carcinoma and an ischemic necrotic nodule. Usually the ischemic masses are multiple. The fluid in the masses is dark, resembling India ink, and is diagnostic if it can be recovered.

HYDATID DISEASE.—Hydatid disease in the chest is often found as a pulmonary mass especially on chest surveys for tuberculosis. Patients are usually asymptomatic. In the United States the disease is common in Indians in the Southwest and Northwest and in Eskimos in the Northwest and Alaska.

It is reported that the lower lobes of the lungs are most often involved,[4,7] but in our experience there was equal distribution between the upper and lower lobes among 50 personally reviewed cases. About 25% of cases are multiple. The well-known water lily sign is present only after rupture of a cyst, at which time the patient becomes symptomatic.

There is no characteristic roentgen pattern (Figs. 145–147). The usual appearance is that of a sharply circumscribed ovoid mass in the lung. If observed in survey radiographs of Eskimos or Indians, a high index of suspicion of Echinococcus disease should be maintained.

PLASMA CELL TUMORS.—Plasma cell tumors do occur in the mediastinum and lung, although rarely. They seem to be primary growths rather than secondary deposits from the bone marrow. There are no specific roentgen patterns (Fig. 150). In the lung parenchyma they appear as solitary pulmonary nodules, usually with sharply marginated edges and with no clues to indicate their malignant nature. In the mediastinum they may appear as soft tissue masses along the trachea and major bronchi.

The best treatment seems to be surgical removal, with an excellent prognosis. The incidence of development of generalized plasma cell lesions is essentially unknown since few lesions have been reported. The histologic appearance is that of plasma cell tumors elsewhere.

LIPOMAS.—Lipomas are similar to fibromas and cause no symptoms, but they may cast a less dense shadow than one would expect from their size in roentgenograms (Fig. 143). Rarely, if ever, are they obstructing, and they are almost always an incidental finding in chest roentgenograms. With a change in the melting point of the fat these may be called hibernomas containing fat similar to the hibernating glands of mammals (Fig. 144).

LIPOSARCOMA.—Liposarcomas are most common in later life but have been reported in all age groups. They may be multicentric in origin but do metastasize especially to the lungs and liver. Differentiation between metastatic lesions and other primary tumors may be difficult (Figs. 141 and 142). These tumors may reach large size before detection and grow by infiltrating extensions. When well differentiated they contain large amounts of adult fat, so may cast only a faint shadow in the roentgenogram. Large tumors occupying an entire hemithorax have been overlooked because of the faintness of the shadow. Conversely, some masses are well circumscribed with a preponderance of fibrous stroma and may appear as dense as other pulmonary nodules. Especially difficult to localize are some of these lesions occurring near the chest wall.

Surgical removal is the treatment of choice. About 40% metastasize.

ANGIOMYOMATOUS HYPERPLASIA.—This is an unusual condition of the chest having the roentgen appearance of nodular pulmonary disease and pleural effusions, the latter being chylous in nature. The microscopic appearance in the lung is that of many small cystic spaces connected with bronchioles. Diffuse hyperplasia of smooth muscle cells is present in the interstitial tissues of the lungs, in the walls of bronchi, bronchioles and lymphatics. In many areas tumorlike nodules of smooth muscle are interlaced with slitlike spaces resembling vascular channels. Bronchopulmonary and mediastinal lymph nodes as well as the thoracic duct may show smooth muscle proliferation.

The reported cases all have had an associated chylothorax leading to a postulated sequence of events:[2] Chylous fluid empties into the chest from some type of thoracic duct injury or obstruction resulting in chylomediastinum and chylothorax. Chyle stasis in the mediastinum and lungs and along pleural surfaces results in smooth muscle proliferation and hyperplasia secondary to lymphatic obstruction. Microscopic emphysema develops secondary to a decrease in, or injury to, intra-alveolar elastic tissue.

In spite of the tumorlike appearance and poor prognosis, these lesions have been regarded as muscular hyperplasia rather than neoplasia.

FIBROMA.—These are unusual tumors which are benign, usually are related to the main bronchi and may occur as endobronchial lesions or in adjacent parenchyma (Fig. 152). Rarely are they pedunculated. Symptoms, when present, are long-standing. Bleeding is rare. Prognosis is excellent.

BIBLIOGRAPHY

1. Boyden, E. A.: The distribution of bronchi in gross anomalies of the right upper lobe, particularly lobes subdivided by the azygos vein and those containing pre-epiarterial bronchi, Radiology 58:797, 1952.
2. Laipply, T. C., and Sherrick, J. C.: Intrathoracic angiomyomatous hyperplasia associated with chronic chylothorax, J. Lab. Invest. 7:387, 1959.
3. Liebow, A. A.: Pathology of carcinoma of the lung as related to the roentgen shadow, Am. J. Roentgenol. 74:383, 1955.
4. McPhail, J. L., and Arora, T. S.: Intrathoracic hydatid disease, Dis. Chest 52:772, 1967.
5. Michelson, E., and Salik, J. O.: The vascular pattern of the lung as seen on routine and tomographic studies, Radiology 73:511, 1959.
6. Molnar, W., and Riebel, F. A.: Bronchography: An aid in the diagnosis of peripheral pulmonary carcinoma, Radiol. Clin. North America 1:303, 1963.
7. Nicks, R.: Thoracic hydatid cysts, M. J. Australia 1:999, 1967.
8. Shanks, S. C., and Kerley, P. (ed.): *A Text-book of X-ray Diagnosis* (3rd ed.; Philadelphia: W. B. Saunders Company, 1962), Vol. II.

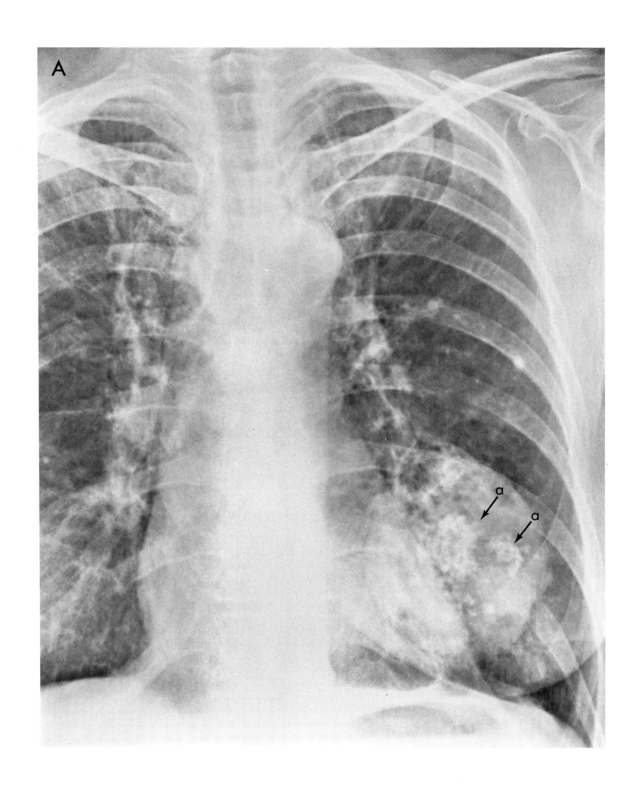

Figure 126.—Hamartoma of the left lower lobe.

A, posteroanterior radiograph: Showing old fibrotic and calcific changes in both upper lobes and several small calcified lesions in the midportion of the left lung. A solitary, large, spherical, sharply marginated lesion is present in the left lower lobe. This contains rather large, speckled, popcorn areas of calcification (**a**) throughout.

B, magnification of the left lower lobe lesion.

The size, shape, location and diffuse distribution of the calcification indicates that this is a benign process, probably a hamartoma. A more characteristic appearance of calcification in hamartoma is shown in Figure 53.

A 63-year-old woman entered the hospital with central nervous symptoms of chronic brain syndrome and an old history of tuberculosis. The course was rapidly downhill. At autopsy the lesion in the left lower lobe proved to be a hamartoma.

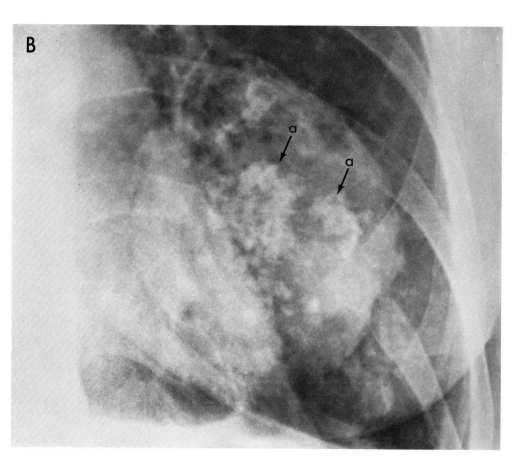

Figure 126 · Hamartoma / 353

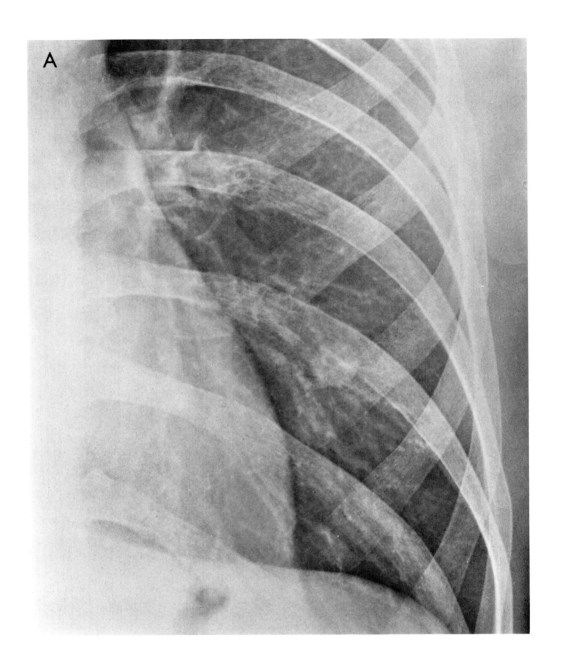

Figure 127.—Hamartoma.

A, close-up of a posteroanterior radiograph: Revealing a 1 cm solitary spherical parenchymal nodule in the left lower lobe. It contains no calcification. There is no radiographic means of differentiating between a benign and malignant process in this case.

B, close-up of a posteroanterior radiograph: Showing a sharply outlined round mass overlying the anterior end of the left third rib. There is no radiographic clue to its nature.

A 20-year-old seaman was completely asymptomatic when he came up for his annual physical examination. The lesion was removed by wedge resection and proved to be a hamartoma.

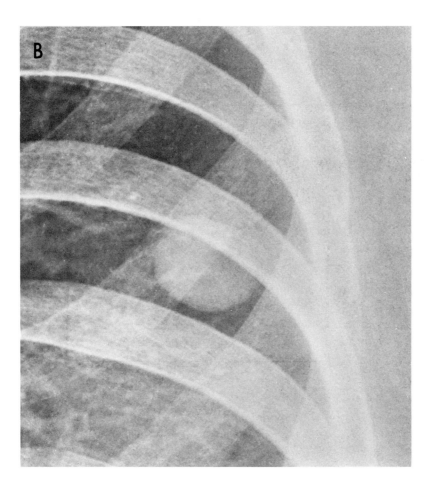

Figure 127 · Hamartoma / 355

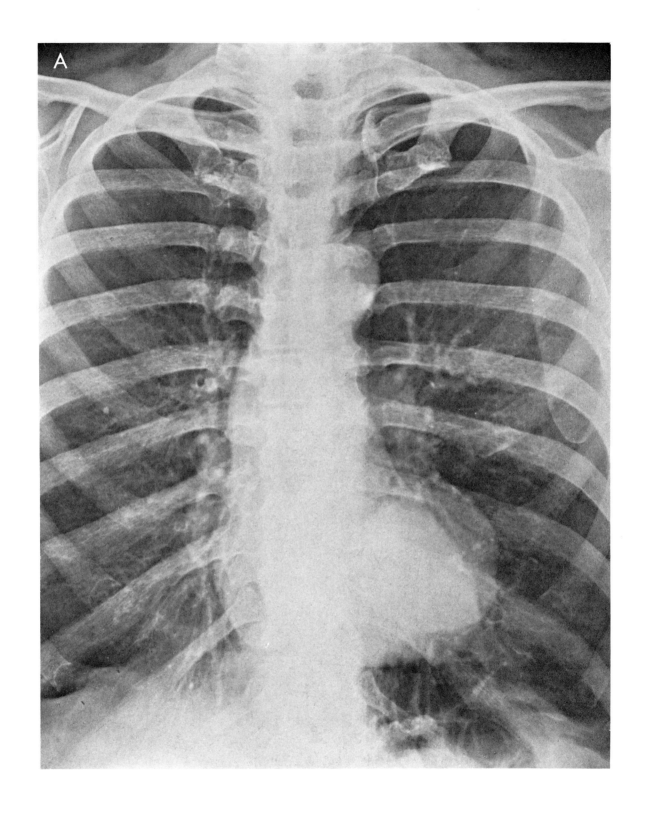

Figure 128.—Hamartoma.

A, posteroanterior radiograph: Revealing a sharply outlined spherical lesion which is seen through the heart in the left lower lobe. The fact that it is a distinct shadow attests to its location behind the heart.

B, lateral exposure: Demonstrating the lesion behind the heart and overlying the spine. It contains a speckled, popcornlike calcification (**arrow**).

C, body-section radiograph through the central portion of the mass: Clearly delineating the shape and density of the calcification (**arrow**). Calcifications of this nature are highly suggestive of hamartoma.

This abnormality was detected when the patient, an asymptomatic 45-year-old man, had a minifilm survey. On resection of the left lower lobe a hamartoma was found (pathologic diagnosis).

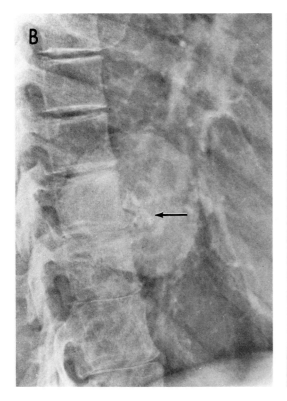
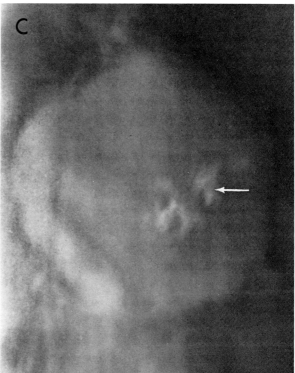

Figure 128 · Hamartoma / 357

Figure 129.—Bronchial adenoma.

A, posteroanterior radiograph: Demonstrating a linear atelectatic area in the right upper lobe with a round mass (**x**) in the superior portion of the right hilar area. Narrowing of the main stem bronchus and loss of pulmonary vessel outlines in the hilus near the junction of the mediastinum are the major features of the lesion.

B, close-up of the significant area in **A.**

C, lateral exposure: Delineating a round mass (**x**) obscuring the normal tracheal bifurcation and air shadows. The pulmonary hilar vessels (**y**) lie anterior to the mass. The linear atelectasis so clearly seen in **A** is barely perceptible in this projection (**arrow**).

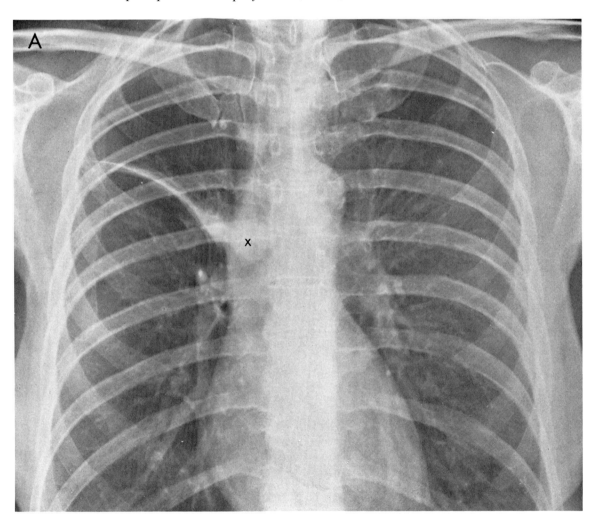

A 25-year-old woman had a rather high-pitched wheeze of uncertain duration. She had no other symptoms and results of routine laboratory studies were within normal limits. Bronchoscopy and biopsy revealed an adenoma in the main stem bronchus causing considerable occlusion of the right upper lobe bronchus. She refused thoracotomy. In the next 10 years the adenoma was periodically cored from the main stem bronchus and upper lobe. Ultimately it was impossible to remove more tissue and complete collapse of the right lung ensued.

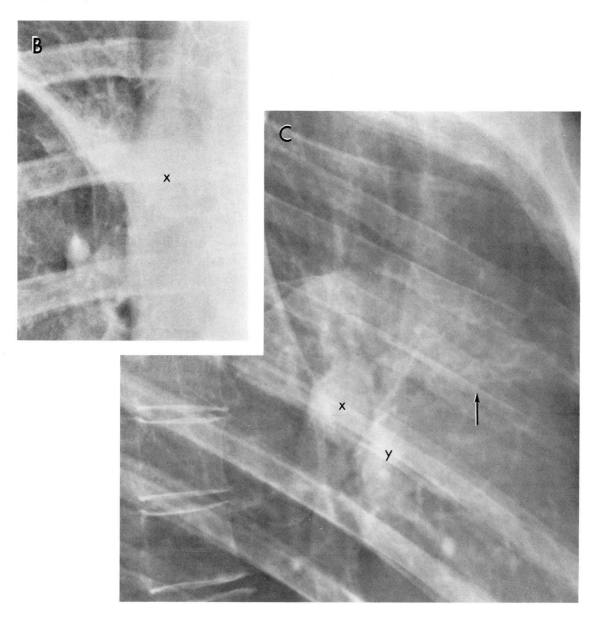

Figure 129 · Bronchial Adenoma / 359

Figure 130.—Bronchial adenoma.

A, posteroanterior radiograph: Revealing some tenting in the left hilar area (**a**) and a central, sharply marginated shadow adjacent to the main left pulmonary artery with linear extension into the left upper lobe (**b**).

B, lateral projection: Showing a sharp-edged linear shadow extending into the anterior segment of the left upper lobe in part superimposed on a vessel (**c**). The shadow in the superior portion of the hilus represents superimposed vessel and mass (**d**).

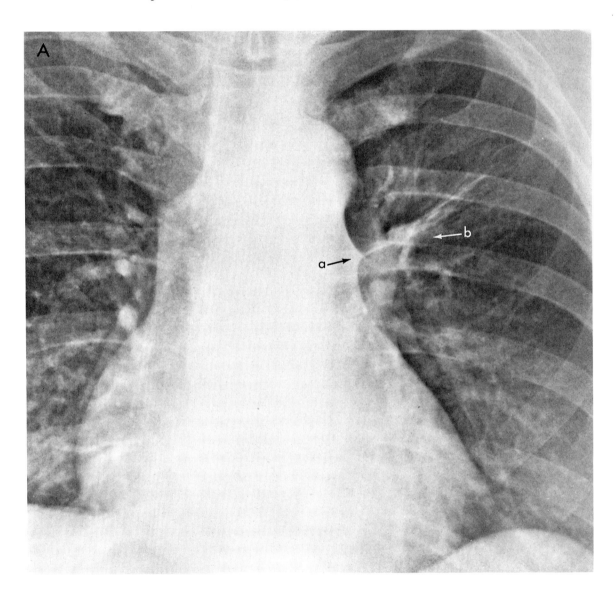

A 60-year-old man was examined because of an inspiratory wheeze that was quite apparent on physical examination. No other abnormalities were found. Bronchoscopy disclosed a lesion in the left upper lobe bronchus. Biopsy and some coring of the lesion led to a diagnosis of bronchial adenoma. While awaiting operative removal the patient had a massive coronary occlusion, and it was thought unwise to operate on him at this time. Five years later bronchial obstruction required coring of the lesion, but the patient's precarious cardiac status made thoracotomy unwise. Two years later he was doing well but again showed evidence of some increase of tumor size.

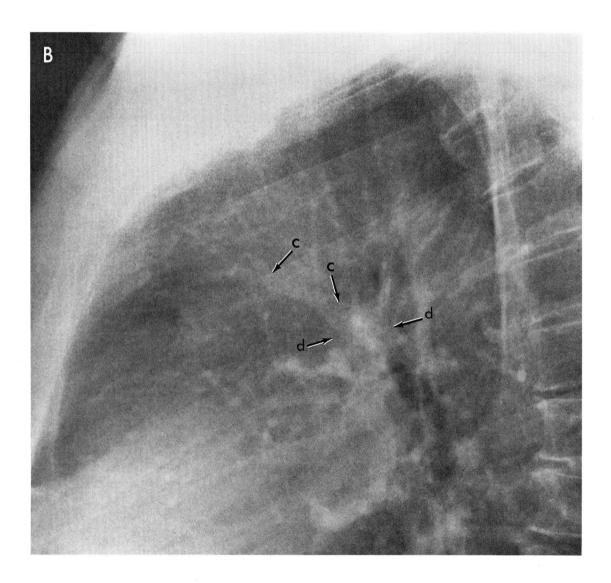

Figure 130 · Bronchial Adenoma / 361

Figure 131.—Diffuse alveolar cell carcinoma.

A, posteroanterior radiograph: Demonstrating diffuse miliary nodules evenly distributed throughout both lungs. These can be separated from vascular channels. No dominant mass is present.

B, magnification of a portion of **A.**

A 55-year-old man with a nonproductive cough and weight loss consulted his physician. Lung biopsy revealed diffuse alveolar cell carcinoma.

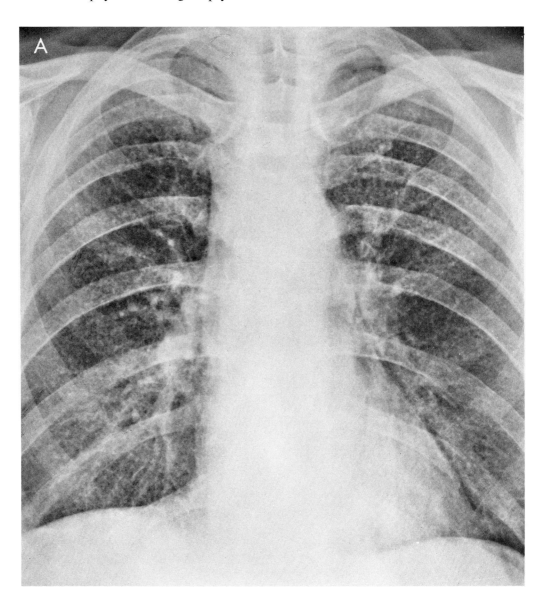

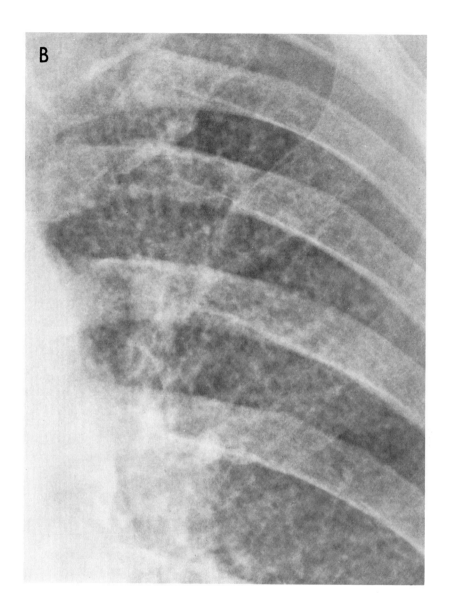

Figure 131 · Alveolar Cell Carcinoma / 363

Figure 132.—Diffuse alveolar cell carcinoma.

A, posteroanterior radiograph: Revealing diffuse, shaggily margined nodular lesions throughout major portions of both lungs, more pronounced in the lower lobes on each side. Hilar vessels are prominent bilaterally, but no adenopathy is seen.

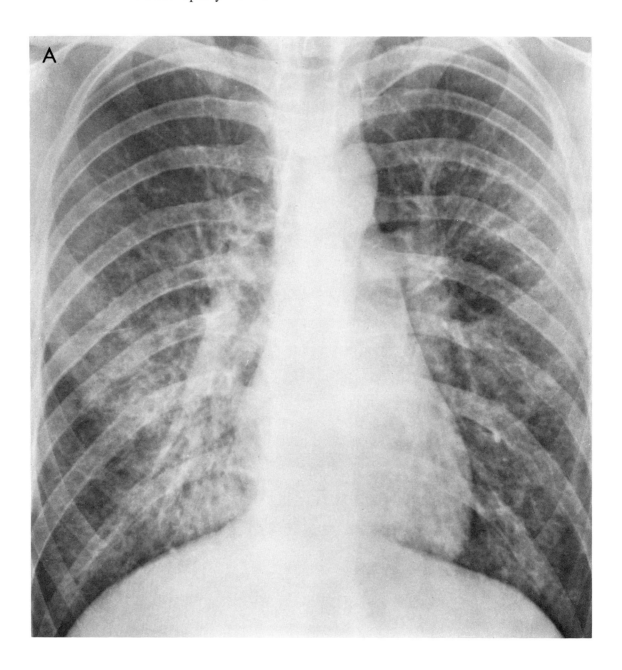

B, close-up of the left lower lobe in **A:** Accentuating the nodular lesions.

A 45-year-old man had had increasing cough and productive sputum for several months, with apparent loss of 10 lb. during this period. Moderate amounts of sputum were produced without hemoptysis. Otherwise his history was normal, and results of routine laboratory studies were within normal limits. Physical changes were confined to the chest. Histologic diagnosis of lung biopsy tissue was diffuse alveolar cell carcinoma.

Comment: Radiographically such lesions can resemble many other malignant as well as benign processes.

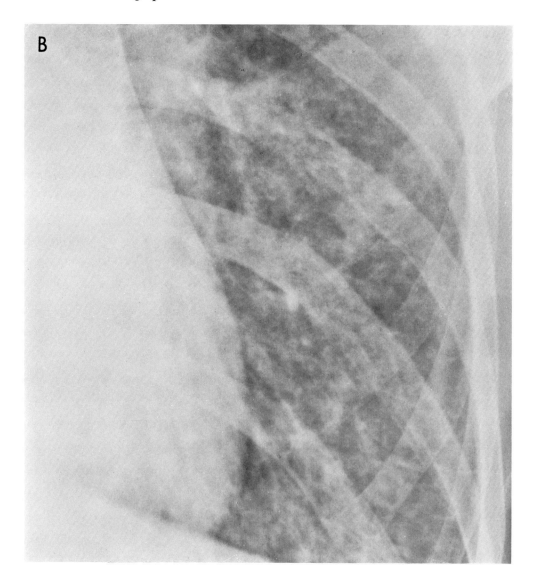

Figure 132 · Alveolar Cell Carcinoma / 365

Figure 133.—Primary adenocarcinoma of the left upper lobe.

A, posteroanterior radiograph: Showing a rather discretely outlined ovoid lesion (**x**) in the interspace between the anterior ends of the left second and third ribs.

B, magnification of the lesion in **A:** Revealing a suggestion of umbilication (**a**); one of the nearby vessels is elevated (**b**). There is no evidence of hilar nodal enlargement. One can outline clearly the vascular structures in the hilar area.

C, lateral projection: Revealing the ovoid character of the lesion, which is somewhat elongated, not spherical. It overlies several large pulmonary veins and alters their clear projection (**arrows**). No adjacent or inherent calcification is apparent. All evidence points to a malignant process.

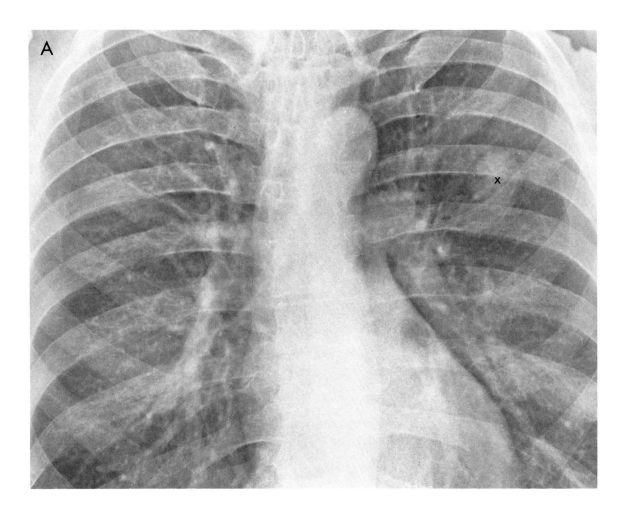

366 / **Parenchymal Tumors**

A 48-year-old man, a nonsmoker, consulted his physician because of several episodes of hemoptysis, but no other symptoms. Left upper lobectomy and pathologic study revealed a primary adenocarcinoma of the left upper lobe without nodal extension.

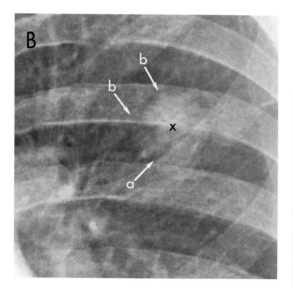

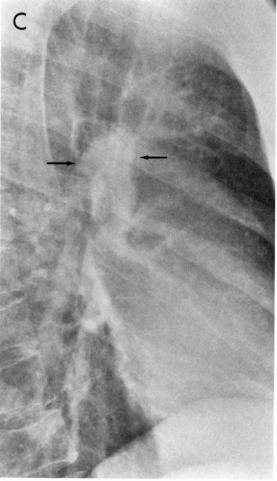

Figure 133 · Adenocarcinoma: Left Upper Lobe / 367

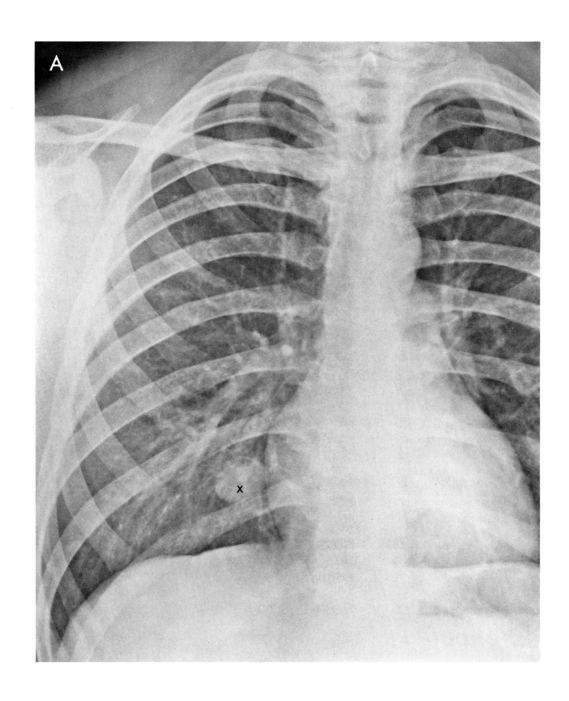

Figure 134.—Bronchiectatic cavity in the right lower lobe.

A, posteroanterior radiograph: Revealing a sharply outlined spherical lesion (**x**) adjacent to the cardiac shadow in the right lower lobe. Clear separation between the margin of the right cardiac border and the lesion indicates its posterior location.

B, magnification of the lesion in **A:** Showing somewhat exaggerated lower lobe markings adjacent to the nodule (**x**) and also farther laterally in the right lower lobe. A denser area overlying the midportion of the shadow is a vessel seen on end (**a**). At **b** a small air–fluid level is faintly visible.

A 20-year-old student had a chest roentgen examination because of recurrent respiratory infections which had increased in frequency since admission to college. Bronchography was not performed but lower lobectomy revealed extensive bronchiectatic changes. The lesion demonstrated radiographically was a bronchiectatic fluid-filled cavity.

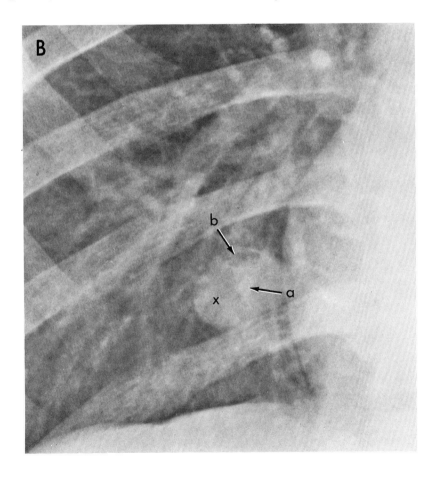

Figure 134 · Bronchiectatic Cavity / 369

Figure 135.—Multiple arteriovenous malformations.

A, posteroanterior radiograph: Revealing multiple sharply outlined ovoid masses (**x**) in the right lower lobe. They seem to be continuous with pulmonary vessels extending from the right hilar area.

B, posteroanterior radiograph made at the same time as **A,** with an increase of intrathoracic pressure induced by having the patient blow against a mercury manometer through the open glottis. The manometer is seen over the left shoulder (**arrow**). The patient maintained 10 mm Hg pressure while the radiograph was being exposed. There is demonstrable decrease in size of the masses (**x**), suggesting their vascular nature.

C, venous angiogram: Showing contrast medium in the superior vena cava (**y**) and in the pulmonary arteries filling multiple distended and tortuous masses (**x**) in the right lower lobe.

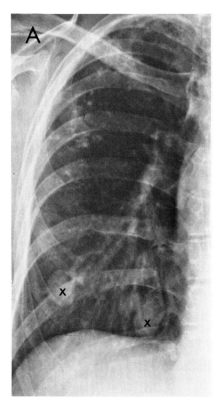
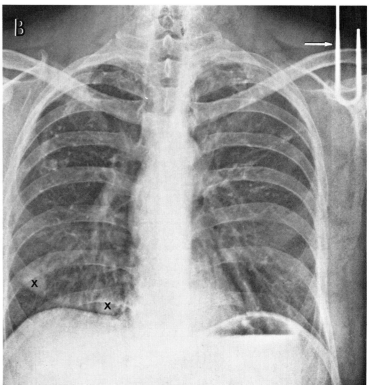

Comment: If an arteriovenous malformation is suspected, pulmonary angiography is a necessary supplementary procedure because these abnormalities are usually multiple and smaller communications are often found in unexpected areas of the lung.

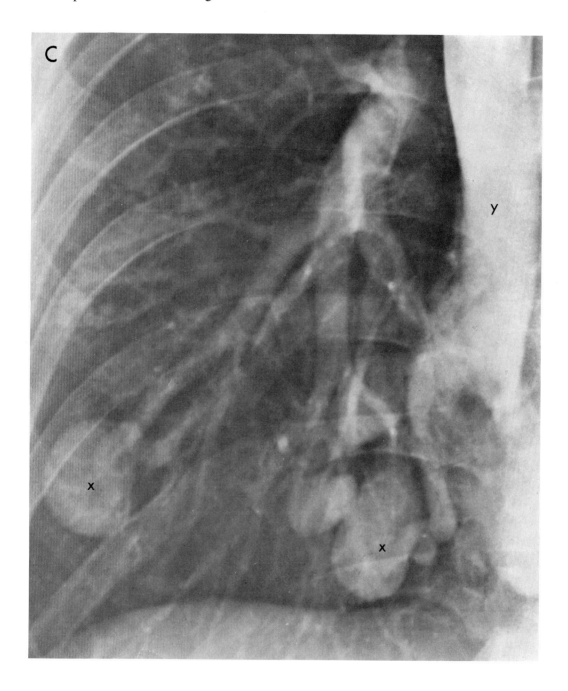

Figure 135 · Multiple AV Malformations / 371

Figure 136.—Multiple arteriovenous malformations.

A, posteroanterior radiograph: Revealing an ovoid lesion (**x**) in the region of the right nipple shadow. Because this was confusing in the initial study, round metallic washers were placed over each nipple, indicating in this view that the nodular lesion is above the nipple.

B, close-up of the lesion in **A:** Demonstrating several large, tortuous vascular channels (**arrows**) intimately related to the ovoid area (**x**) in the right lower lobe.

C, body-section radiograph: Delineating a single large ovoid lesion (**x**) with closely allied large vessels (**arrows**) leading to it. A second smaller round shadow lies above the major one.

D, body-section radiograph, more anterior than **C:** Showing a tadpole-like shadow (**arrow**) with an intimately related vessel.

E, venous angiogram: Outlining the multiplicity of the pulmonary vascular malformations. No rapid pulmonary venous filling is evident, indicating the slow flow and lakelike nature of the multiple lesions, which occupy both middle and lower lobes of the right lung.

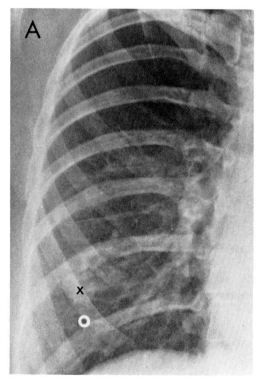
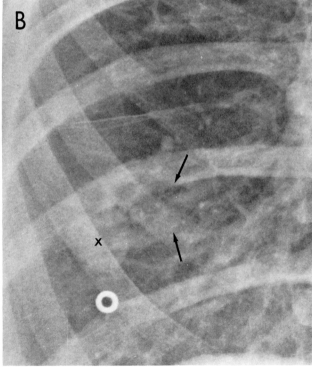

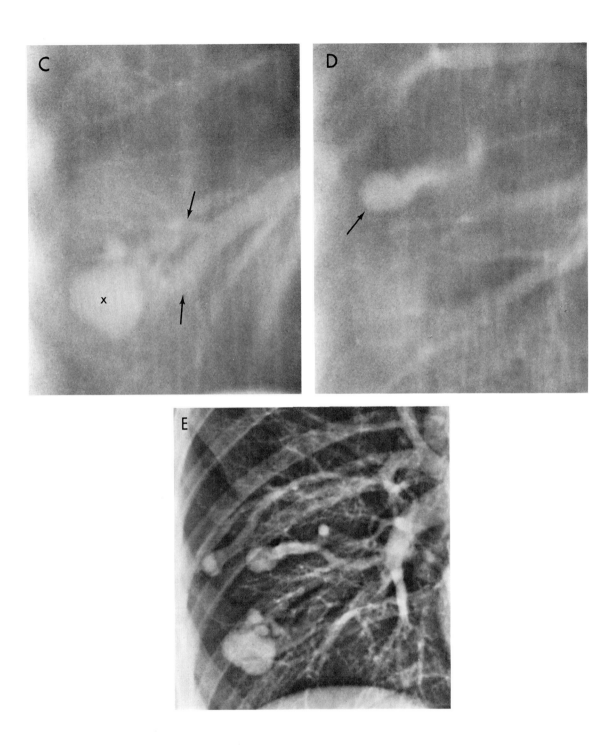

Figure 136 · Multiple AV Malformations / 373

Figure 137.—Bronchopulmonary sequestration.

A, posteroanterior radiograph: Revealing a rather sharply marginated, elongated ovoid lesion (**x**) of varying density in the right lower lobe. There is no evident distortion or communication between the surrounding vessels and no apparent calcification.

B, close-up of the lesion in **A.**

C, body-section radiograph through the mass (**x**): Not significantly informative but indicating a more diffuse nature rather than a solitary shadow. There is a seemingly intimate relationship of a pulmonary vessel at the upper margin (**arrow**).

(Continued.)

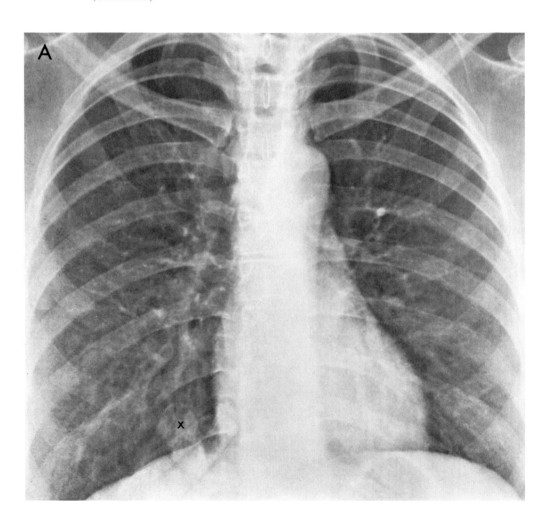

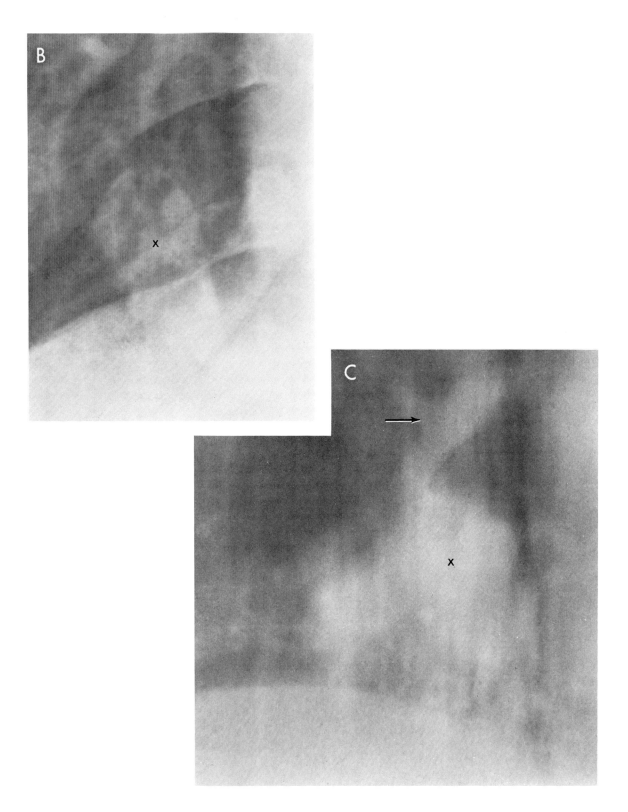

Figure 137 · Bronchopulmonary Sequestration / 375

D, selective arteriogram of the vessel arising from the aorta (**arrow**): Indicating the true nature of the lesion, which represents a bronchopulmonary sequestration.

When a 24-year-old woman was examined because of recurring respiratory infections, the abnormality was discovered in the right lower lobe. A bronchogram revealed no abnormalities in the bronchial system. On operative removal the large arterial vessel was found arising directly from the aorta. The large vessel seen in the body-section radiograph (**C**) was a draining pulmonary vein.

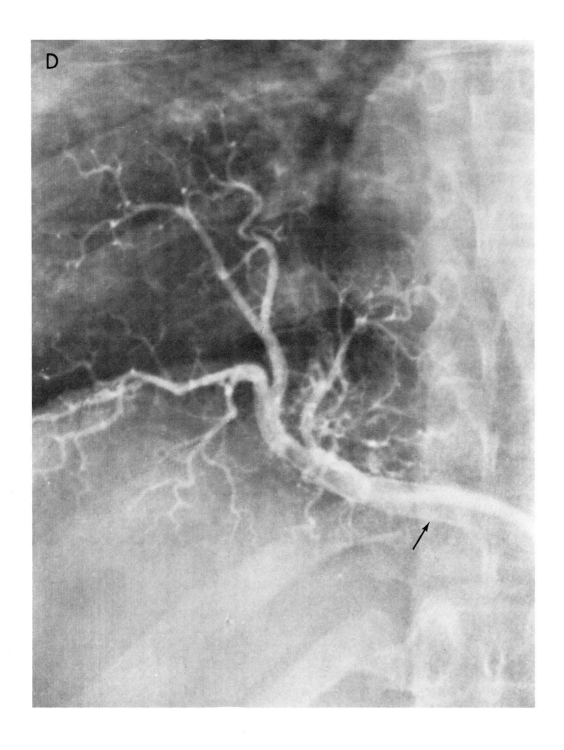

D

Figure 137 · Bronchopulmonary Sequestration / 377

Figure 138.—Lipoid pneumonia.

A, posteroanterior radiograph: Showing a roughly marginated ovoid lesion in the right paracardiac area (**x**). Normal blood vessels can be seen through the shadow. A second lesion lies below and medial to the ovoid mass (**y**).

B, close-up of the lesions in **A.**

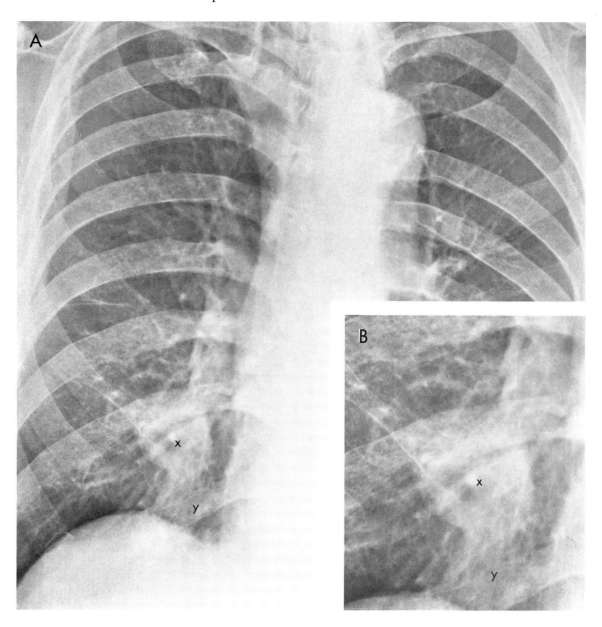

C, lateral projection: Showing the lesion (**x**) in the right middle lobe close to the oblique fissure. Its ill-defined rough margins blend into the surrounding lung. Several calcifications are adjacent to, but not part of, the mass.

D, close-up of lesion in **C.**

A mentally retarded man 45 years old, in a nursing home, had been given mineral oil for constipation over a period of years. An annual chest radiographic survey disclosed the abnormal shadow in the right hemithorax. The patient was asymptomatic. At operation, lipoid granuloma was found.

Comment: The history and demonstration of double lesions should make one suspect the lipoid nature of the process.

Figure 138, courtesy of Dr. Walter Miller, City Health Center, Seattle, Wash.

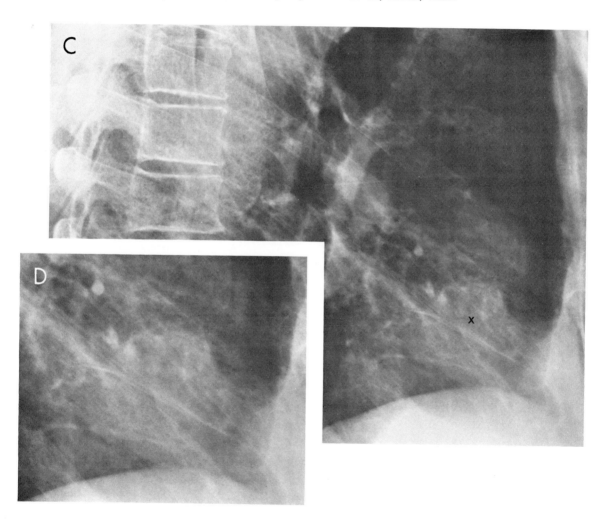

Figure 138 · Lipoid Pneumonia / 379

Figure 139.—Conglomerate mass of silicosis.

A, posteroanterior radiograph: Revealing a shaggily marginated lesion in the posterior portion of the right upper lobe (**x**) with a small calcification at its top (**arrow**) and hyperaeration superior to it (**y**). A smaller lesion with regular, fairly sharp margins is present in the left apex (**a**).

B, lateral projection: Showing the lesion in the posterior segment of the right upper lobe, with a flatter appearance (**arrows**) than one would expect from its size in the posteroanterior exposure. Linear streaking (**b**) is also more apparent, extending up from the hilus. The esophageal appearance of narrowing is artifactual.

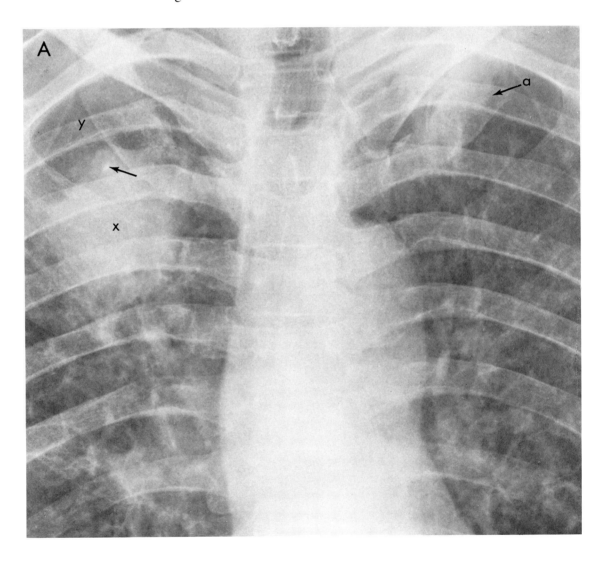

A 55-year-old worker in the sand glass industry had been followed for a number of years with survey chest radiographs. In a relatively short time changes appeared in his chest radiographs; he had an episode of blood-streaked sputum at the time of this study but no other clinical findings. His exposure to finely ground silica was sufficiently heavy and prolonged to produce silicosis. Suspicion that the lesion might be a neoplasm rather than a conglomerate mass of silicosis led to its excision. It proved to be a conglomerate mass of silicosis.

Comment: Review of a large number of patients with conglomerate masses of silicosis and a lesser number having silicosis and carcinoma suggests that conglomerate masses tend to be flatter and more irregular, viewed in lateral projections, than do neoplasms of similar size. In general, neoplasms tend to be more similar in size in various projections. Irregular apparent extensions into surrounding pulmonary tissue are alike in the two diseases.

Figure 139, courtesy of Dr. Eugene Pendergrass, University of Pennsylvania Hospital, Philadelphia.

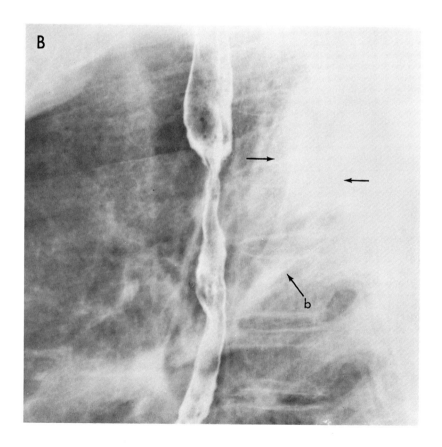

Figure 139 · Silicosis / 381

Figure 140.—Ischemic necrosis in a silicotic conglomerate mass.

A, posteroanterior radiograph: Showing diffuse, small nodular lesions throughout both lungs with massive conglomerate shadows (**y**) characteristic of pneumoconiosis. A large cavity (**x**) with shaggy walls and a fluid level (**arrow**) is present in the right upper lobe.

B, lateral exposure: Showing the cavity (**x**), fluid level (**arrow**), and a confluence of several superimposed conglomerate masses (**y**).

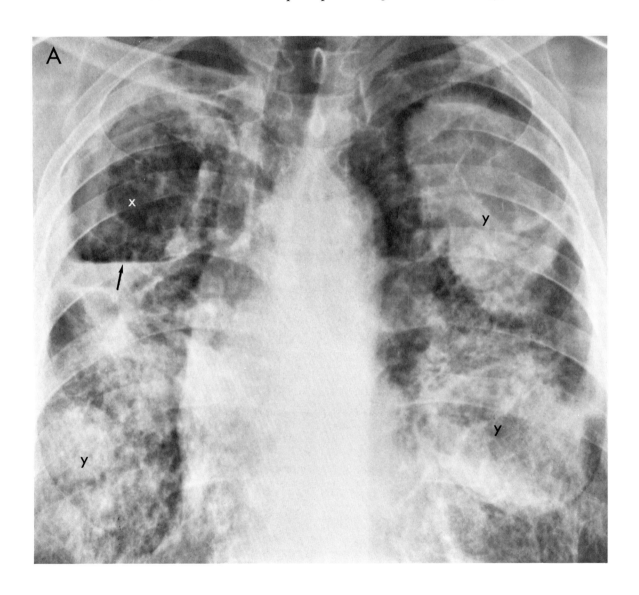

A 60-year-old asymptomatic hard coal miner had been followed radiographically for a number of years. On needle aspiration of the necrotic area, India ink-like material was obtained from the cavity. It was sterile and contained no malignant cellular material. Because of previous experience with such conglomerate masses, the condition was thought to be ischemic necrosis in a large conglomerate mass, not a neoplasm. Subsequent radiographic study over a period of years revealed filling and emptying of the ischemic necrotic area without a change of symptoms.

Comment: Considerable difficulty may be experienced in differentiating such masses from neoplasms. However, in a patient with an adequate history of exposure to dust and with other conglomerate masses, each of which is flatter in one projection than in another, one seems justified in concluding that the lesions represent ischemic necrosis rather than neoplasms.

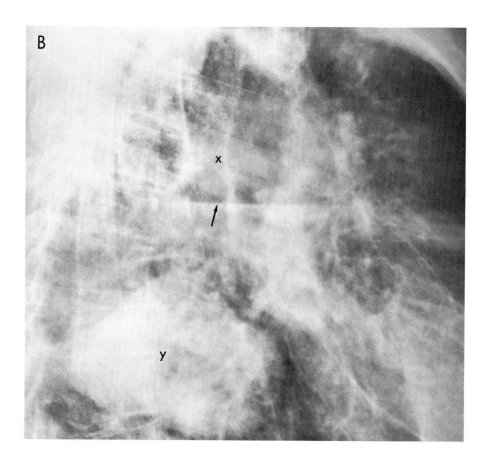

Figure 140 · Ischemic Necrosis in Silicosis / 383

Figure 141.—Liposarcoma.

A, close-up of a posteroanterior radiograph: Showing a large mass occupying the apex and upper portion of the right hemithorax and extending to the thoracic inlet. The inferior margin contains a thin rim of calcification (**arrow**). The trachea and esophagus are slightly displaced to the left. Bony structures are intact and hilar vessels obscured but not displaced.

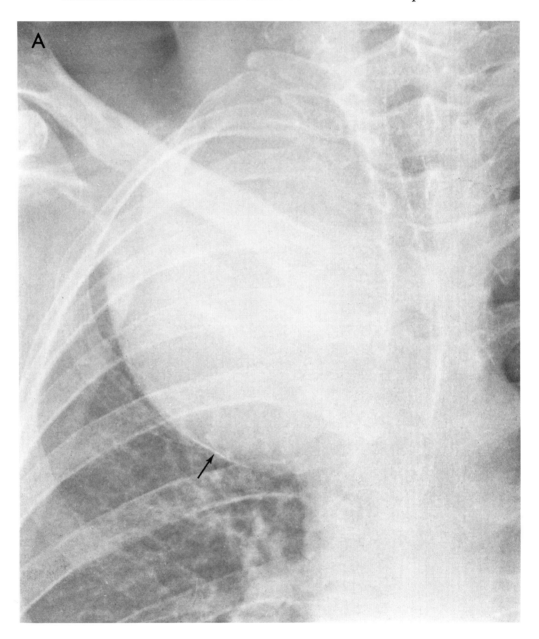

B, lateral projection: Revealing a slightly more posterior position of the mass (**arrows**) and a little anterior displacement of the trachea and esophagus. On fluoroscopy no motion of the mass occurred with deglutition.

A 54-year-old man was examined because of vague gastrointestinal complaints. The chest mass was discovered on routine chest examination. On lobectomy (right upper lobe) pathologic diagnosis was xanthogranuloma. About six months after removal of the mass the patient had a small recurrent pulmonary nodule. It was excised; this time the pathologic diagnosis was liposarcoma. Review of the initially excised material led to a similar pathologic opinion.

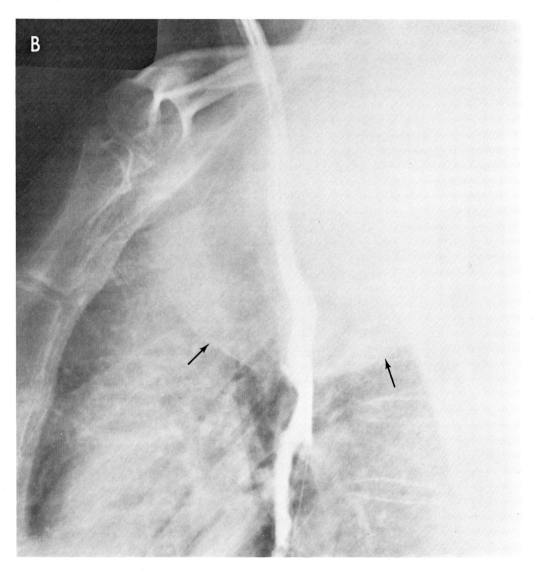

Figure 141 · **Liposarcoma** / **385**

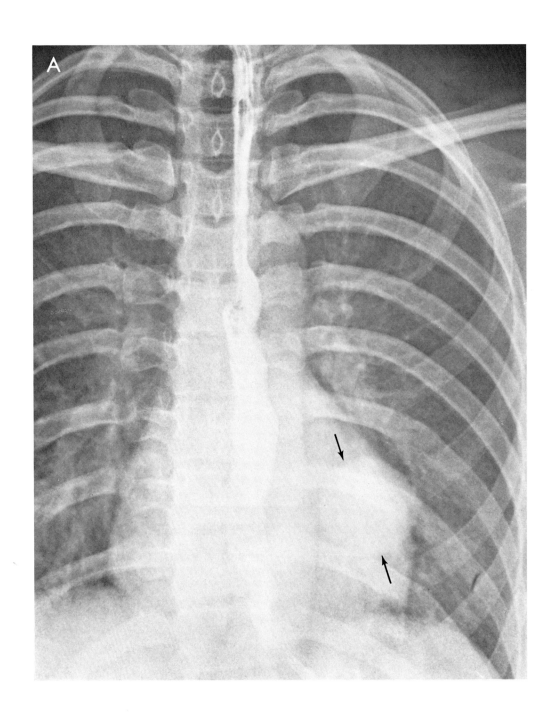

Figure 142.—Liposarcoma of the lung.

A, posteroanterior radiograph: Revealing a golf ball-sized mass seen through the left side of the heart. The sharp outlines of the mass through the cardiac shadow indicate its posterior location (**arrows**).

B, body-section radiograph: Demonstrating the sharply circumscribed nature of the mass in the left lower lobe with no apparent vascular distortion or communication.

A 24-year-old woman complained of rather severe midthoracic back pain after playing golf. As part of the clinical examination her physician asked for radiographic study of the chest, at which time the abnormality was discovered. The patient then confessed to having had a 35 mm film of the chest made four years before. Comparison of the two studies revealed the same mass in the earlier film. The patient herself now elected to have the lesion removed. A left lobectomy was performed and pathologic study revealed a primary liposarcoma of the lung. Ten years later the patient was well.

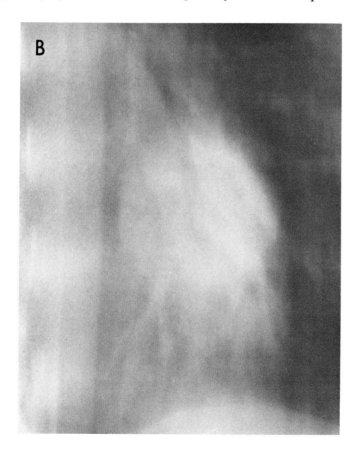

Figure 142 · Liposarcoma / 387

Figure 143.—Intrapulmonary lipoma.

A, posteroanterior radiograph: Revealing a smooth-edged, slightly ovoid, sharply marginated mass (**x**) extending to the right of the cardiac border.

B, lateral projection: Delineating the spherical nature of the mass (**x**) overlying the cardiac shadow. The density seems less than one would expect in a mass of this size and is the only clue to its fatty nature.

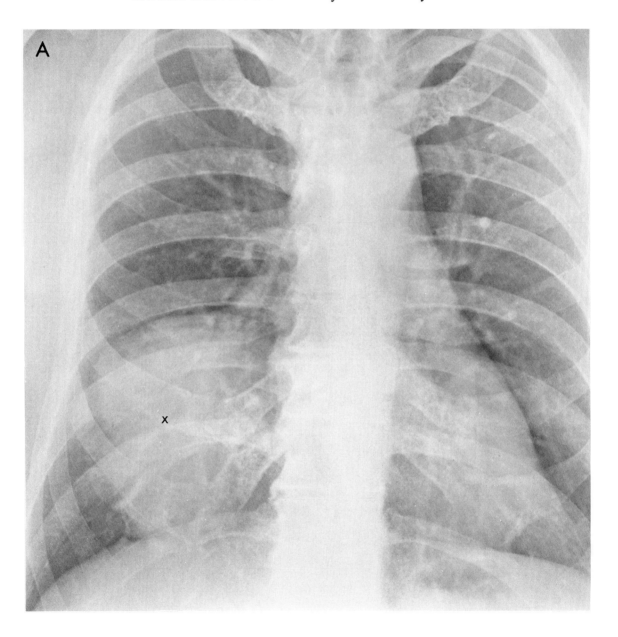

A 55-year-old man was studied because of fatigue and some weight loss. He had no chest symptoms and results of all clinical studies were within normal limits. At thoracotomy a large, soft mass was found adjacent to the pericardium and peeled readily from it. Pathologic diagnosis was lipoma.

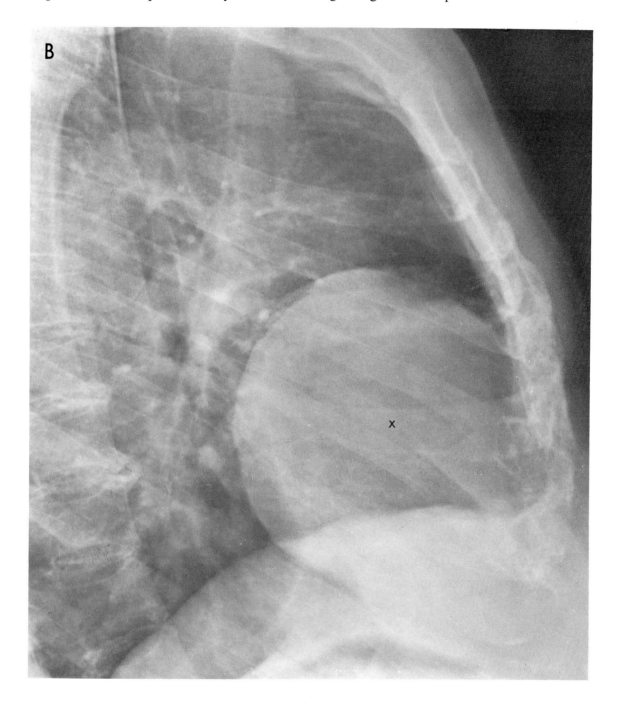

Figure 143 · Intrapulmonary Lipoma / 389

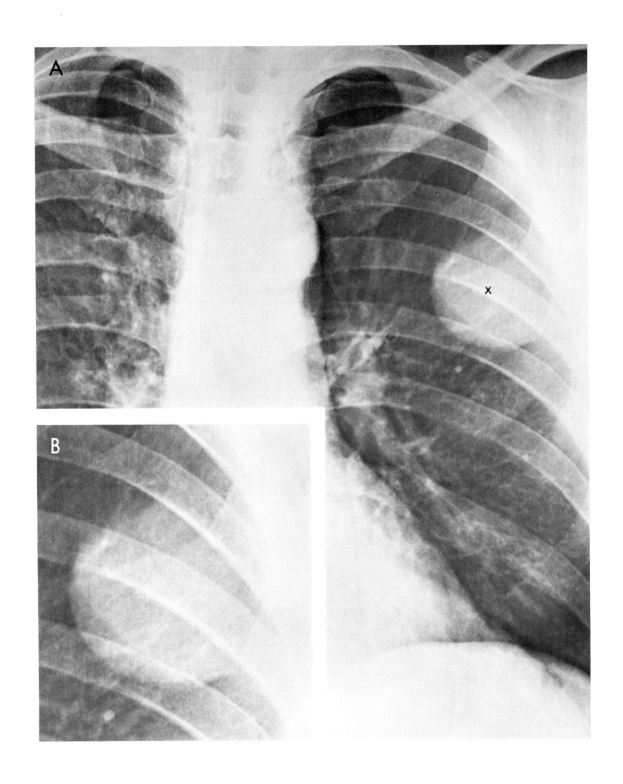

Figure 144.—Hibernoma.

A, posteroanterior radiograph: Revealing a solitary mass (**x**) with a sharply marginated medial border. The lateral margin gradually blends into the density of the chest wall. No bony erosion is visible in the adjacent ribs.

B, close-up of the lesion in **A.**

C, lateral view: Demonstrating the posterior position of the mass (**x**).

In a 45-year-old man the abnormality was discovered in a 35 mm survey film. When interviewed he was asymptomatic and had no other known disease. At thoracotomy a dark fatty mass found in the pulmonary parenchyma of the apical segment of the left lower lobe was removed by wedge resection. The tumor contained an abnormal type of fat; pathologic diagnosis was hibernoma.

Figure 144, courtesy of Dr. Walter Miller, City Health Center, Seattle, Wash.

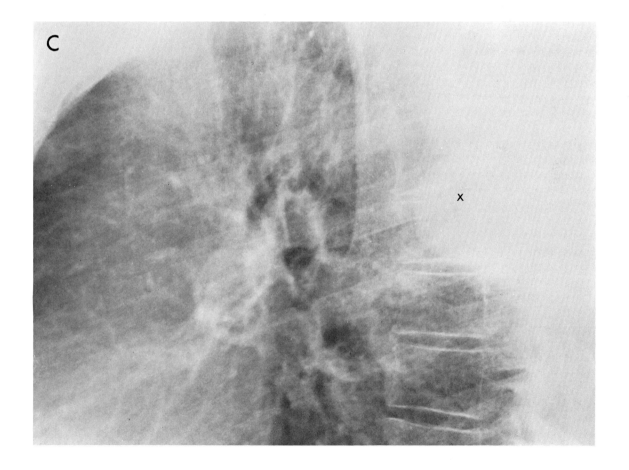

Figure 144 · Hibernoma / 391

Figure 145.—Hydatid cyst of the left lower lobe.

A, posteroanterior radiograph: Revealing a spherical, slightly lobulated, smooth-edged mass in the left lower lobe (**x**). A portion of the left mid-cardiac border is blurred but visible (**a**), suggesting the posterior adjacent position of the lesion.

B, lateral projection: Confirming the spherical nature of the mass abutting on the posterior cardiac margin (**arrows**). No characteristic calcifications or other helpful diagnostic clues are visible.

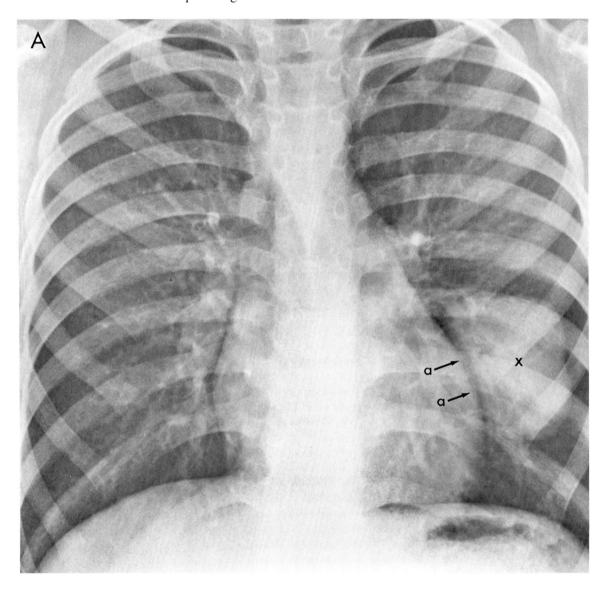

The patient, a 12-year-old asymptomatic Eskimo boy, had a chest survey performed by the U.S. Public Health Service in Alaska. At this time the abnormality was discovered. On removal the mass proved to be a hydatid cyst.

Figure 145, courtesy of Dr. Walter Miller, City Health Center, Seattle, Wash.

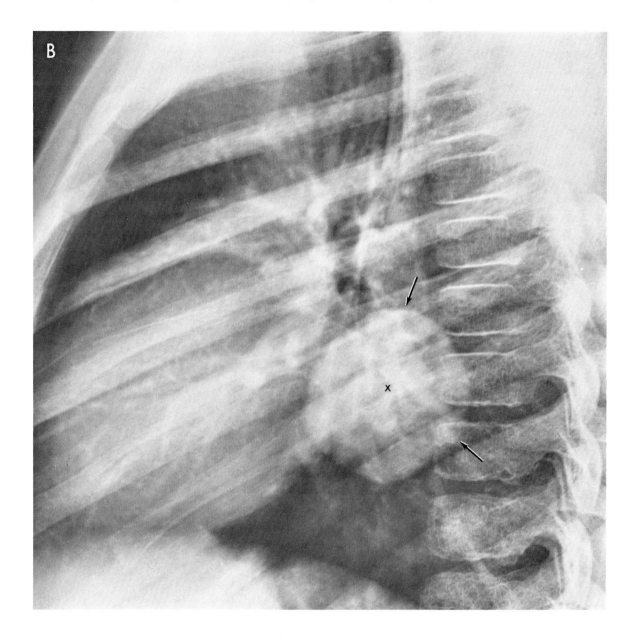

Figure 145 · Hydatid Cyst / 393

Figure 146.—Hydatid cyst.

A, posteroanterior radiograph: Portraying a huge mass with sharp superior and inferior margins extending laterally to the chest wall. The cardiac outline is visible adjacent to the lower edge medially (**a**), but the aortic knob and left hilar vessels are lost through the density of the mass (**b**).

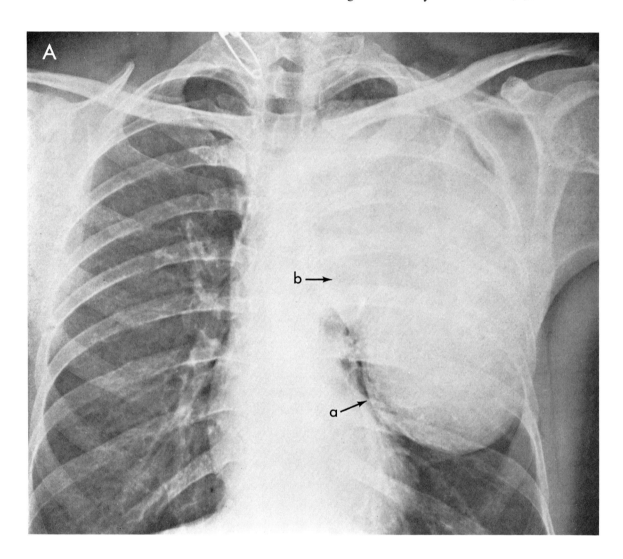

B, lateral projection: Clearly demonstrating the huge, slightly lobulated, elongated, ovoid mass with smooth margins. There is no vascular displacement or disruption.

A 42-year-old Eskimo had a Public Health survey chest radiograph, at which time a large mass was discovered. On removal it proved to represent a large hydatid cyst.

Figure 146, courtesy of Dr. Walter Miller, City Health Center, Seattle, Wash.

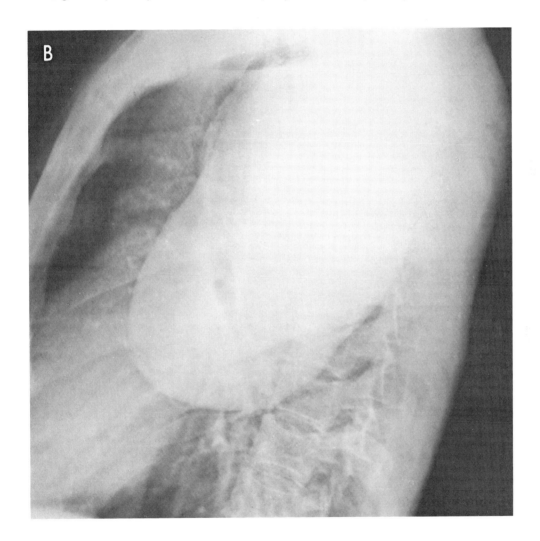

Figure 146 · Hydatid Cyst / 395

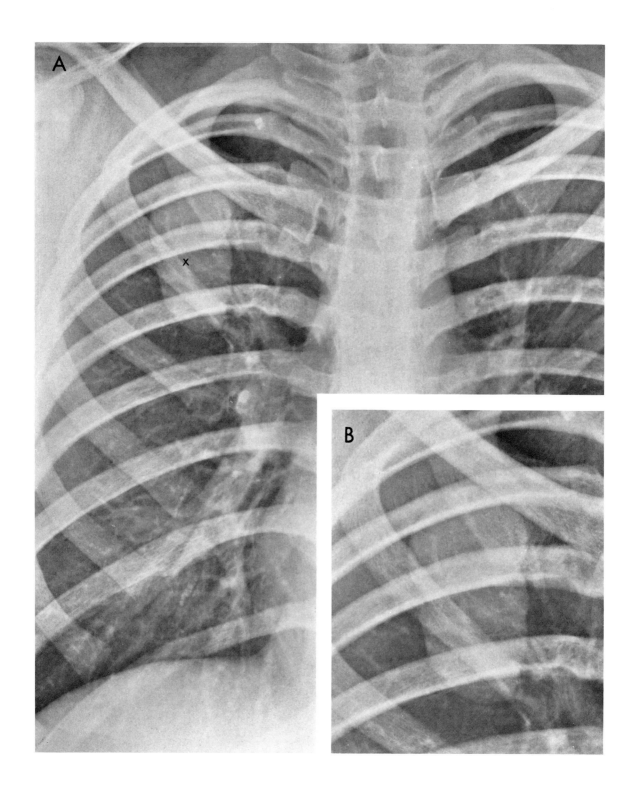

Figure 147.—Hydatid cyst of the right upper lobe.

A, posteroanterior radiograph: Showing a slightly wavy, sharp-edged ovoid mass in the right upper lobe (**x**). No associated abnormalities are present and no calcium is visible. The adjacent vessels and hilar structures as well as the bones appear to be normal.

B, close-up of the lesion in **A.**

C, a lateral body-section radiograph: Demonstrating the lobulated lesion (**x**) in the posterior portion of the right upper lobe. No bone change is evident.

A 40-year-old asymptomatic Alaskan Eskimo had a survey chest radiograph made by the Public Health Service, at which time the abnormal shadow was found. Right upper lobectomy and pathologic study revealed Echinococcus disease.

Figure 147, courtesy of Dr. Walter Miller, City Health Center, Seattle, Wash.

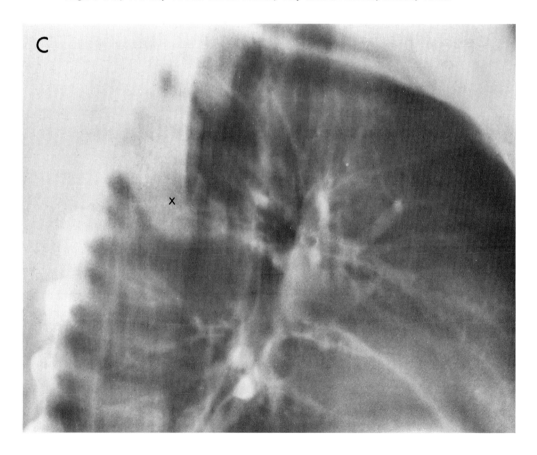

Figure 147 · Hydatid Cyst / 397

Figure 148.—Hyperplastic lymph node.

A, posteroanterior radiograph: Revealing a sharply outlined ovoid mass (**x**) closely aligned to the pulmonary artery leading to the right lower lobe. It is slightly kidney-shaped and contains no calcification. No significant distortion of the adjacent vessels is present.

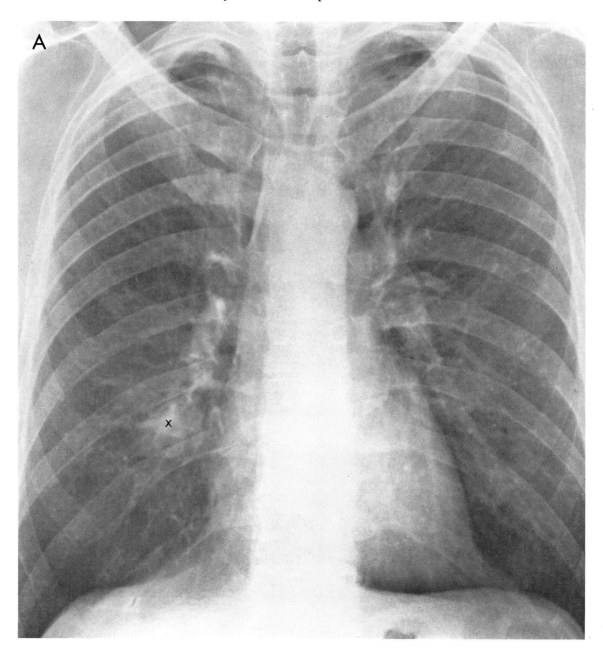

B, close-up of the lesion in **A.**

C, a body-section radiograph through the mass: Delineating margins of the kidney-shaped shadow adjacent to a right lower lobe pulmonary artery with slight medial bowing of an adjacent vessel (**arrow**). Impingement on surrounding bronchi could not be demonstrated.

A 40-year-old asymptomatic man had a routine chest study as part of a general physical examination. At thoracotomy, what appeared grossly to be a large lymph node was peeled from the right hilar area. The pathologic diagnosis was hyperplastic lymph node. The suggested prognosis was excellent; when seen five years later, the patient had remained healthy.

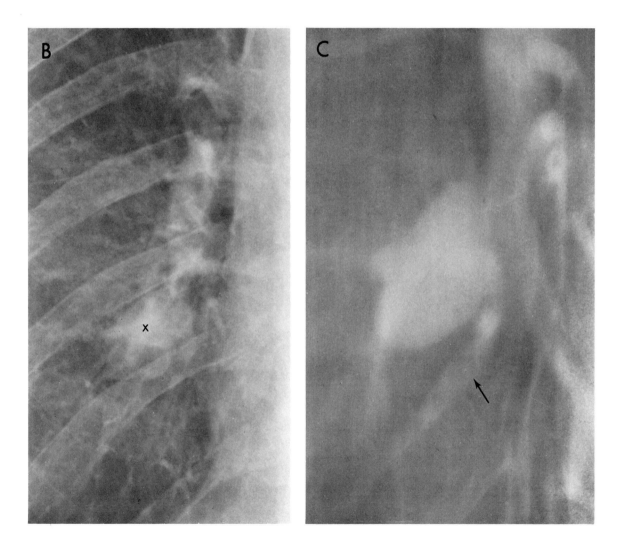

Figure 148 · **Hyperplastic Lymph Node** / **399**

Figure 149.—Pulmonary plasmacytoma.

A, posteroanterior radiograph: Revealing a solitary spherical nodule (**x**) in the right lower lobe. In body-section radiographs also, the abnormality was seen to be sharply circumscribed with no evidence of calcification within or adjacent to it. No other abnormalities were detected.

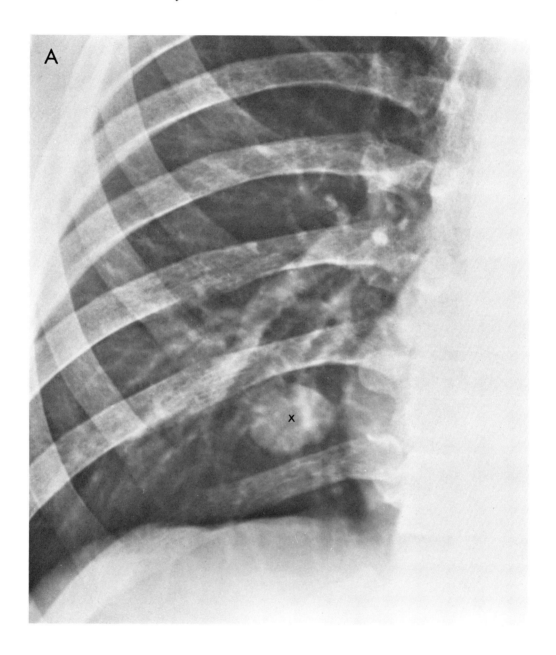

B, lateral study: Demonstrating the posterior location of the mass (**x**) and several normal vessels overlying it.

A 50-year-old man who was going through a standard executive medical examination had a nodule detected in the survey radiograph of his chest. He had no pulmonary symptoms and no history of pulmonary disease. On removal, the nodule proved to be a solitary pulmonary plasmacytoma. This was the only lesion detected and the patient was well when last seen three years later.

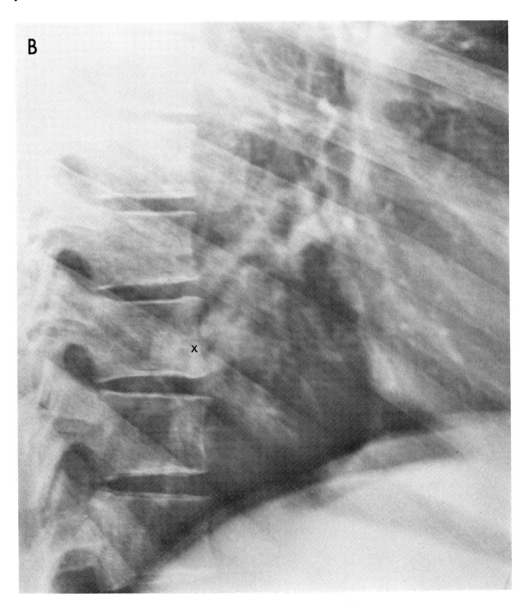

Figure 149 · Pulmonary Plasmacytoma / 401

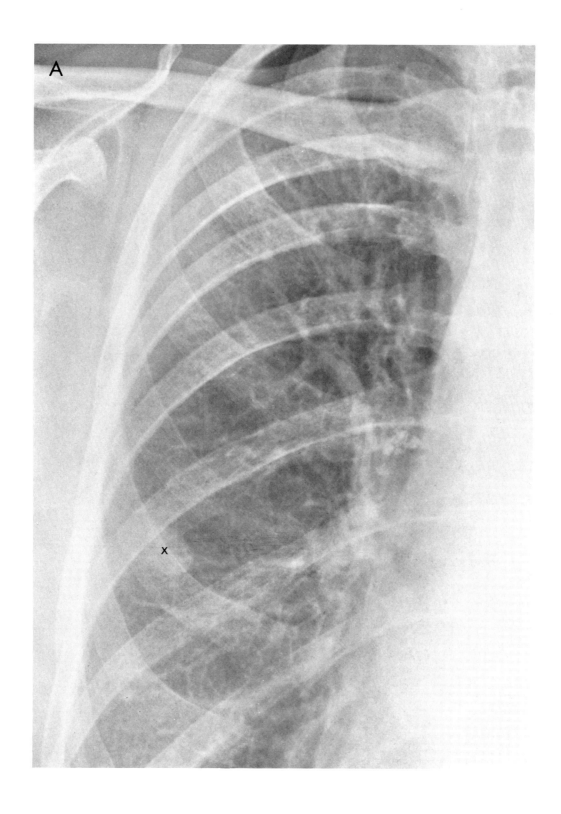

Figure 150.—Chemodectoma of the right lung.

A, posteroanterior radiograph: Revealing an ovoid, sharply marginated nodule (**x**) in the right lower lobe. No helpful hints as to its etiology are present despite the increased vascularity in the right upper lobe.

B, body-section radiograph through the nodule (**x**): Demonstrating the sharply marginated borders and absence of calcification within the nodule.

A 37-year-old asymptomatic woman had a chest survey at a city health clinic. The lesion was removed by wedge resection. Pathologic diagnosis was chemodectoma.

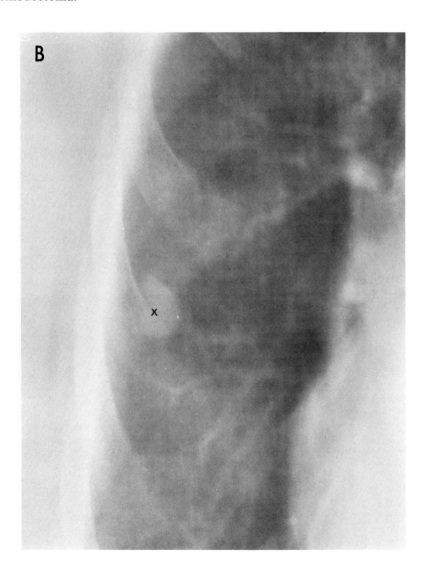

Figure 150 · **Chemodectoma** / **403**

Figure 151.—Angiomyomatous hyperplasia.

A, posteroanterior exposure: Revealing diffuse, roughly marginated parenchymal nodular lesions from 2–3 mm in size which, on close inspection, appear to be somewhat coalescent. The nodules are diffusely distributed in both lower lobes but are somewhat more pronounced on the right side. The appearance is suggestive of metastatic disease. However, the unequal distribution between the lungs and the greater preponderance in the lower lobes is unusual for either a blood-borne or a lymphatic metastatic process.

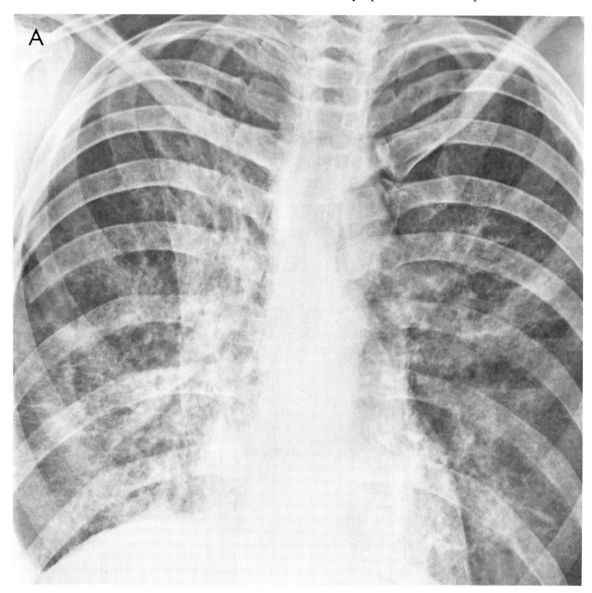

B, close-up of lesions in the right midlung field in **A.**

A 27-year-old woman presented herself with a large mass involving the left buttock. This was ill-defined and had the consistency of adjacent soft tissues. The lesion was removed and proved to be a large liposarcoma. At this time, radiographic findings in the chest were thought to be normal.

The radiographs shown here were obtained approximately six months after resection of the mass from the buttock. At this time the patient was having considerable respiratory difficulty and was somewhat anoxic. There was no unusual sputum production. Cytologic study of the sputum did not reveal malignant cells. A blood-stained chylous effusion that required repeated aspirations was present. An abdominal cystic mass also contained bloody chylous fluid. Treatment of various types was completely unsuccessful, and the course was steadily downhill. Autopsy disclosed extensive distribution of the lesions throughout both lungs, but relatively free areas were present in both upper lobes. The pathologic conclusion was angiomyomatous hyperplasia.

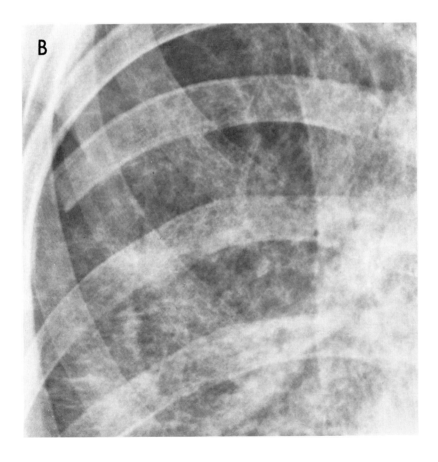

Figure 151 · Angiomatous Hyperplasia / 405

Figure 152.—Pulmonary fibroma.

A, posteroanterior radiograph: Delineating a rounded, sharp-edged mass (**arrows**) superimposed on the left cardiac border (**a**). No calcification is visible and the related vessels appear to be normal.

B, close-up of the lesion in **A.**

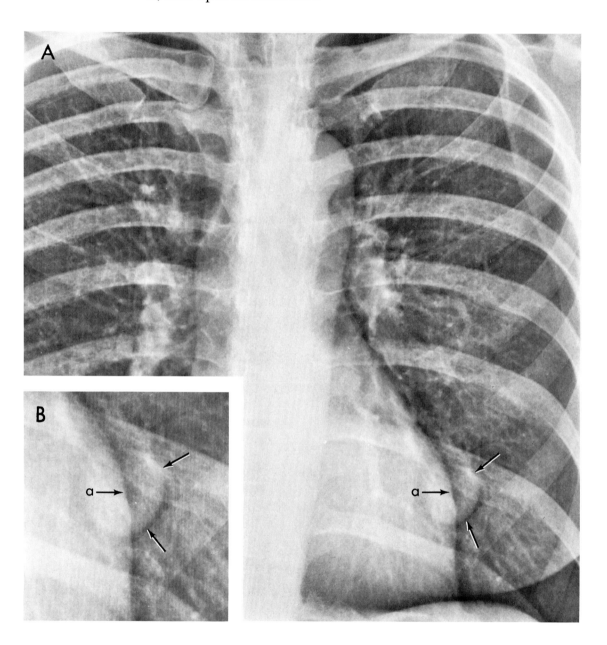

C, lateral radiograph: Showing the spherical nature of the mass (**x**) close to the cardiac shadow and in the region of the interlobar fissure between the left upper and lower lobes.

A 40-year-old asymptomatic man was found to have a nodule on a chest survey by the municipal health clinic. He had no symptoms. Thoracotomy and removal of the mass revealed its close approximation to the interlobar fissure, but it appeared to extend into or be part of the lung. Pathologic diagnosis was pulmonary fibroma.

Figure 152, courtesy of Dr. Walter Miller, City Health Service, Seattle, Wash.

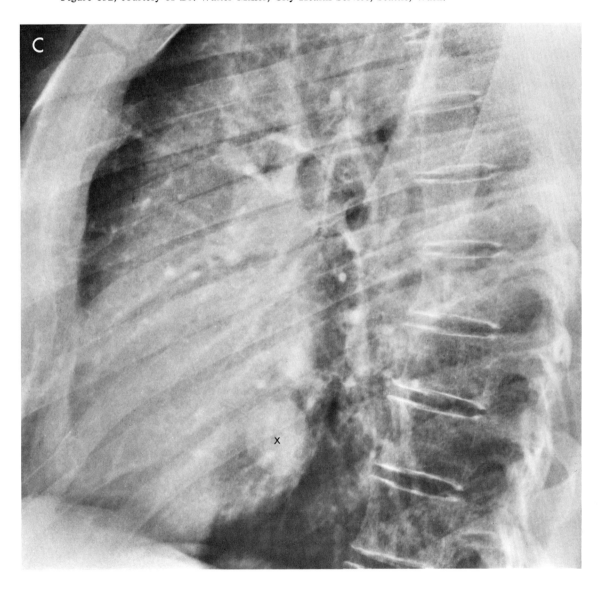

Figure 152 · Pulmonary Fibroma / 407

Figure 153.—Primary amyloid tumor of the lung.

   A, posteroanterior radiograph: Showing a shaggy, thick-walled cavity in the left lung (**arrow**) with a suggestion of a fluid level within it. Adjacent vessels appear normal.

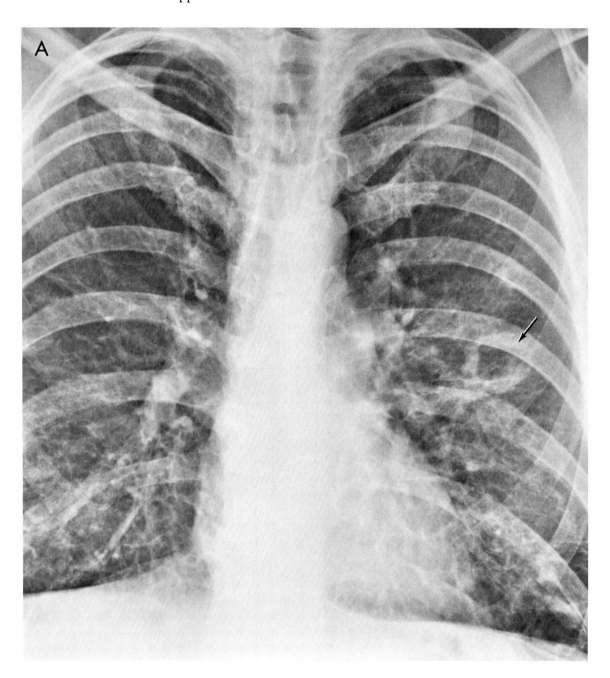

B, close-up of the lesion in **A.**

C, lateral body-section radiograph: Showing the lesion to better advantage and emphasizing its thickened walls with local parenchymal extensions (**arrows**).

A 60-year-old man was examined because of slight cough and some blood-tinged sputum. Bronchoscopy disclosed no abnormality. Left lower lobectomy and pathologic analysis revealed characteristic amyloid tumor of the lung.

Figure 153, courtesy of Dr. Walter Miller, City Health Service, Seattle, Wash.

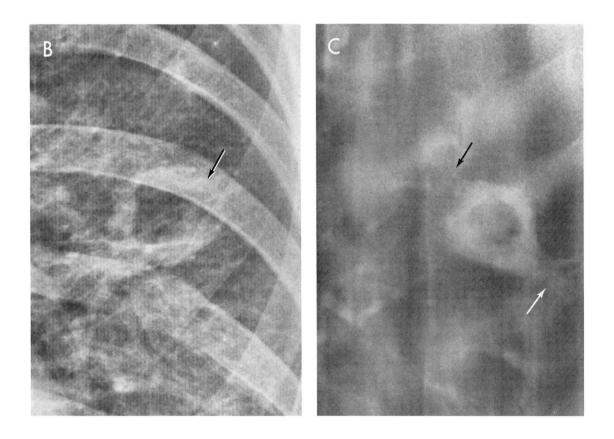

Figure 153 · Amyloid Tumor of Lung / 409

PART 6

Tumors of the Pleura and Chest Wall

Types and Characteristics

LOCALIZED PLEURAL tumors may include fibromas, neurofibromas, lipomas, fibrosarcomas and probably chondromas and chondrosarcomas.

MESOTHELIOMAS.—These are the most common tumors in this area. They may be of two types: a localized, usually large, smoothly demarcated tumor (Figs. 154 and 156), and a more diffuse, spreading tumor (Fig. 155) extending platelike over pleural surfaces, especially along diaphragmatic and basal pleura with a frequently associated bloody effusion (Fig. 157). Both may be associated with occupation, especially asbestosis exposure. The flat spreading type of tumor tends to be more locally invasive and slowly progressive with a poor prognosis. The only treatment, if discovered early, is removal. If not removed, the average survival is about one year; with pleurectomy or pleuropneumonectomy survival may be three to six years.

The more common local solitary type tends to grow slowly and may reach large size before being discovered. Microscopically, these may appear to be benign or malignant, but with removal there is usually an excellent result with no recurrence.

FIBROSARCOMAS.—The mesenchymal tumors may occur anywhere. They are designated by the pathologists according to the predominant cell type such as chondrofibrosarcoma, myxofibrosarcoma and so on. They are usually very slow growing, late to metastasize, may occur at any age and have no characteristic roentgen pattern when they occur in the chest (Figs. 158 and 159). Origin may be from the various structures in the chest wall, mediastinum and possibly interstitial lung tissue.

ANGIOSARCOMAS.—These are uncommon malignant, vascular tumors which usually occur in children or young adults, often developing in muscle. Their vascular nature may be obvious clinically if they lie near the skin surface, but when deep they may not be suspected prior to surgery. Occasionally, vascular hums can be detected on auscultation. If the vascular nature is suspected, angiography is of help in determining the extent and possibility of successful removal. Occasionally large vascular channels may be seen in plain roentgenograms of the chest. However, these lesions, when they occur primarily in the chest, arise from the chest wall (Fig. 162).

A similar tumor, the hemangiopericytoma (Fig. 163), was described by Stout.[9] These too may be benign or malignant and have no characteristic roentgen pattern. Differentiation between these and other vascular tumors is for the pathologist. The clinical course is about the same and early removal seems the only successful method of treatment, although some response of the local tumor may be obtained by radiation therapy.

Benign vascular tumors may contain phleboliths demonstrated by roentgen methods. This may be the only diagnostic clue in such lesions.

METASTASES TO PLEURAL SURFACES.—A variety of tumors spread to pleural surfaces by direct extension or lymphatics. Most of the time the first indication of extension is development of a pleural effusion. Unless one takes special pains, the metastatic deposits will be obscured by the fluid. If one wants to demonstrate nodules, artificially induced pneumothorax followed by decubitus, erect, Trendelenburg and sometimes horizontal lateral exposures may be necessary to demonstrate them. For the most part, no specific characteristics suggest the primary site if it is unknown. Rarely, tiny round bubblelike deposits can be demonstrated on the diaphragmatic pleura and adjacent lower thoracic pleura as typical extension from ovarian carcinoma. This is one of the few diagnostic indications of a primary tumor.

Neurogenic tumors (Fig. 160), lipomas (Fig. 161), hibernomas (Fig. 144), liposarcomas (Fig. 141), benign angiomas, leiomyoma and leiomyosarcoma may all involve the chest wall. Their characteristics are described in Part 4, Mediastinal Tumors. Bone tumors and primary breast tumors are not included in this volume.

BIBLIOGRAPHY

1. Abrams, H. L.: *Angiography* (Boston: Little, Brown & Company, 1971).
2. Berne, A. S., and Heitzman, E. R.: The roentgenologic signs of pedunculated pleural tumors, Am. J. Roentgenol. 87:892, 1962.
3. Finby, N., and Steinberg, I.: Roentgen aspects of pleural mesothelioma, Radiology 65:169, 1955.
4. Fraser, R. G., and Pare, J. A. P.: *Diagnosis of Diseases of the Chest* (Philadelphia: W. B. Saunders Company).
5. Herlitzka, A. J., and Gale, J. W.: Tumors and cysts of the mediastinum, Arch Surg. 76:697, 1958.
6. Lillington, G. A., and Jamplis, R. W.: *A Diagnostic Approach to Chest Diseases* (Baltimore: Williams & Wilkins Company, 1965).
7. Simon, G.: *Principles of Chest X-ray Diagnosis* (New York: Appleton-Century-Crofts, Inc., 1971).
8. Shanks, S. C., and Kerley, P. (ed.): *A Text-book of X-ray Diagnosis* (3rd ed.; Philadelphia: W. B. Saunders Company, 1962), Vol. II.
9. Stout, A. P.: Tumors of the Soft Tissues, In *Atlas of Tumor Pathology*, Sect. VII, fasc. 5 (Washington, D. C.: Armed Forces Institute of Pathology).

Figure 154.—Fibrous mesothelioma.

A, posteroanterior radiograph: Revealing a precisely marginated ovoid mass in the right upper lung field in the region of the oblique fissure. There are no additional clues to its nature.

B, lateral projection: Showing the ovoid mass intimately related to the oblique fissure between the right upper and lower lobes. The heart and lungs are within normal limits.

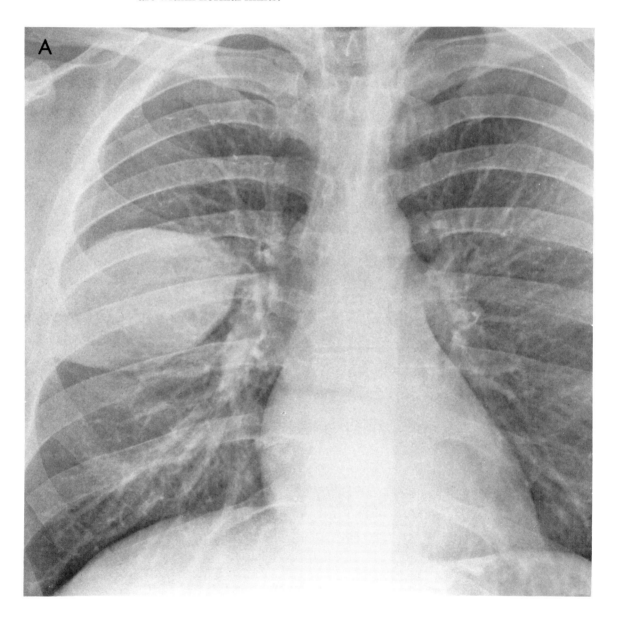

A 37-year-old executive had an annual physical examination at which time the abnormality was detected in the radiograph of his chest. There was no previous history of industrial exposure nor were any significant findings in the past history or routine laboratory studies detected. Because of a questionable history of an acute respiratory infection, nothing was done for about eight weeks. In this time interval the shadow was completely unchanged.

Thoracotomy disclosed a tumor in the fissure between the upper and lower lobes which was attached by a very thin layer of connective tissue. The mass was shelled out readily and on microscopic examination proved to be a mesothelioma.

Figure 154, courtesy of Dr. Peter Arger, University of Pennsylvania Hospital, Philadelphia.

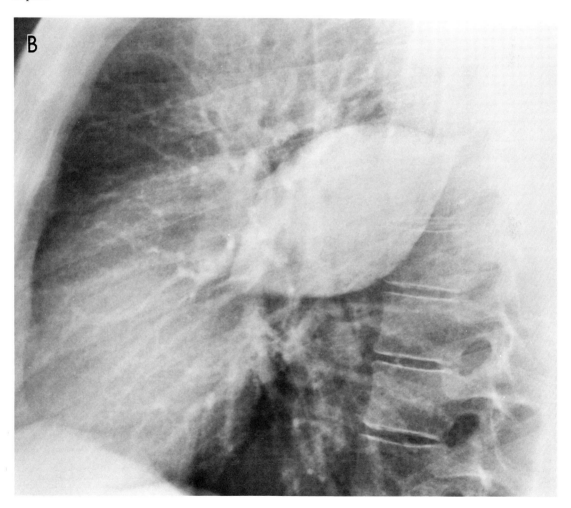

Figure 154 · Mesothelioma / 415

Figure 155.—Mesothelioma.

A, posteroanterior radiograph: Revealing a shaggy mass (**x**) projecting from the mediastinum into the right lung. Prominent pulmonary markings are present throughout both lungs but are somewhat more exaggerated in the bases, especially on the right side.

B, lateral projection: Showing the mass (**arrows**) overlying the transverse arch of the aorta (**y**). Again, the diffuse shaggy markings adjoining the edge of the lesion are apparent.

C, close-up of the lesion in **A:** In which the ascending aorta is barely perceptible through the mass. On close examination much of the ragged lateral edge (**arrow**) of the mass appears to be continuous with the adjacent distorted pulmonary markings rather than being a part of the mass itself.

A 50-year-old shipyard worker had a 35 mm survey chest film in which the abnormality was discovered. He was asymptomatic, although he had worked with asbestos for some years. The tumor was removed at thoracotomy. Pathologic diagnosis was mesothelioma.

Figure 155, courtesy of Dr. Walter Miller, City Health Center, Seattle, Wash.

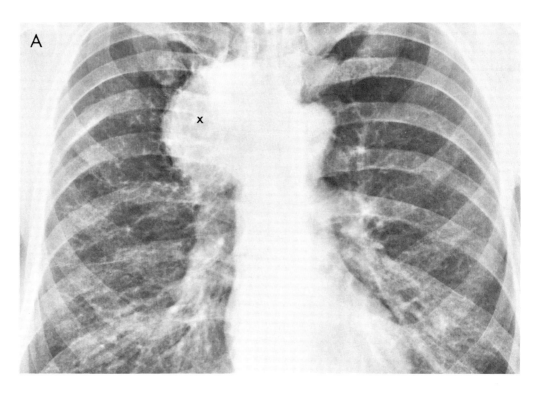

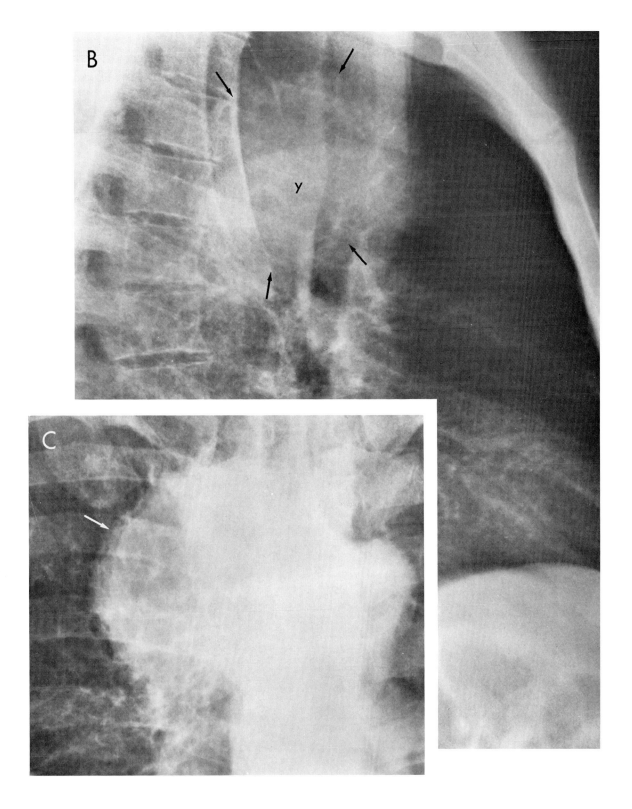

Figure 155 · Mesothelioma / 417

Figure 156.—Asbestosis and mesothelioma.

A, posteroanterior radiograph: Revealing a large lobulated mass with sharp margins situated laterally in the right midlung field. There is a short segment of dense calcification (**arrow**) in the right hemidiaphragm. Note the fibrosis in the right lower lobe (**y**).

B, oblique exposure tangential to the mass: Making it obvious that the lobulated mass originates in the pleura and extends inward.

This 55-year-old man had worked with asbestos for a number of years. He was examined because of dyspnea. Biopsy of the mass revealed mesothelioma.

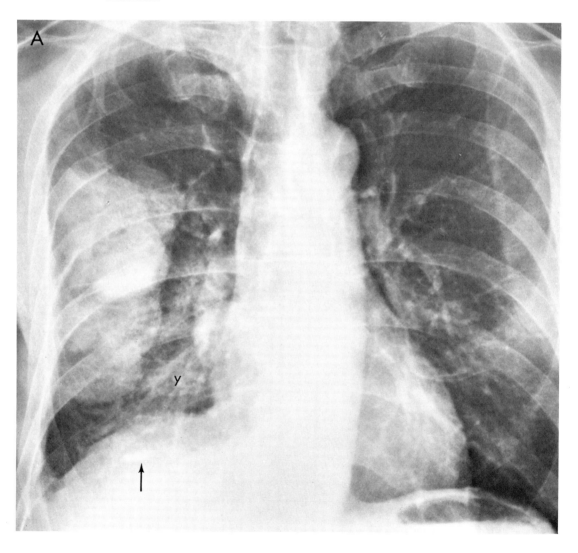

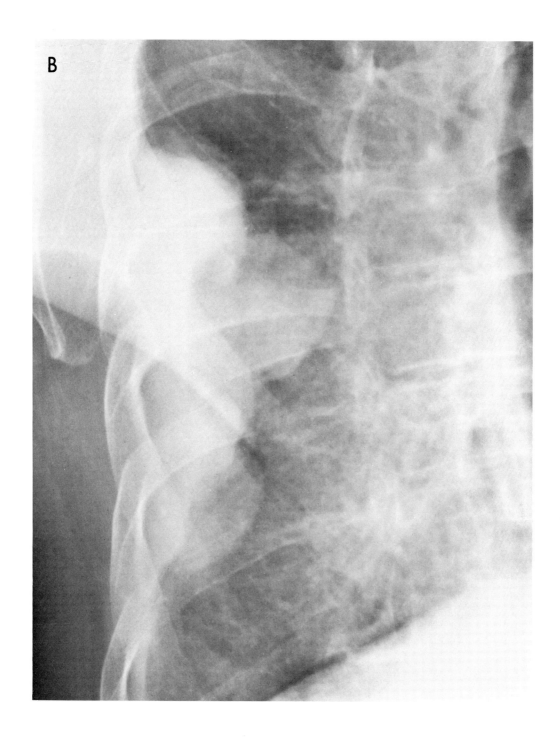

B

Figure 156 · Asbestosis & Mesothelioma / 419

Figure 157.—Asbestosis and mesothelioma with pleural effusion.

A, posteroanterior radiograph: Showing pleural effusion with marked pleural thickening in the left apex (**a**). There is diffuse interstitial fibrosis in the right lower lung field, and a short segment of calcification is visible in the right diaphragm (**b**).

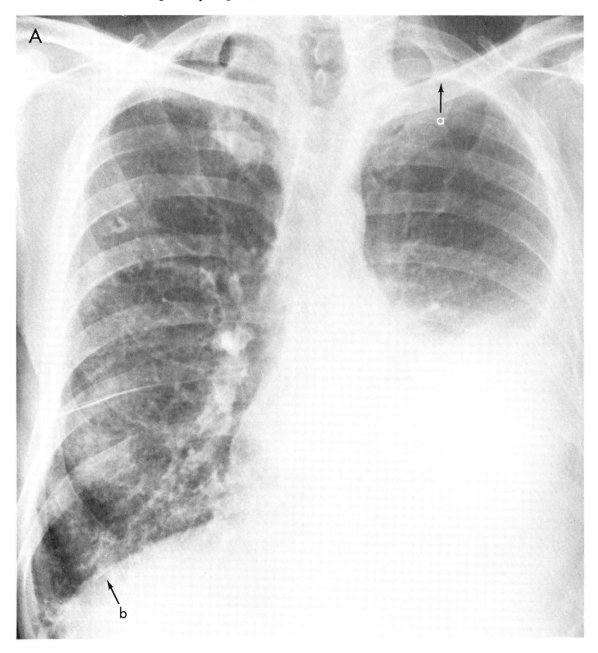

B, close-up of the right lower lobe in **A:** Note the calcification in the right diaphragm (**b**).

C, following thoracentesis and instillation of a small amount of air in the left hemithorax: Demonstrating pleural nodules (**arrows**) and considerable pleural thickening.

This 60-year-old man had worked in an asbestos plant for many years. He consulted his physician because of mild dyspnea and pain in the left shoulder. Pleural biopsy revealed a mesothelioma.

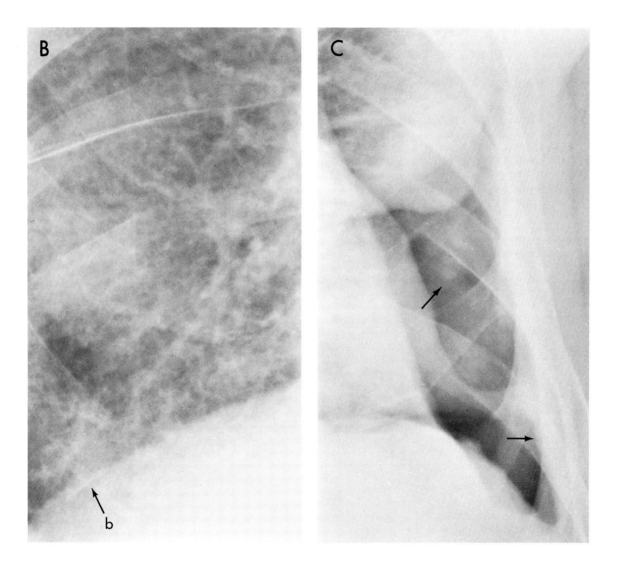

Figure 157 · Asbestosis & Mesothelioma / 421

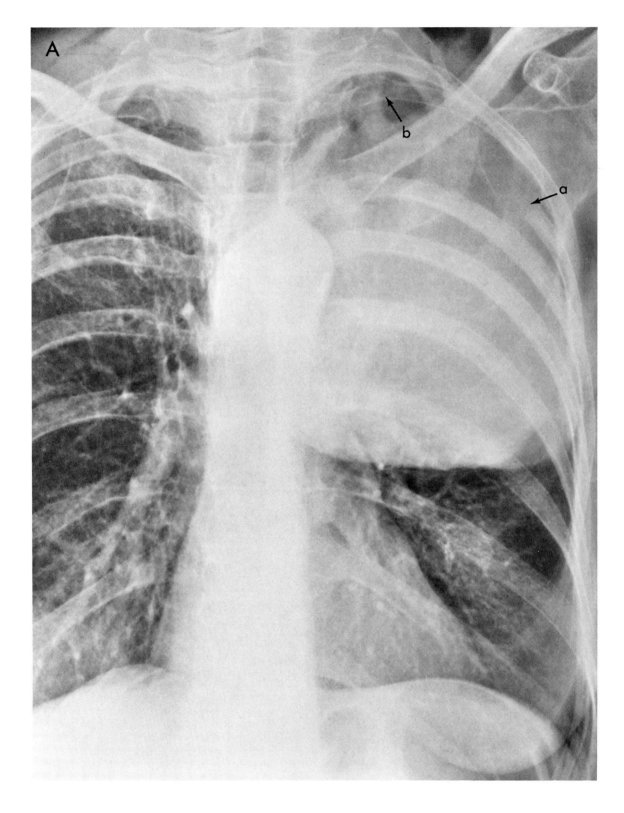

Figure 158.—Fibrosarcoma of the chest wall.

A, posteroanterior radiograph: Revealing a huge mass projecting intra-thoracically, with extensive destruction of the left fourth rib (**a**) and less evident destruction of the third rib posteriorly (**b**). The density of the mass is greater than that of the cardiac shadow; it contains no calcification.

B, lateral projection: Delineating the sharp margins and great size of the tumor. A significant concave border between the mass and the posterior chest wall (**arrow**) provides a clue to the extrapulmonary nature of the lesion.

A 70-year-old woman complained of weight loss and some discomfort in the posterior part of the left hemithorax. Biopsy revealed a fibrosarcoma of the chest wall. Radiation therapy led to some reduction of size of the tumor.

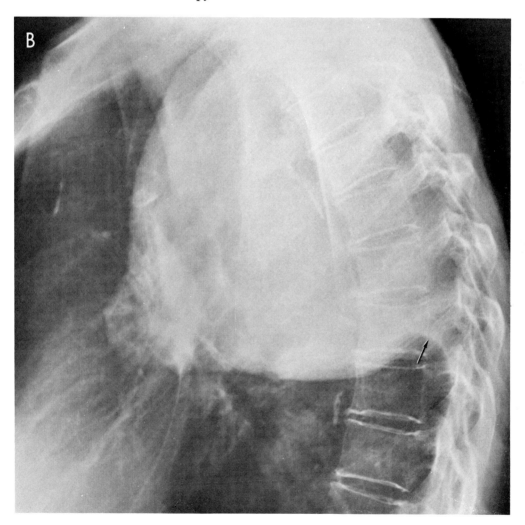

Figure 158 · Fibrosarcoma of Chest Wall / 423

Figure 159.—Fibrosarcoma of the chest wall.

A, posteroanterior radiograph: Revealing a smooth-edged ovoid mass with concave edges (**arrows**), indicating the extrapulmonary nature of the tumor. There is no esophageal or tracheal displacement. The rib cage and spine appear to be intact. There was no motion during swallowing.

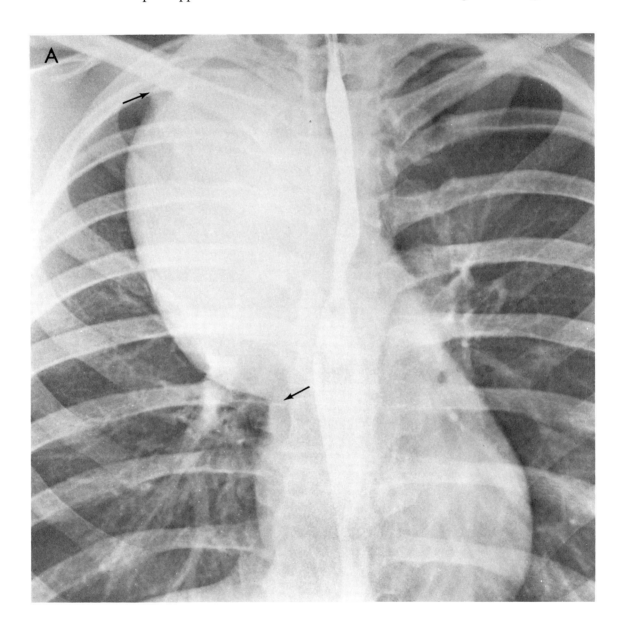

B, postoperative posteroanterior radiograph 30 months after **A:** Disclosing recurrence of the mass (**x**) at the initial site of resection plus several metastatic nodules in the right lung (**arrows**).

A 19-year-old asymptomatic youth had a routine chest x-ray study on entrance to college, when the large mass was detected. Removal and pathologic study indicated that it was a fibrosarcoma apparently arising from the chest wall. Thirty months later there was recurrence with metastases. All of the lesions continued to enlarge despite chemotherapy, and the patient died three years after the initial resection. Review of the material by a number of pathologists resulted in a consensus diagnosis of fibrosarcoma.

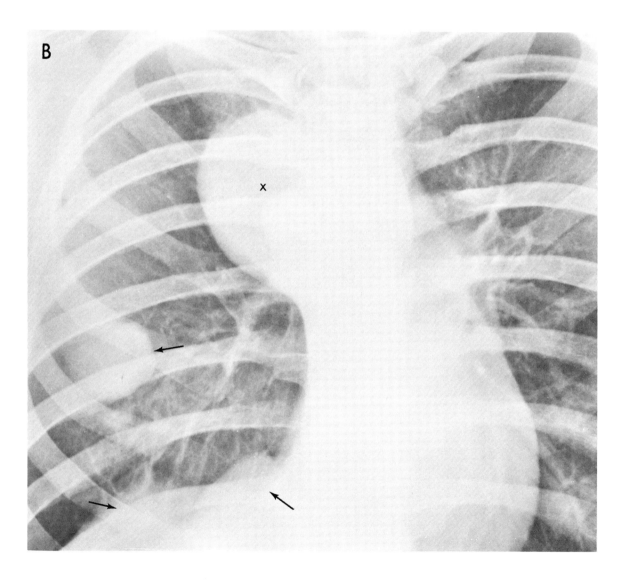

Figure 159 · Fibrosarcoma of Chest Wall / 425

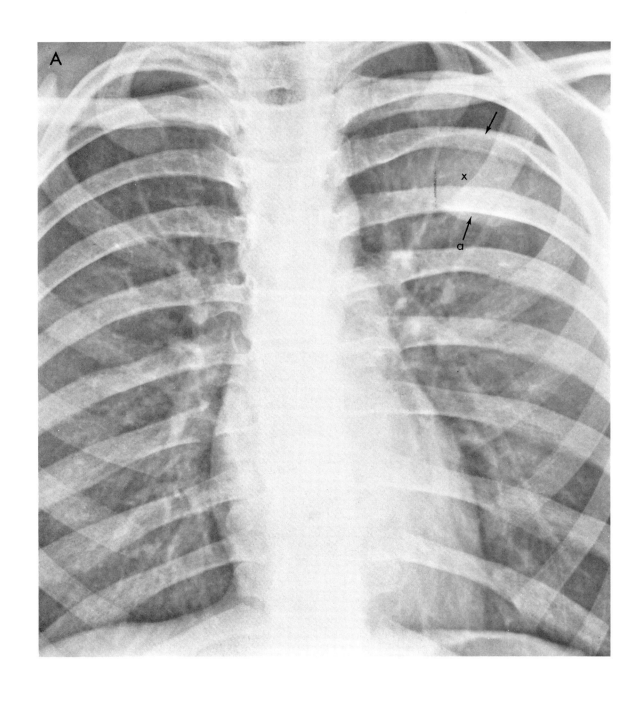

Figure 160.—Neurofibroma of an intercostal nerve.

A, posteroanterior radiograph: Revealing a soft tissue mass (**x**) adjacent to a smooth elliptical erosion of the undersurface of the posterior portion of the left fourth rib (**arrow**). The lateral margins are vague but the inferior margin is sharp (**a**).

B, close-up of the lesion in **A.**

C, oblique projection: Demonstrating the edges of the lesion (**x**). Note the convex lower margin (**arrow**), suggesting the extrapleural origin of the lesion.

A 13-year-old child had central nervous symptoms which proved to be due to a cerebellar astrocytoma. Prior to craniotomy the chest lesion was found; it was thought to be of neurogenic origin. The child had no chest complaints. On removal of the chest lesion, pathologic diagnosis was neurofibroma.

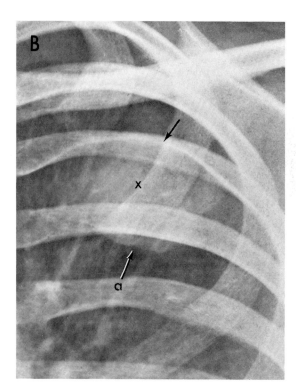
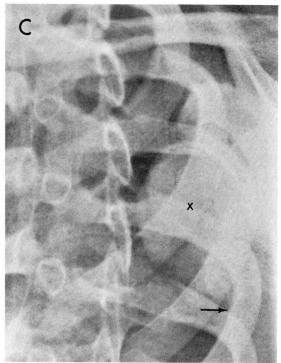

Figure 160 · Neurofibroma / 427

Figure 161.—Lipoma of the lateral chest wall.

A, posteroanterior radiograph: Showing a sharply marginated soft tissue mass somewhat less dense than the aortic and cardiac shadows adjacent to the left lateral chest wall. Note the concave blending of the margins of the shadow with the chest wall (**arrows**); this indicates the extrapulmonary nature of the lesion. The density of the shadow is somewhat less than one would expect with a fluid-filled cystic area or the usual neoplastic lesion of this size. No adjacent rib erosion is visible.

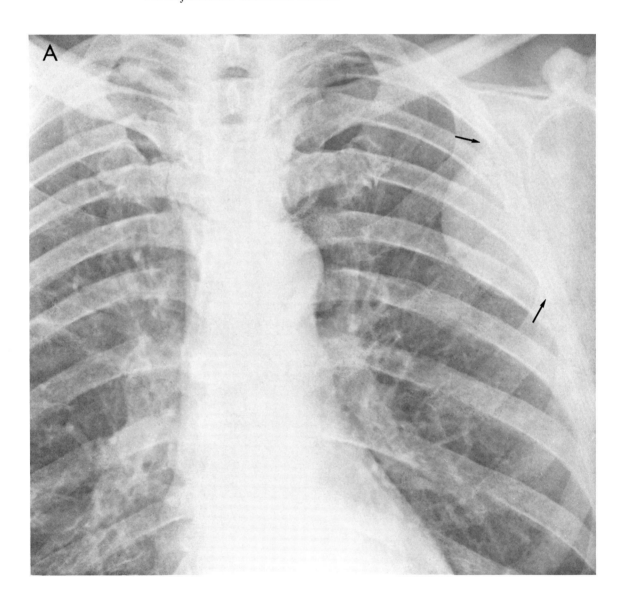

B, lateral projection: Delineating the very sharp outlines of the mass (**x**). The density is less than one would expect in a solid mass of this size and shape.

A 45-year-old man entered the hospital for a hernia repair. Surgery disclosed an extrapleural mass projecting from the chest wall. Pathologic diagnosis was lipoma.

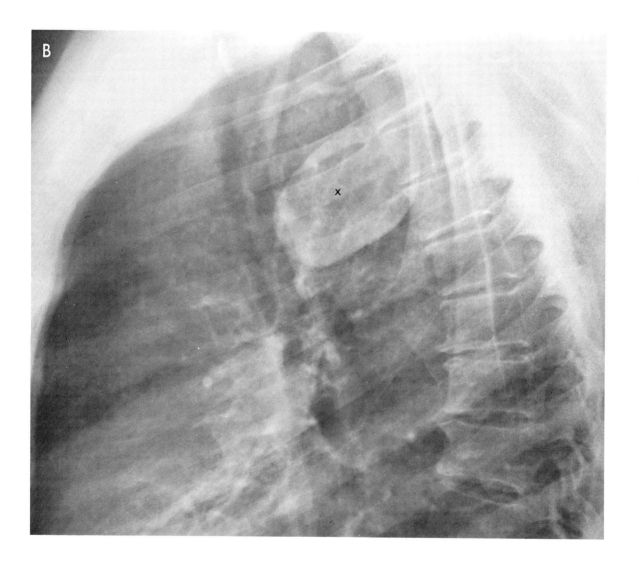

Figure 161 · Lipoma of Chest Wall / 429

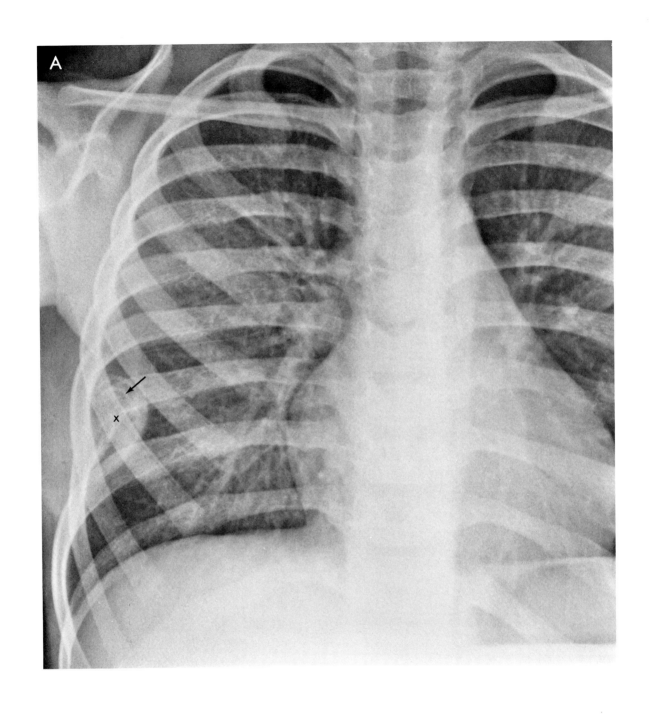

Figure 162.—Hemangiosarcoma of the chest wall.

A, posteroanterior radiograph: Revealing a sharply marginated mass (**x**) adjacent to the right eighth rib in the midaxillary line. Rib destruction (**arrow**) is evident, with only a shell remaining in the area of the soft tissue mass. The involved portion of the rib seems slightly expanded.

B, soft tissue tangential radiograph of the chest wall: Demonstrating the mass (**x**) extending into the lateral soft tissues with a line of fat overlying it (**arrow**). The deeper portion is invading the rib (**a**), which is destroyed. The lesion does not appear to involve the underlying lung.

A 4-year-old boy had a lump along the right lateral chest wall that had been discovered by his mother when giving him a bath. There was a very questionable history of injury. The mass was not tender, quite firm but not bone hard, and seemed movable over the rib rather than fixed to it. The mass and adjacent rib were removed. Pathologic diagnosis was hemangiosarcoma.

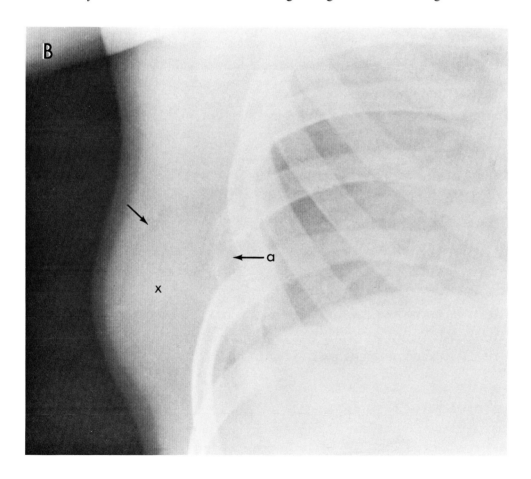

Figure 162 · Hemangiosarcoma of Chest Wall / 431

Figure 163.—Hemangiopericytoma.

A, posteroanterior radiograph: Showing a smooth-edged mass (**x**) extending above and below the thoracic inlet on the left with tracheal deviation to the right and a slight impression on the air column.

B, body-section exposure through the mass: Demonstrating calcifications in the inferior portions of the lesion (**arrow**). Bone erosion (**a**) in the lower cervical spine is obvious. Also clearly illustrated is the tracheal displacement and decreased size of the air column (**y**).

C, body-section radiograph through the cervical spine: Emphasizing the bone erosion, which is sharp and fragmented (**arrows**).

D, myelogram: Showing compression and displacement of the cervical spinal cord (**b**).

(*Continued.*)

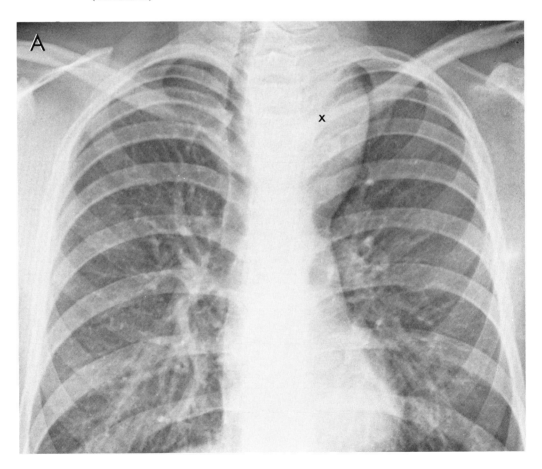

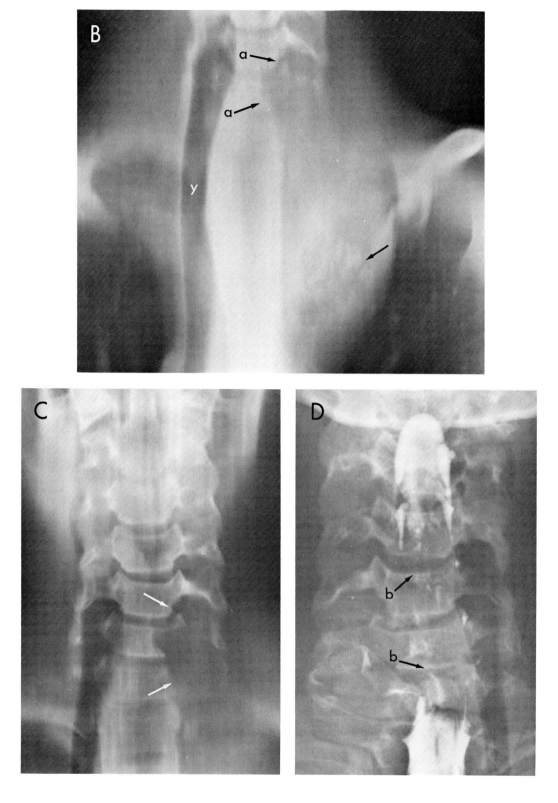

Figure 163 · Hemangiopericytoma / 433

Figure 163 (cont.).—Hemangiopericytoma.

E, left subclavian arteriogram: Revealing an extensive vascular lesion with tumor vessels.

F, later phase of the arteriogram: Revealing a tumor stain (**x**).

A 16-year-old boy had had pain and numbness in the left shoulder for about eight weeks. Physical examination revealed weakness and loss of reflexes of the left arm. A fixed mass was found in the left supraclavicular region. Laboratory studies were not helpful. Attempted removal of the main portion of the mass revealed an extensive vascular lesion. Pathologic diagnosis was hemangiopericytoma.

Figure 163, courtesy of Dr. R. Abell, Ann Arbor, Mich.

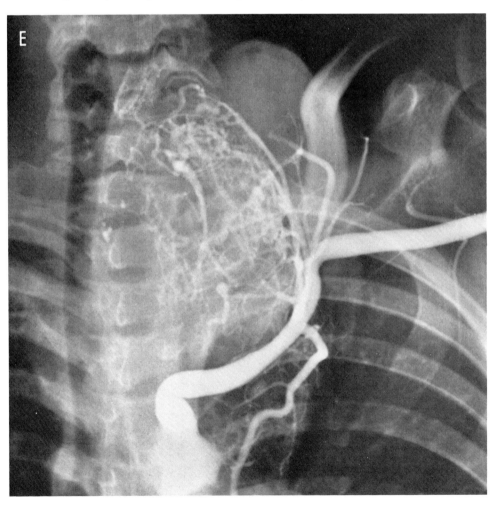

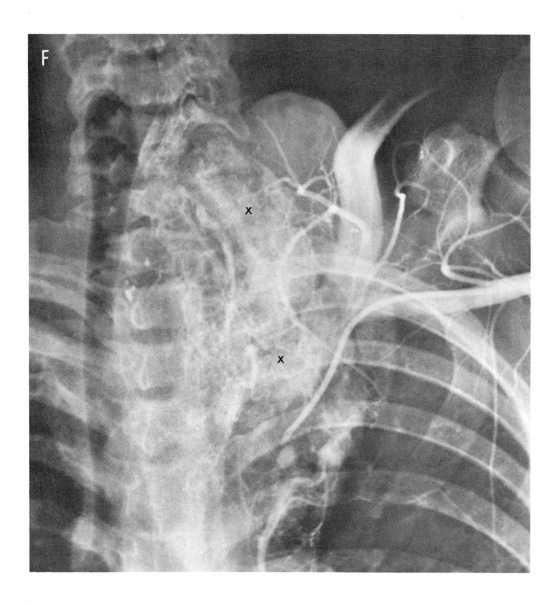

Figure 163 · Hemangiopericytoma / 435

Figure 164.—Phantom tumor.

A, posteroanterior radiograph: Revealing cardiac enlargement, pulmonary vascular fullness and blunting of each costophrenic angle. In addition, there is an obvious mass (**x**) adjacent to the right hilar area. Note the pulmonary vessels visible through the base of the mass (**y**), suggesting its posterior relationship to the pulmonary hilar vessels. The margins are sharp but somewhat undulating.

B, posteroanterior projection 48 hours after digitalization and beginning of diuresis: Showing the cardiac outline significantly smaller, the blunting of the costophrenic angles disappearing and the mass almost completely gone.

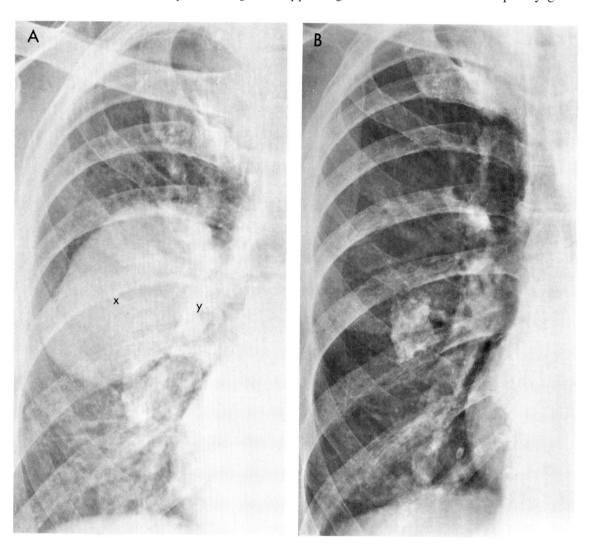

C, lateral projection: Demonstrating the ovoid outline of the mass (**x**), seen in **A,** which lies along the path of the oblique fissure and posterior to the hilar vessels. A second ragged-edged density (**arrow**) lies anteriorly which is unrelated to the large mass.

Figure 164, courtesy of Dr. Walter Miller, City Health Center, Seattle, Wash.

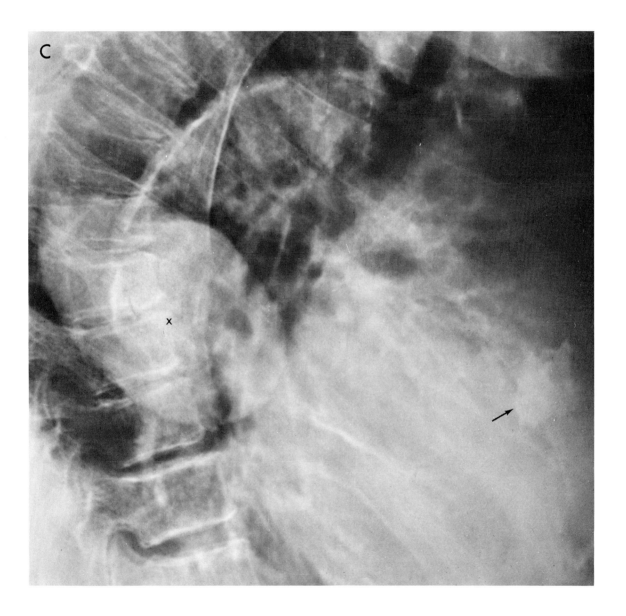

Figure 164 · Phantom Tumor / 437

Figure 165.—Extrapleural fluid collection.

A, posteroanterior radiograph: Revealing a sharply outlined mass (**x**) in the posterior mediastinum and blending with the apical pleural shadow above and the aortic arch below.

B, lateral projection: Showing the convex posterior margin of the mass (**x**) lying adjacent to lung (**arrow**) interposed posteriorly. The upper margins of the mass are lost in the surrounding adjacent soft tissues.

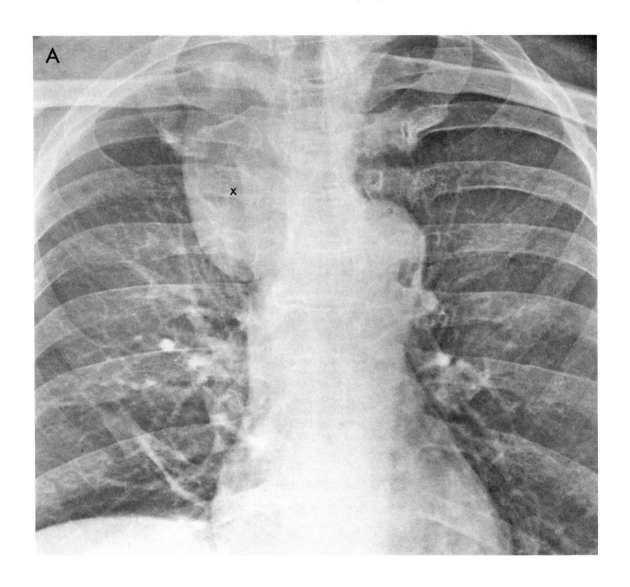

A 45-year-old man with severe essential hypertension and no pulmonary complaints was treated by thoracic sympathectomy. The mass, which was noted following sympathectomy, gradually became smaller and disappeared in several weeks after medical treatment.

Comment: Although this picture is characteristic of an extrapleural fluid collection after sympathectomy, the convex lower margin is unusual for an extraparenchymal, extrapleural lesion, which usually has a concave margin where it abuts the chest wall.

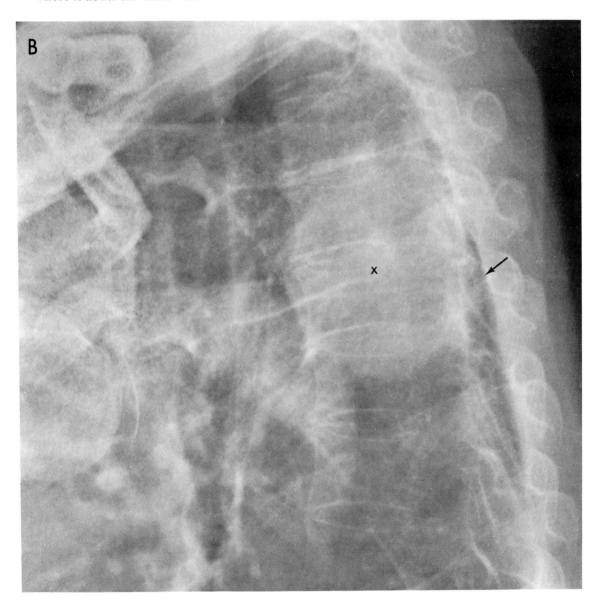

Figure 165 · Extrapleural Fluid Collection / 439

Figure 166.—Loculated fluid in the bed of a resected granuloma.

A–C, roentgen studies after resection of a granuloma.

A, posteroanterior radiograph of the right half of the chest: Showing a centrally placed, sharply marginated loculated mass (**x**) in the region of the oblique and horizontal fissures. An associated loculated area extends farther laterally (**y**). The silhouette seen through the cardiac outline indicates its posterior location (**arrow**).

B, lateral radiograph: Demonstrating the lesion (**x**) in the area of the oblique fissure extending to the junction with the horizontal fissure posteriorly (**arrow**). The mass retains its sharp margins and the lobulated appearance.

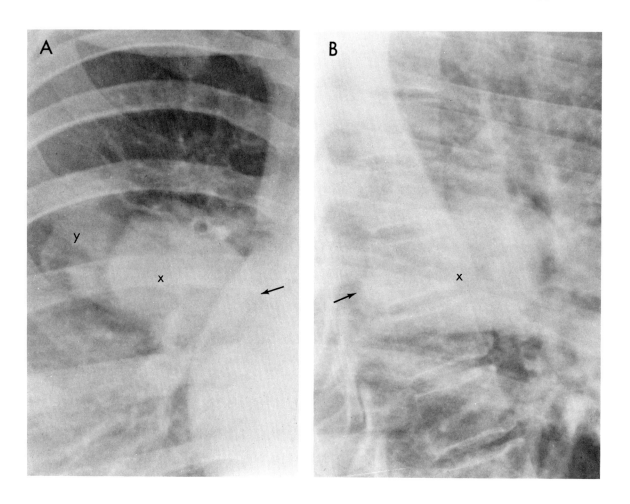

C, anteroposterior body-section radiograph through the mass: Revealing its sharply marginated borders with a clear area (**a**) between its two components (**x** and **y**) and along the medial edge (**b**).

A 35-year-old asymptomatic woman had a shadow detected in a 35 mm film survey. Further study showed it to be in the right upper lobe adjacent to the junction of the oblique and horizontal fissures. The lesion was resected, and microscopic examination revealed a granuloma. On recurrence of the mass, shown in the studies illustrated here, clear serous fluid was obtained on needle aspiration and the lesion disappeared.

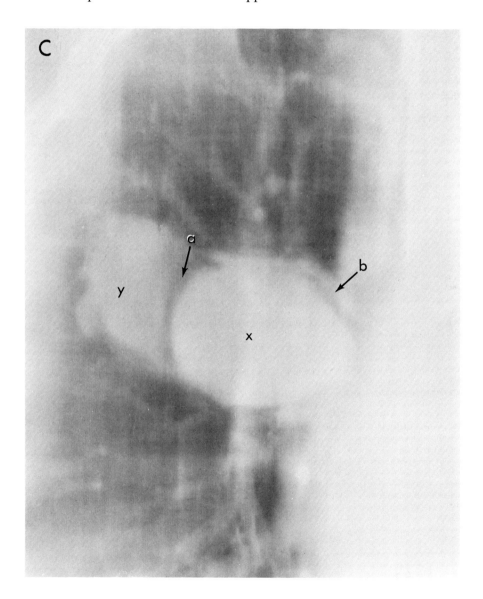

Figure 166 · Fluid in Bed of Resected Granuloma / 441

PART 7

Metastatic Tumors

Sources and Characteristics

METASTATIC TUMORS to the chest extend by any of the three basic mechanisms: direct extension, lymphatic and lymph node spread, and blood-borne deposits. Similarities are present within each group, but slight variations in expected patterns can indicate to the careful observer the probable site of origin when the primary source is unknown. For example, blood-borne metastases from a variety of tumors are characterized by multiple, diffuse, spherical, sharply marginated nodules in both lungs (Figs. 167–169). If only one or two large spherical nodules are present in one or both lungs, the primary source is usually the kidney, thyroid, gastrointestinal tract or some unusual site such as the sweat glands (Fig. 187).

The rate of growth of such spread is usually quite rapid, but with tumors marked by a few large deposits or from unusual sites, as the sweat gland and the salivary gland carcinomas (Figs. 187 and 189), growth may be very slow over a period of many years.

Blood-borne metastatic lesions may remain dormant in the lung for long periods of time and appear years after removal of a primary malignant neoplasm from any one of many sources. Occasionally metastatic foci simulate primary tumors of the lung (Fig. 178). When they do, removal may result in long-term survival, presumably influenced by the excision.

Lymphangitic extension is typical of primary neoplasms in the gastrointestinal tract, especially the stomach (Figs. 181 and 182), but also may occur from gallbladder and colon malignancies. Many other primary neoplasms may extend to the chest in a similar fashion. Likely types are tumors of the breast and thyroid and the various lymphomas. In each, the roentgen appearance is that of a linear increase in perivascular soft tissues with a fanlike extension from the hilar areas (Fig. 177). The summation of multiple thickened lymphatic channels, each channel itself below the visual threshold, initially creates the visual impression of linear shadows in the deeper anterior-posterior portions of the lung. As the tumors grow, lymphatic channels enlarge enough to be seen individually. Small nodules created at the junction of the neoplasm-filled lymphatics create nodular shadows, again most prominent in central pulmonary areas (Figs. 173 and 175).

Nodal enlargements in the mediastinum and hilar areas are nonspecific and resemble such enlargements from any cause.

A variety of metastatic lesions may cavitate, but the classic ones are of squamous cell origin (Figs. 183 and 184). A mass of almost any size may excavate in the center. Typically the wall is thick and shaggy, as found in the primary cavitating neoplasms; however, on occasion thin-walled lesions are seen. The margins may be sharply spherical or develop pseudopods, as in some breast lesions extending to the lung. Cavitation has been reported in Hodgkin's disease, lymphosarcoma, metastatic lesions from the kidney and gastrointestinal tract, squamous cell lesions of any origin, osteogenic sarcomas and other mesodermal tumors.

Metastatic tumors from the breast present an unusual variety of patterns, only a few of which are illustrated here. For the most part, when these tumors spread, one at first finds either bone or soft tissue lesions (Fig. 170). Later in the course, spread may be to any tissue, including bone, mediastinal tissues and lung. As a result, in some patients with extension one finds predominant bone lesions which may involve the thoracic spine and rib cage alone or together, without pulmonary or mediastinal lesions. Such deposits may be osteolytic, osteoblastic, or both. The earliest manifestation may be a solitary lesion, but often the first indication is a ground-glass change in density from the normal bony rib cage. This means that *one must always compare the newest radiograph with the oldest ones,* and not with the immediately previous ones. Pathologic rib fractures occasionally are an initial manifestation of tumor spread. Pulmonary and mediastinal extension can be found together and initially may be discovered as solitary or multiple soft tissue masses. When in lung parenchyma, masses may be spherical with sharp margins, as is true of the usual blood-borne metastatic lesion. If there is more than one mass, the sizes may vary, suggesting differing ages of spread. Frequently, however, the margins are ragged and ill defined, but still seemingly are blood-borne.

Spread by way of lymphatics may involve the mediastinum as masses within lymph nodes in mediastinal and hilar areas on one or both sides or initially on the side opposite that of the primary tumor. Invasion of the pericardium is seen with or without resultant effusion and occasional myocardial extension. The classic lymphangitic spread of neoplasm may be found fanning out from the hilar areas. Multiple pleural nodulation of any size may be seen frequently with pleural effusion. Artificially induced pneumothorax utilizing decubitus studies may help in demonstrating such suspected nodules.

Occasionally direct extension from supraclavicular nodal metastases is seen extending into the lung apices or directly invading a first rib or nearby vertebral body.

Ancient pulmonary, pleural or chest wall disease can result in additional variations in patterns and can influence the location of spread as well as the character of extension.

No further discussion of various other metastatic nodules seems necessary, as almost any primary neoplasm may spread to the chest in the ways already discussed.

BIBLIOGRAPHY

1. Rubin, P.: *Solitary Metastases* (Springfield, Ill.: Charles C Thomas, Publisher, 1968).
2. Shanks, S. C., and Kerley, P. (ed.): *A Text-book of X-ray Diagnosis* (3rd ed.; Philadelphia: W. B. Saunders Company, 1962, Vol. II).

Figure 167.—Metastatic seminoma.

Posteroanterior exposure: Revealing sharply demarcated spherical nodular lesions diffusely distributed in both lungs characteristic of a blood-borne metastatic process. Variations in the size of nodules indicate showers of metastatic foci of different ages.

A 26-year-old man had a testicular inner mass removed from an undescended testicle six months prior to the present radiographic study. At this time some cough and dyspnea were present. Autopsy revealed diffuse metastatic lesions of varied size in both lungs. Microscopically these were similar to the primary testicular seminoma.

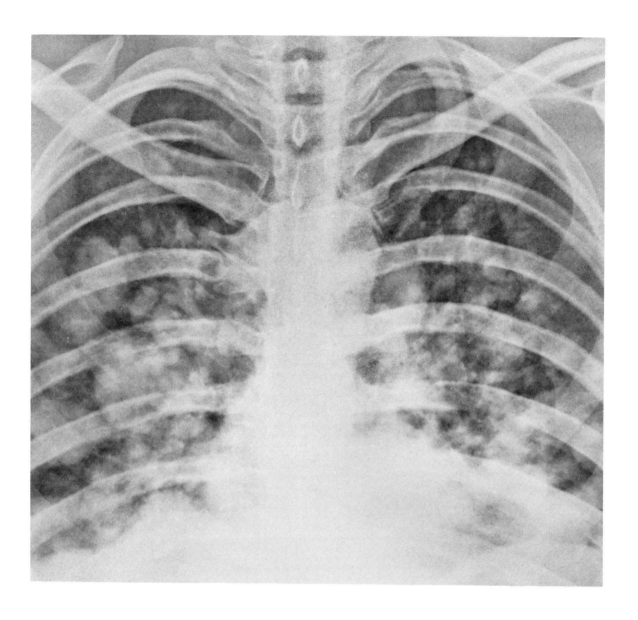

Figure 167 · Metastatic Seminoma / 449

Figure 168.—Metastatic seminoma.

Posteroanterior radiograph: Showing sharply outlined large spherical lesions (**x**) in the lower portion of the left lung and at least one large lesion in the right lung (**arrow**). No small lesions are visible, suggesting that the visible lesions may be of about the same age.

A 22-year-old man was first seen because of a somewhat painful and enlarged testicle. Radiographs of his chest at that time were thought to be normal. Removal of the testes and pathologic study revealed a rather characteristic seminoma. The illustrated study was made six months following orchidectomy and retroperitoneal node resection. Postoperative radiation therapy was not given. The metastatic lesions continued to develop in spite of chemotherapy and the patient died some three months following this radiographic study.

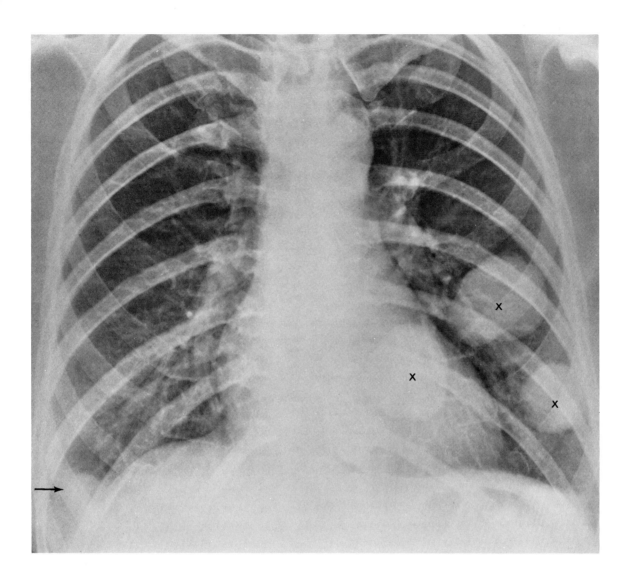

Figure 168 · Metastatic Seminoma / 451

Figure 169.—Metastatic choriocarcinoma testis.

Posteroanterior radiograph: Demonstrating smooth, sharp-edged spherical masses of different size diffusely distributed in each lung. The differences in size suggest showers of metastatic cells at various intervals.

A 24-year-old man had an enlarged testicle removed one year prior to this study. At this time he had some weight loss and an annoying cough. Pathologic analysis of the removed testicle disclosed choriocarcinoma. In spite of chemotherapy the course was rapidly downhill. Postmortem study of the pulmonary tissues revealed choriocarcinoma microscopically similar to the original neoplasm.

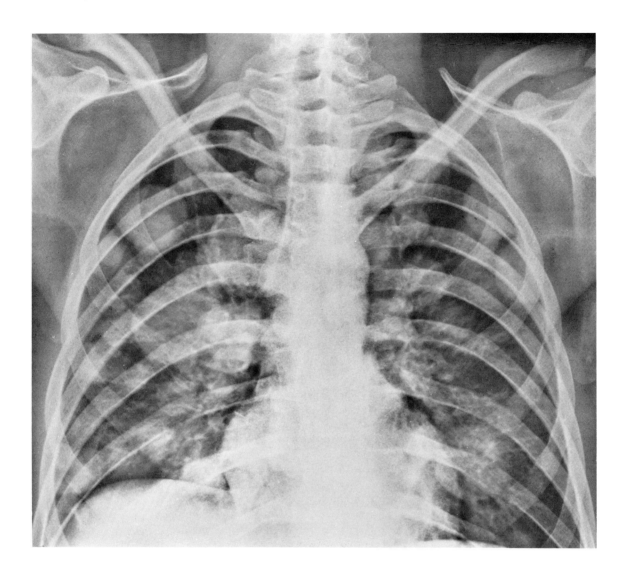

Figure 169 · Metastatic Carcinoma Testis / 453

Figure 170.—Breast carcinoma metastatic to the sternum.

A, posteroanterior radiograph: Revealing a superior mediastinal ill-defined density extending into the right parasternal region (**a**). Note that the right breast shadow is not present.

B, lateral projection: Demonstrating considerable bone destruction of the sternum. A large soft tissue mass is obvious within the chest behind the sternum (**x**), and there is evidence also of a tumor extending into the soft tissues in front of the sternum (**y**). Extremely significant is the manner in which the soft tissues are being stripped or pulled from the surface of the sternum, attesting to the extramediastinal origin of the mass (**arrows**).

A 52-year-old woman had undergone a right radical mastectomy. The present radiographic study was made because of anterior chest pain.

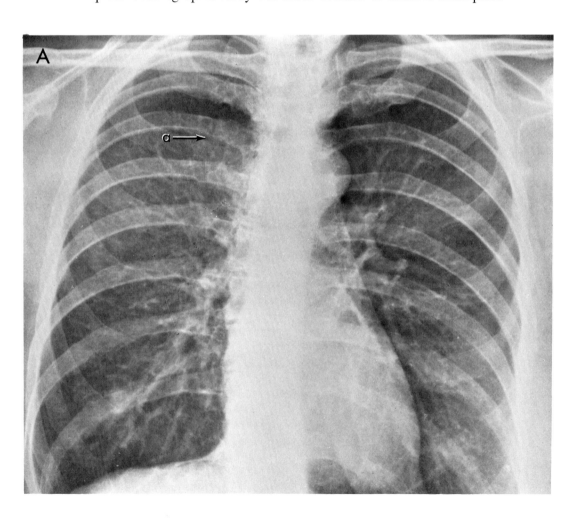

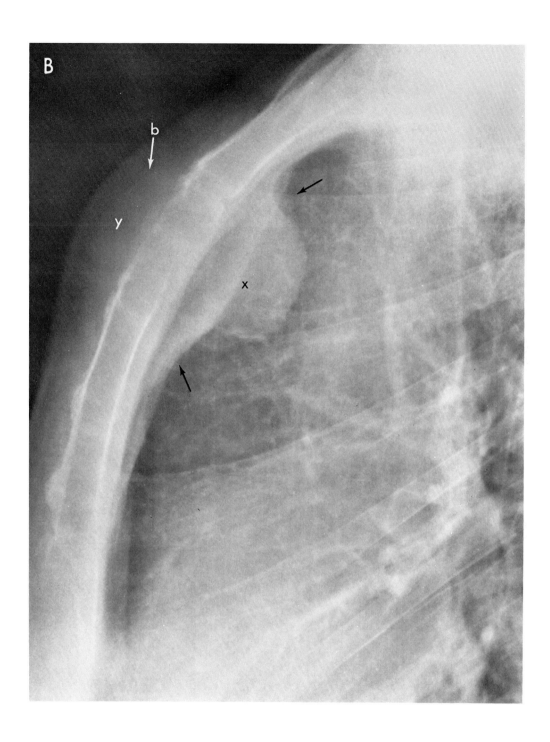

Figure 170 · Breast Carcinoma to Sternum / 455

Figure 171.—Metastatic carcinoma from the breast.

Posteroanterior radiograph: Showing absence of the left breast shadow. A sharp-bordered nodule is clearly seen in the left upper lobe (**x**) and a tiny nodule in the left lower lobe (**arrow**). No other abnormalities are evident. Note the normal vascular outlines in each hilar area that are identified with ease, in contrast to Figure 173.

A 60-year-old woman had had a left radical mastectomy for adenocarcinoma three years previously. The present study was part of a routine follow-up examination; the patient was asymptomatic. Some regression followed chemotherapy.

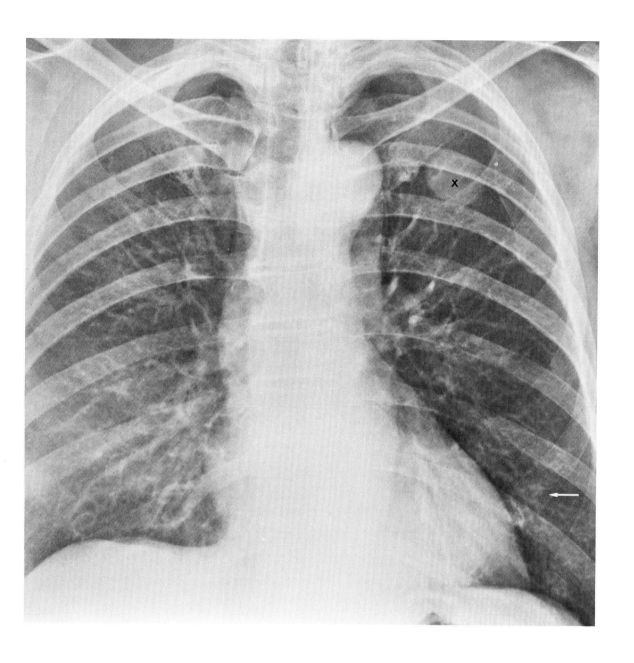

Figure 171 · Breast Carcinoma to Lung / 457

Figure 172.—Metastatic carcinoma from the breast.

A, posteroanterior radiograph: Showing absence of the left breast shadow. Two very sharply marginated nodules are visible in the right lung (a) and a third nodule, of irregular shape, in the left lung. No other lesions can be identified.

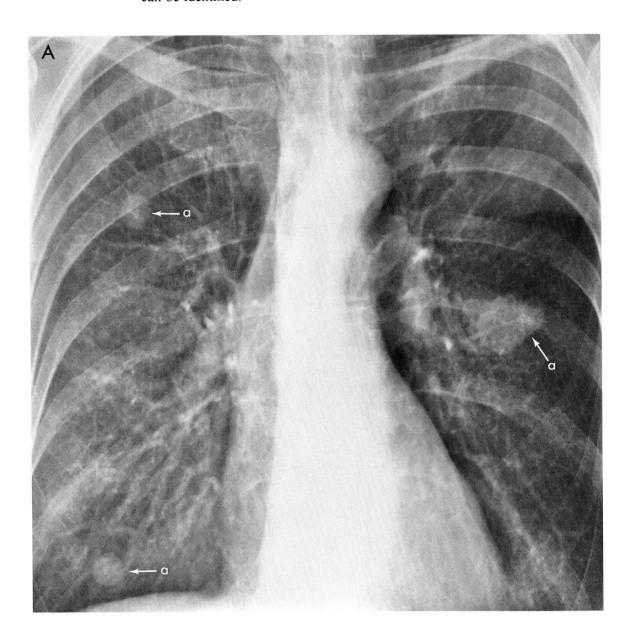

B, posteroanterior radiograph made 8 months after **A** (following therapy): Demonstrating marked regression of the nodules, which have almost completely disappeared in the right lung (**a**) and much reduced in the left (**b**).

A 57-year-old woman had had a left radical mastectomy for adenocarcinoma of the breast some 18 months prior to **A.** On discovery of the pulmonary nodules she received chemotherapy which led to the marked regression of the nodules. These eventually returned, but the initial response was most dramatic.

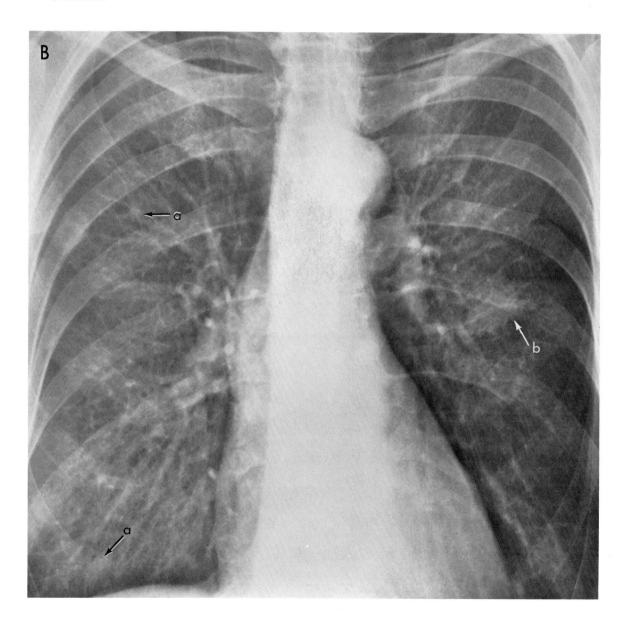

Figure 172 · Breast Carcinoma to Lung / 459

Figure 173.—Metastatic carcinoma from the breast.

Posteroanterior radiograph: Revealing absence of the right breast shadow. Diffusely distributed throughout both lungs are innumerable small irregularly marginated nodules, seemingly more numerous in the central positions of both lungs (**x**), especially on the right. This may be due to an additive subliminal visual effect analogous to that seen with pneumoconiotic nodules superimposed on each other.*

There is complete loss of normal vascular definition in the right hilar region with soft tissue changes tending to blend all the vascular outlines into an ill-defined mass (**y**). The left hilar vascular structures too are ragged in outline, but without a definite mass. These changes indicate additional metastatic disease with a solid sheet of tumor invading the right hilar and paracardiac areas.

A 55-year-old woman had had a right radical mastectomy for adenocarcinoma 28 months prior to this examination. She then complained of an annoying cough, dyspnea on exertion and weight loss. Radiation therapy to the chest relieved the cough somewhat, but additional hormone therapy was not very successful in controlling the steady progression of the disease.

---

* Newell, R. R., and Garneau, R.: Threshold visibility of pulmonary shadows, Radiology 56:409, 1957.

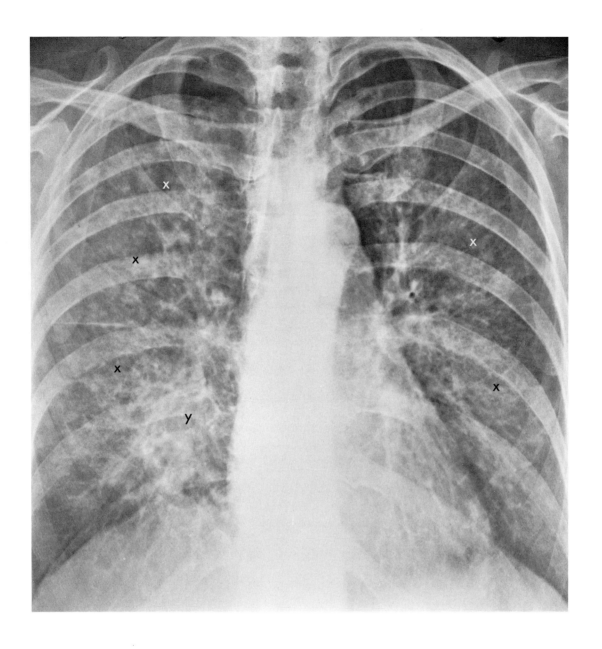

Figure 173 · Breast Carcinoma to Lung / 461

Figure 174.—Metastatic carcinoma from the breast.

A, posteroanterior radiograph: Showing absence of the right breast shadow. A spherical, sharply bordered mass overlies the superior segment of the right lower lobe (**a**). Several small nodules are visible through this mass (**arrows**). Extensive involvement is also apparent in the mediastinum bilaterally (**b**). Note the complete inability to identify normal vascular outlines adjacent to the mediastinum in both lungs.

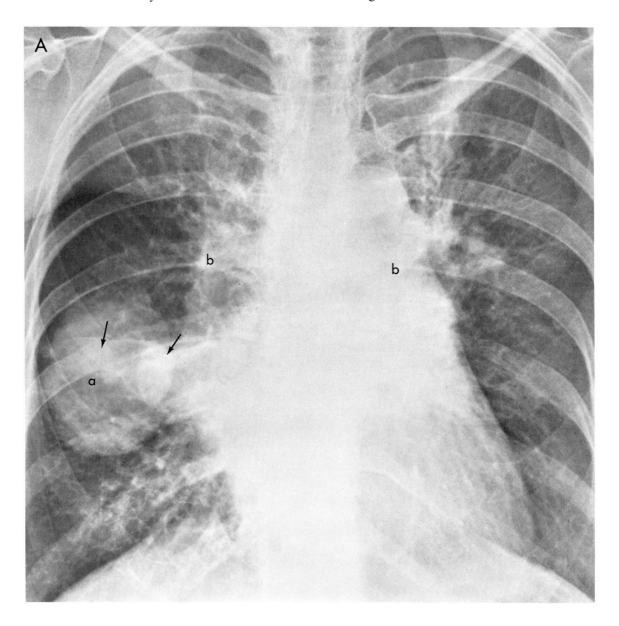

B, lateral projection: Illustrating the superior segmental location and spherical nature of the large mass (**a**). Small satellite nodules lie adjacent to the major mass (**arrows**) and there are extensive mediastinal masses (**b**). Some loss of volume of the anterior segment of the right upper lobe is apparent (**x**).

(*Continued.*)

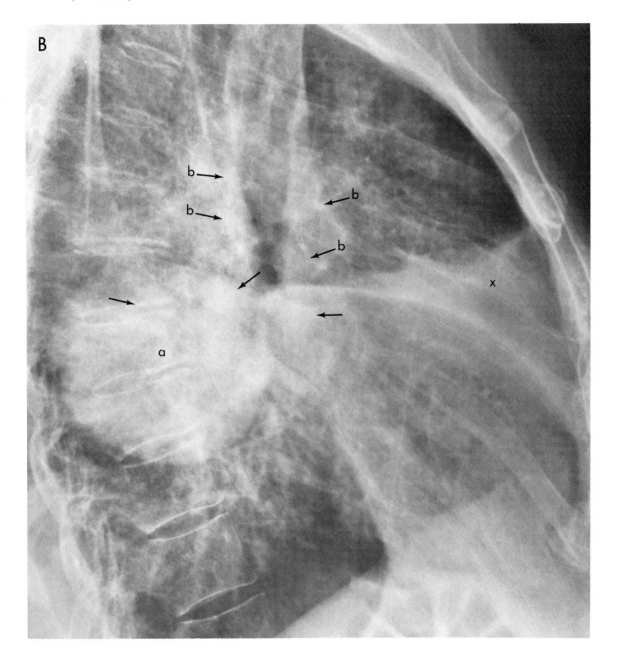

Figure 174 · Breast Carcinoma to Lung / 463

Figure 174 (cont.).—Metastatic carcinoma from the breast.

C, posteroanterior view two weeks after **A** and **B:** Now revealing marked upward shift of the masses in the right lung (**a** and **arrows**), plus a homogeneous shadow of the collapsed right upper lobe (**x**). Some overlying aerated and hyperexpanded portions of the right lung make the shadow of the collapsed right upper lobe less dense.

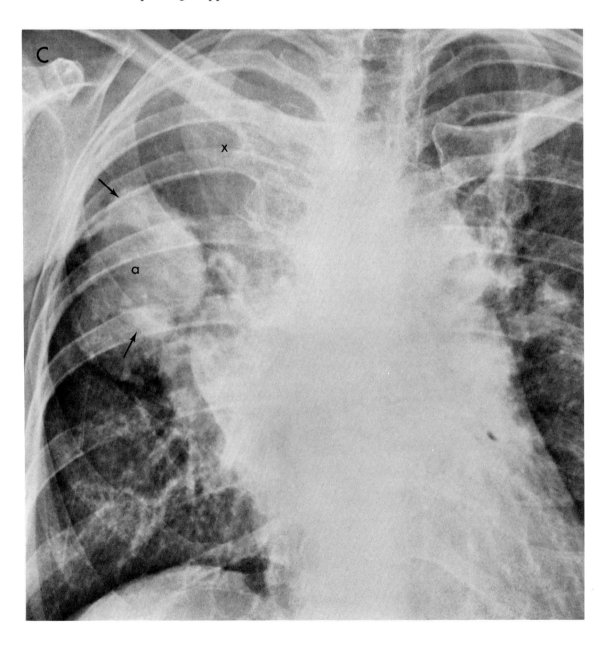

D, lateral radiograph: Showing better the collapse of the upper lobe (**arrows**), and an upward shift of the parenchymal masses, which now overlie the right upper lobe. The hyperaeration of the remaining right lung, which now occupies the space of the collapsed upper lobe, is well seen.

(*Continued.*)

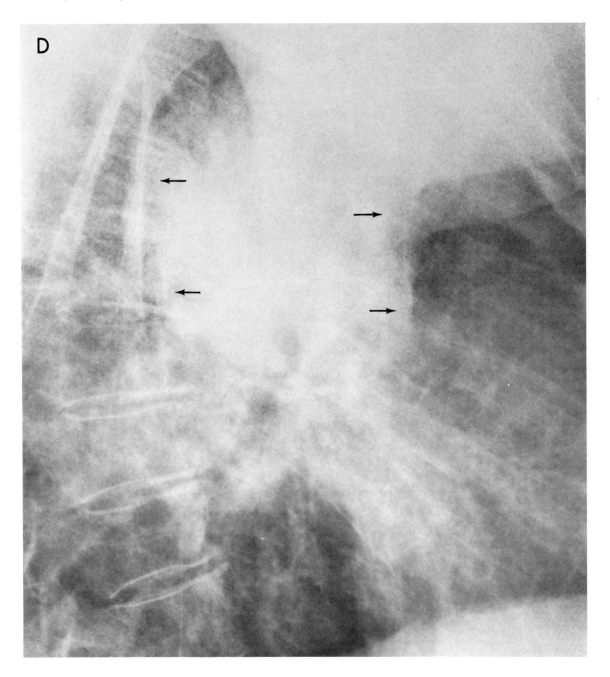

Figure 174 · Breast Carcinoma to Lung / 465

Figure 174 (cont.).—Metastatic carcinoma from the breast.

E, a posteroanterior radiograph six weeks later (after mediastinal radiation therapy): Revealing some decrease in the size of the masses (**a** and **arrows**), the mediastinal tumor, and re-expansion of the right upper lobe.

A 52-year-old woman had had a right radical mastectomy for carcinoma of the right breast three years before the initial study shown here (**A** and **B**). She had these studies because of an annoying cough and wheeze.

Figure 174, courtesy of Dr. Irwin Freundlich, Thomas Jefferson University, Philadelphia.

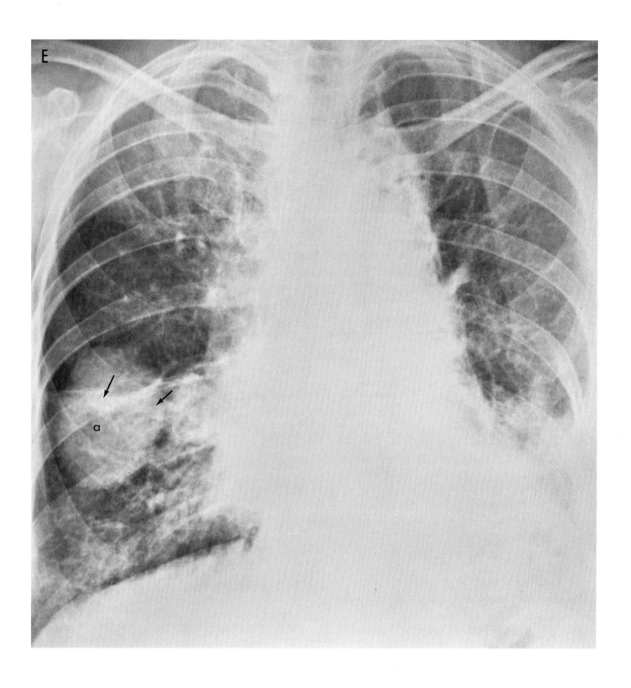

Figure 174 · Breast Carcinoma to Lung / 467

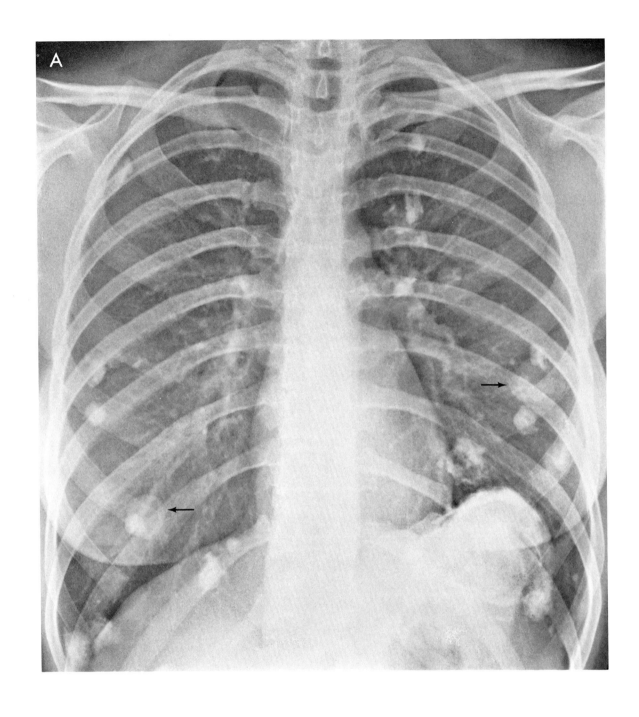

Figure 175.—Metastatic osteosarcoma.

A, posteroanterior radiograph: Revealing many nodules in both lungs. They are quite dense and seem to be producing bone as dense as the adjacent ribs. Note the similarity in size of all of the ossified nodules. Several larger nodules (**arrows**) are not as dense and do not appear to be producing as much bone. Their eccentric calcification and a large soft tissue component suggest recent tumor growth, with the nodules of a second metastatic process of a completely different age superimposed on the older calcified nodules.

B, close-up of the nodules in the right lung: Demonstrating most effectively the two components of one of the large nodules—the older calcified segment (**a**) and the evidence of most recent growth (**b**).

A 19-year-old girl had an osteosarcoma of the left knee removed by an above-knee amputation. These chest studies were made six months later. At autopsy, the bone-producing character of the lesion was confirmed microscopically.

Figure 175, courtesy of Dr. Jack Edeiken, Thomas Jefferson University, Philadelphia.

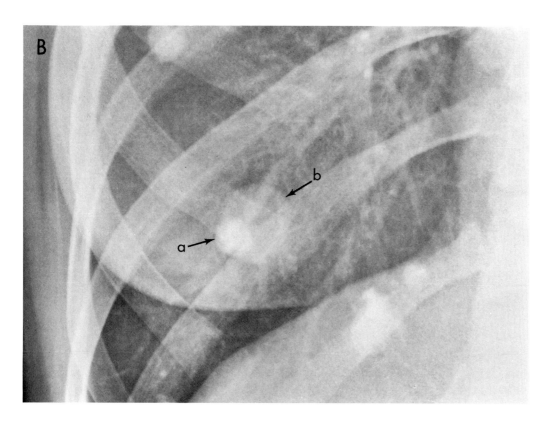

Figure 175 · Metastatic Osteosarcoma / 469

Figure 176.—Metastatic follicular thyroid carcinoma.

A, posteroanterior radiograph: Revealing diffuse nodules scattered throughout both lungs; they seem more numerous in the inferior two-thirds of both sides of the chest. Because there is only slight variation in the size of the nodules, one may consider them to be of similar age.

B, close-up of the right lower lobe in **A:** Demonstrating the general uniformity in size of the nodules. The areas of mottling (**arrows**) represent superimposed nodules which suggest coalescence.

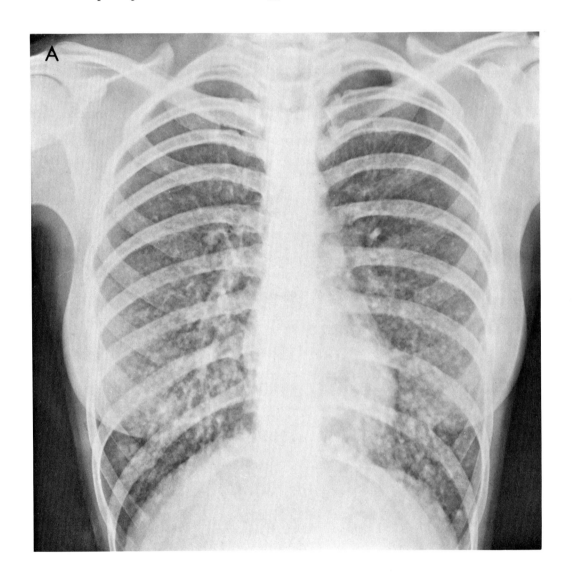

In this 24-year-old woman multiple pulmonary metastatic deposits developed about six months after thyroidectomy for a follicular thyroid carcinoma. At the time of these chest studies she had an annoying, hacking, nonproductive cough but no other symptoms and no weight loss. Radioactive ^{131}I therapy resulted in complete disappearance of the nodules.

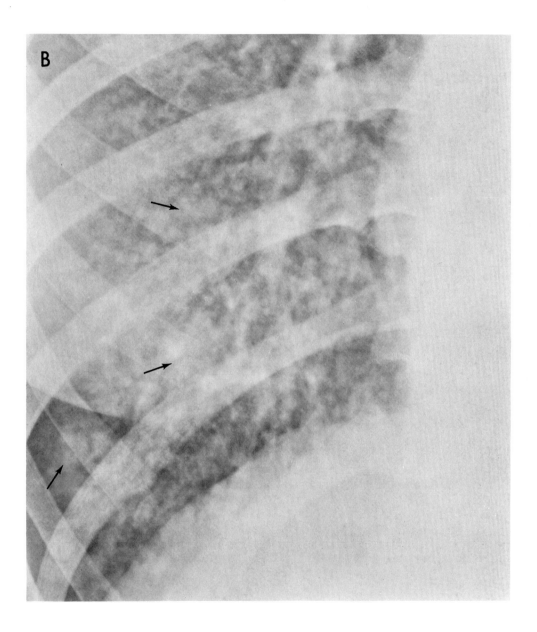

Figure 176 · Metastatic Thyroid Carcinoma / 471

Figure 177.—Metastatic medullary thyroid carcinoma.

A, posteroanterior radiograph: Showing a large midthoracic mass with diffuse shaggy extensions into both lungs. The mass extends from the region of the suprasternal notch to below the midportion of the heart, obliterating all normal hilar vascular shadows bilaterally (**arrows**). The trachea and left main stem bronchus are visible and seem normal. The more distal portions of the main stem bronchi are encroached upon.

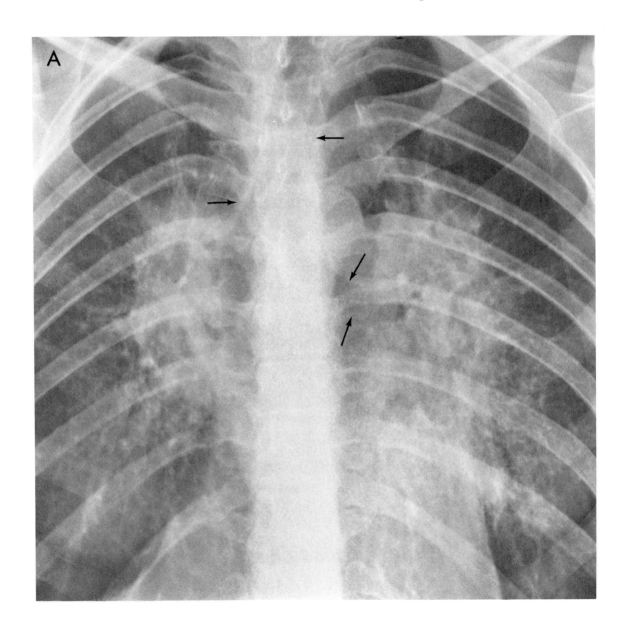

B, close-up of a lateral projection: Demonstrating a long substernal tongue of tumor, seemingly extrapleural (**arrows**). In addition, the shaggy mass (**x**) surrounding the lower trachea and involving the hilum with its dendritic margins (**a**) obliterates all normal vascular and cardiac margins.

A 50-year-old woman had been previously treated for medullary carcinoma of the thyroid. She returned complaining of cough, dyspnea and weight loss. Biopsy of the mediastinal tissue revealed medullary thyroid carcinoma resembling the original tumor.

Figure 177, courtesy of Dr. Gerald D. Dodd, M. D. Anderson Hospital, Houston, Tex.

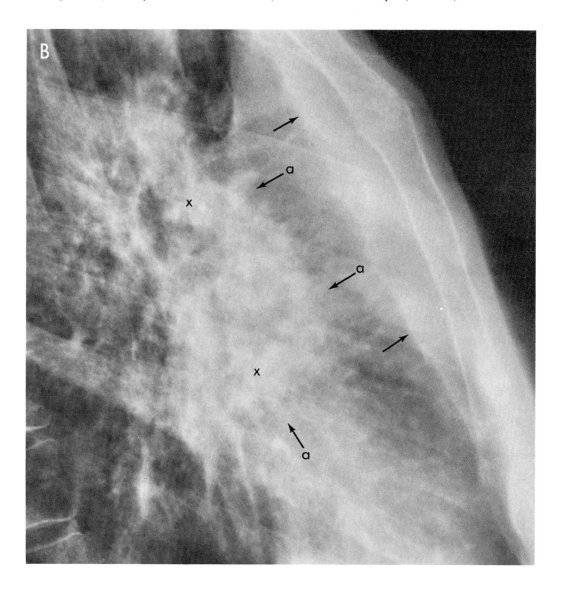

Figure 177 · Metastatic Thyroid Carcinoma / 473

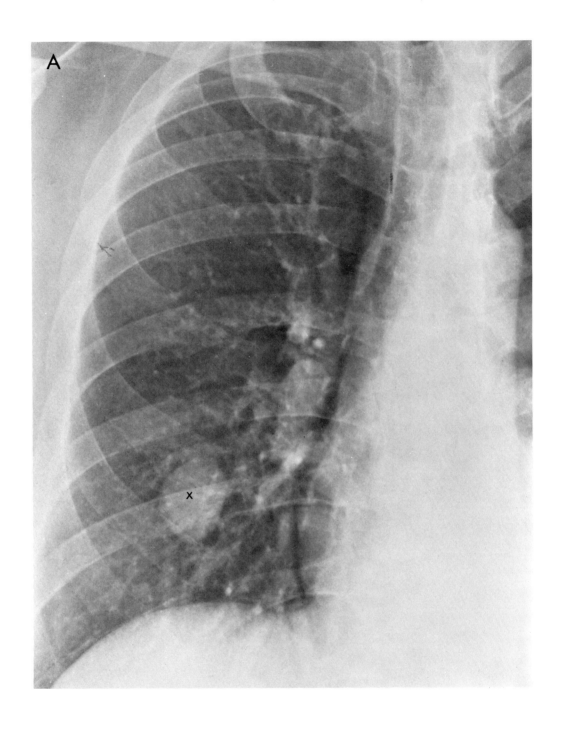

Figure 178.—Solitary metastatic pulmonary nodule from the colon.

A, posteroanterior radiograph: Revealing a solitary, 2 cm, sharply marginated nodule in the posterior portion of the right lower lobe (**x**). No additional nodules were detected in other areas of the lung.

B, body-section projection through the nodule: Demonstrating its fairly well marginated edges. No intrinsic or adjacent calcifications are outlined. Some minor distortion of surrounding vessels is evident (**arrows**).

Random body-section views through portions of the rest of the right lung and the entire left lung revealed no other nodules.

A 55-year-old asymptomatic man returned for a six month follow-up examination after removal of a primary adenocarcinoma of the sigmoid colon. He was completely asymptomatic and results of routine laboratory studies were normal. A right lower lobectomy was performed. Pathologic diagnosis of the nodule was adenocarcinoma, microscopically similar to the previous colonic lesion.

Comment: The radiographic appearance is suggestive of a metastatic nodule, but without the history one could not offer a reasoned opinion as to whether it was a benign or a malignant process.

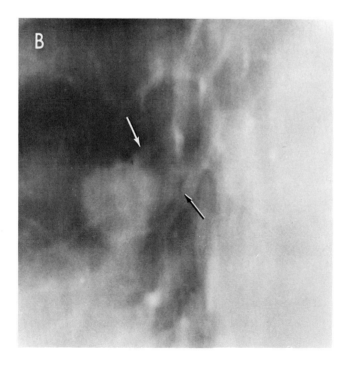

Figure 178 · Metastasis from Colon / 475

Figure 179.—Metastatic melanoma.

Posteroanterior radiograph: Revealing destruction of the left second rib (**a**) and an associated mass (**b**) with classic concave margins indicating its extrapleural origin. In addition, several spherical nodules (**c**) are present in the right upper lobe.

A 40-year-old man complained of some discomfort in the left shoulder which he attributed to bursitis. A melanoma had been removed from the right arm 10 years previously. There were no pulmonary symptoms and a chest radiograph made 1 year previously was normal. Biopsy of the rib lesion revealed a malignant melanoma similar to the tumor removed 10 years previously.

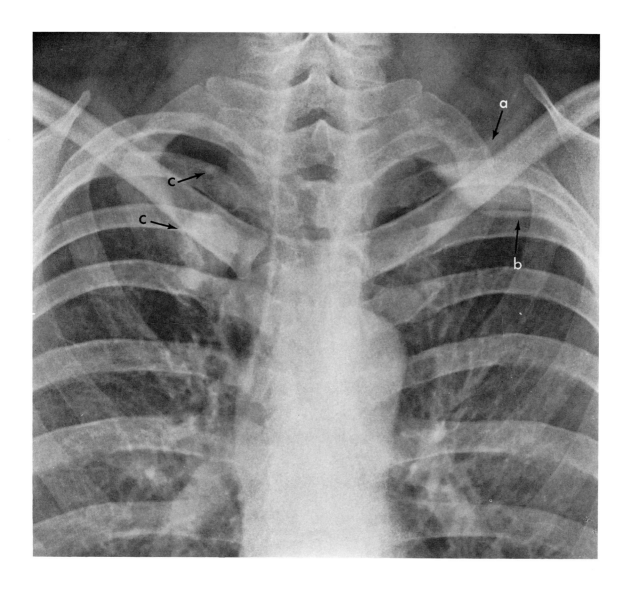

Figure 179 · Metastatic Melanoma / 477

Figure 180.—Metastatic hypernephroma.

A, posteroanterior projection: Revealing sharply demarcated, spherical masses of varied size in both lungs (**arrows**). A faint ill-defined shadow (**x**) extends beyond the large metastatic mass (**z**) which is seen with difficulty in the right upper lobe. Still another sharply marginated mass (**y**) extends from the mediastinum into the right side of the chest along the edge of the trachea.

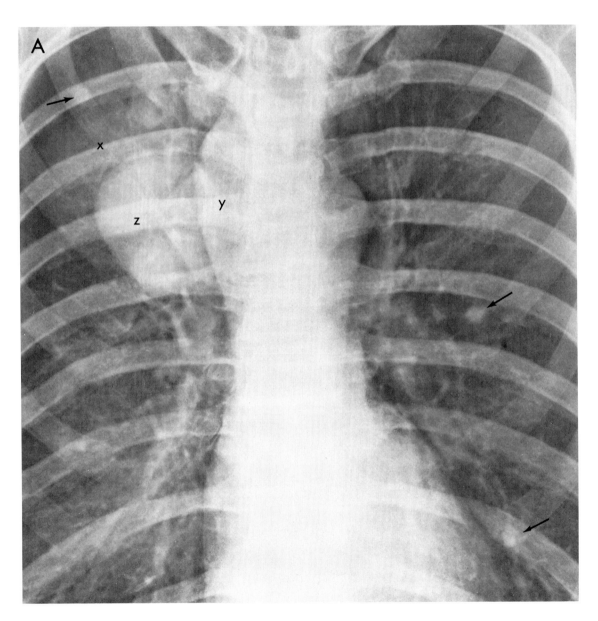

B, lateral radiograph: Showing the mediastinal mass (**y**). The ill-defined right upper lobe mass (**x**) lies against the posterior chest wall. The largest of the spherical masses seen in the right upper lobe in **A** lies posterior to the hilar vessels, obscuring the shadow of the distal trachea and its bifurcation (**z**). Smaller metastatic peripheral nodules are seen at (**a**).

A 48-year-old man had had a primary renal cancer removed two years previously. At the time of this radiographic study he returned because of cough and shortness of breath.

Comment: The peculiar distribution and variation in size of the nodules emphasize the unpredictability of spread and appearance of metastatic renal neoplasms. The size variation suggests that showers of metastatic implants occurred at different times.

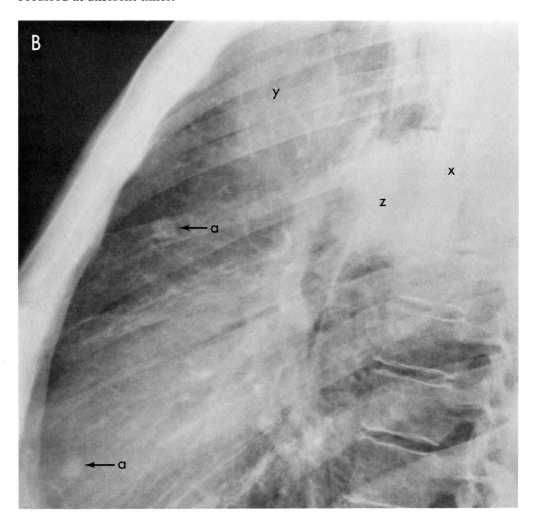

Figure 180 · Metastatic Hypernephroma / 479

Figure 181.—Lymphangitic spread of carcinoma of the stomach.

A, posteroanterior radiograph: Revealing shaggy linear additions to the normal vascular pattern in the middle two-thirds of both lungs where the lesions are accentuated. These shaggy markings extend well into the periphery of both lungs and even into both apices. Minute nodules are visible in the peripheral parenchymal regions and adjacent to some of the linear streaks. Clear delineation of normal vascular shadows in hilar areas is lost.

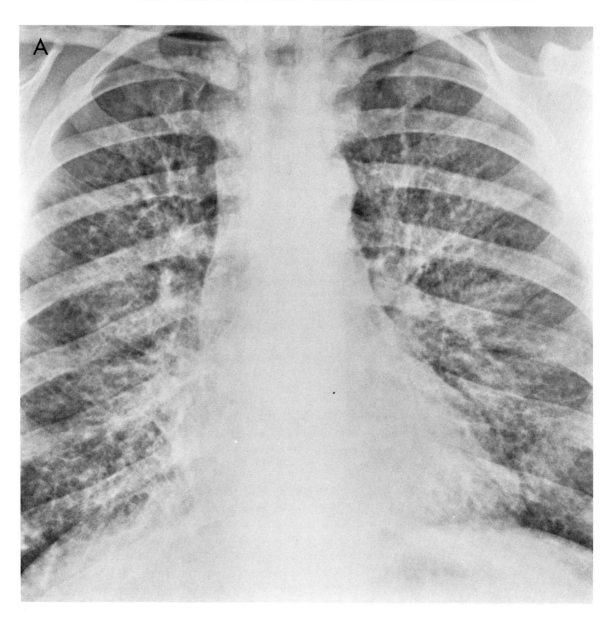

B, close-up of a portion of the right lung in **A:** Showing changes to better advantage.

C, lateral projection: Demonstrating diffusely distributed linear shaggy shadows throughout the lung. In addition, sclerotic metastatic changes are apparent in the upper vertebral bodies of the thoracic spine (**x**).

A 48-year-old man had had an adenocarcinoma of moderate size removed from the stomach two years previously. At the time of this examination he had a dry hacking cough, back pain and weight loss. At autopsy diffuse lymphangitic metastatic lesions were found similar microscopically to the initial primary adenocarcinoma of the stomach.

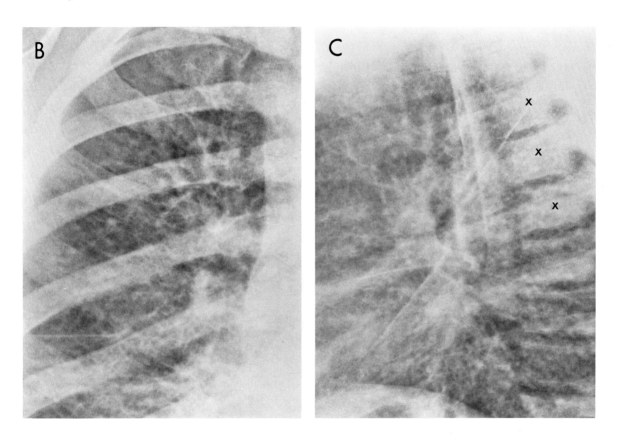

Figure 181 · Metastatic Carcinoma from Stomach / 481

Figure 182.—Lymphangitic spread from carcinoma of the colon.

A, posteroanterior radiograph: Revealing the hilar structures to be unusually prominent bilaterally. Normal sharp vascular outlines are obscured (in the left hemithorax especially) with shaggy edges extending into the lungs bilaterally. No dominant masses are demonstrated.

B, close-up of the left hilar region in **A:** Demonstrating interstitial malignant invasion which has almost totally obscured normal hilar markings.

This 55-year-old man had had resection of an adenocarcinoma of the colon two years prior to this study. Even at that time he complained of chest discomfort and dyspnea; his chest was considered normal preoperatively. Autopsy revealed lymphangitic adenocarcinoma similar microscopically to the initial colonic neoplasm.

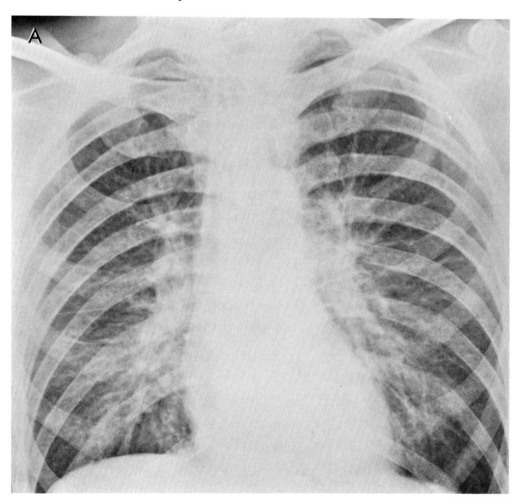

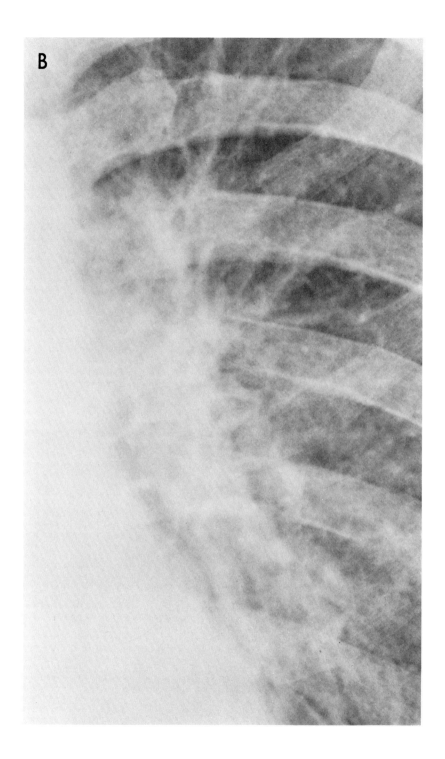

B

Figure 182 · Metastasis from Colon / 483

Figure 183.—Metastatic squamous cell carcinoma from the penis.

A, posteroanterior radiograph: Revealing multiple rounded masses in both lungs. An air–fluid level is present in at least one of the masses (**arrows**). The walls of the cavity are thick and shaggy, characteristic of metastatic squamous cell neoplasm in the chest.

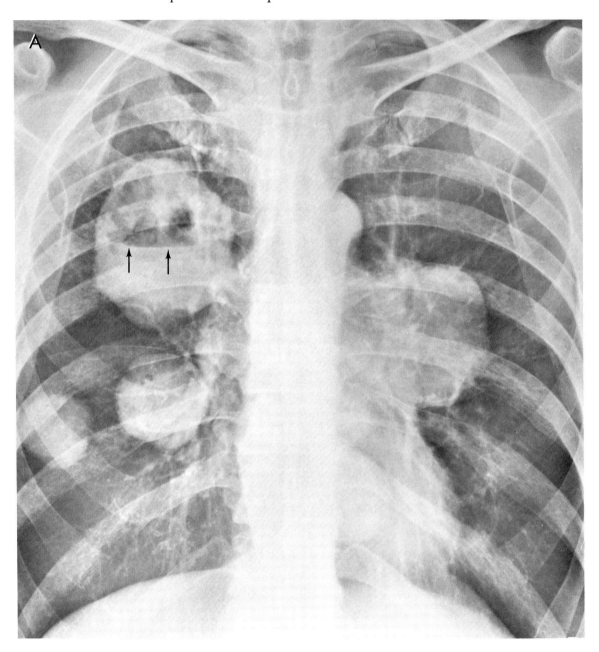

B, lateral projection: Illustrating the spherical nature and diffuse distribution of the pulmonary masses. The shaggy, thick-walled cavity with its air–fluid level in the right upper lobe is clearly depicted (**arrows**).

A 75-year-old man had been treated for a penile squamous cell cancer two years before this radiographic examination. At autopsy, the multiple lesions proved to be squamous cell neoplasms similar in appearance to the original tumor.

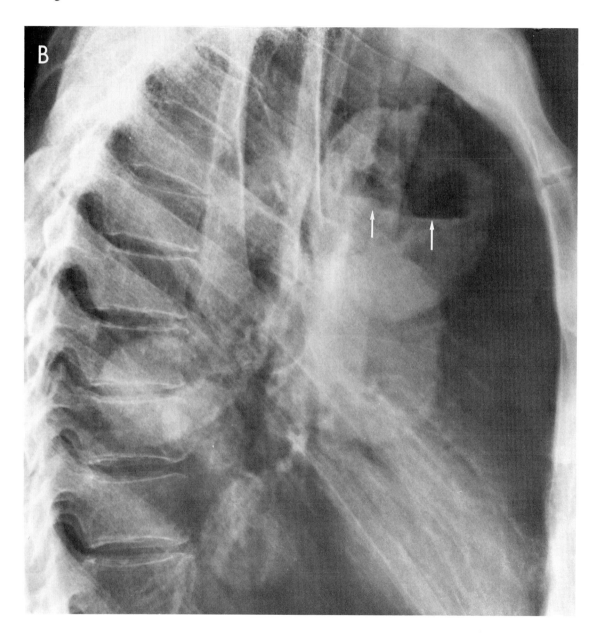

Figure 183 · Metastatic Carcinoma from Penis / 485

Figure 184.—Excavating squamous cell metastatic lesions.

A, posteroanterior radiograph: Revealing a cavitating lesion, with thick walls and a dendritic process extending into the adjacent lung, in the right upper lobe in the fourth anterior interspace (**arrow**). Just above it is a more solid, irregularly marginated lesion in the interspace (**a**).

B, close-up of the lesions in A: Note the dendritic extension from the cavity (**arrow**).

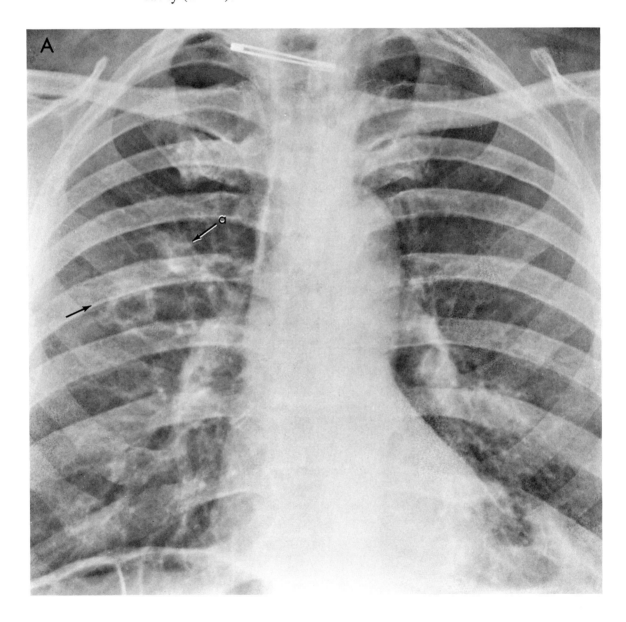

C, radiograph of the lesions in **B** made two months later: Showing an increase in size of the cavity plus thinning of its walls. The more solid lesion (**a**) seems slightly larger.

A 60-year-old man had had a primary buccal mucosal squamous cell lesion treated successfully. About a year later he returned with recurrent disease in the neck, at which time the chest lesions were discovered. These proved to be squamous cell metastatic lesions with a microscopic appearance similar to that of the primary buccal lesion.

Figure 184, courtesy of Dr. Gerald D. Dodd, M. D. Anderson Hospital, Houston, Tex.

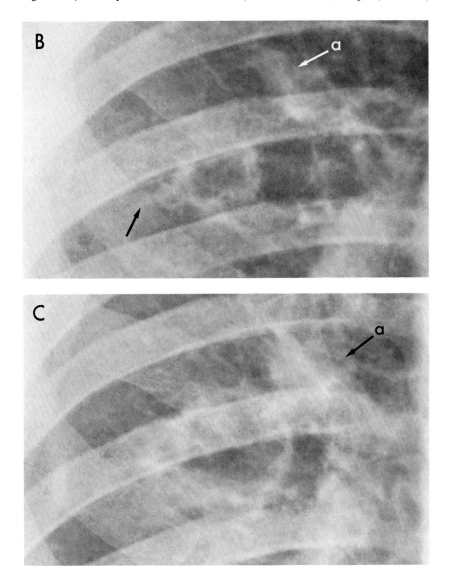

Figure 184 · Excavating Metastatic Lesions / 487

Figure 185.—Metastatic low-grade fibrosarcoma.

A, posteroanterior radiograph: Showing numerous round, sharp-edged pulmonary masses of varied size irregularly distributed throughout both lungs. The larger masses lie in the right lung. Much smaller nodules occupy both hilar regions.

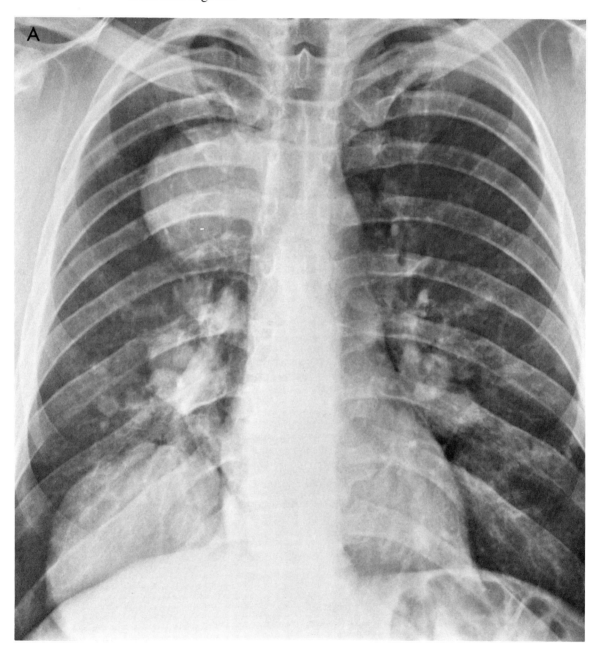

B, posteroanterior radiograph 21 months later: Revealing a little increase in the size of all the lesions but no grossly apparent new foci.

This patient was seen at the age of 14 with a soft tissue mass over the right scapula. When removed it proved to be a fibrosarcoma which the pathologist considered low grade. At that time, results of all studies were within normal limits. **A** was obtained 13 years after removal of the mass. Needle biopsy of one of the large nodules seen in **B** revealed tumor tissue essentially similar to the tissue removed 13 years before.

Figure 185, courtesy of Dr. Walter Miller, City Health Center, Seattle, Wash.

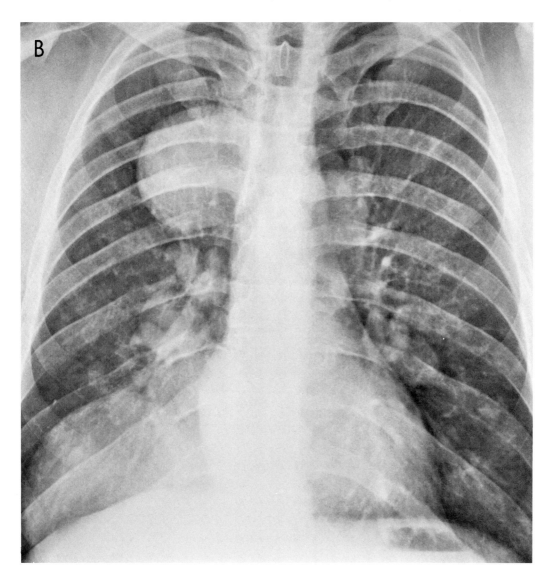

Figure 185 · Metastatic Fibrosarcoma / 489

Figure 186.—Metastatic prostatic carcinoma.

A, posteroanterior radiograph: Showing destructive rib lesions at multiple sites (a). More dense sclerotic lesions are visible in numerous other ribs (b). Nodular sharp-edged masses along pleural edges (d) and irregularly edged pulmonary parenchymal lesions (c) in each lung can be identified.

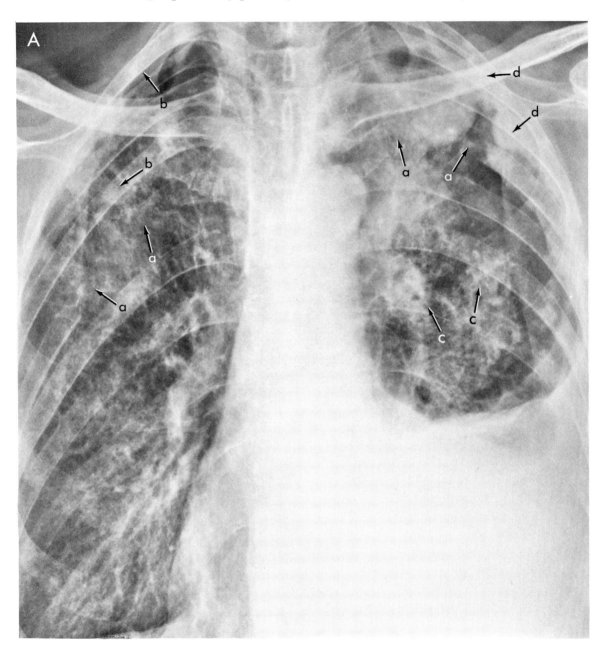

B, close-up of the left upper lung field in **A:** Revealing the destroyed rib (**a**), a pleural metastatic lesion (**d**) and shaggy pulmonary metastatic foci (**c**).

A 72-year-old man known to have had prostatic cancer for five years presented himself because of increasing chest pain, cough and weakness. At autopsy, all of the lesions proved to be similar in microscopic appearance and were identical with the primary prostatic neoplasm.

Comment: Metastatic prostatic cancer seldom causes the variety of lesions seen in this case.

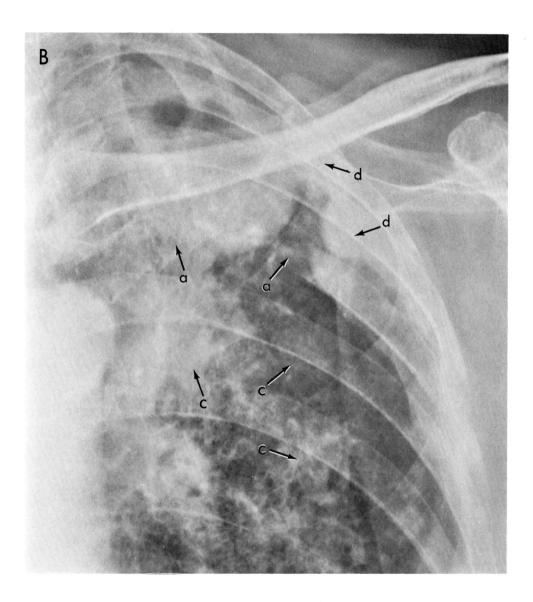

Figure 186 · Metastases from Prostate / 491

Figure 187.—Metastatic sweat gland carcinoma from the hand.

Posteroanterior projection: Revealing multiple spherical masses in both lungs that differ in size. Numerous old rib fractures in the right hemithorax are unrelated to the present disease. No calcifications and no appreciable pulmonary vascular distortions are visible.

A 65-year-old alcoholic woman had firm soft lesions over the distal pads of two fingers of each hand with shiny red skin overlying the lesions. Removal of the first lesion from the little finger of the left hand four years prior to the present study revealed a primary sweat gland carcinoma. Biopsy study of the present finger lesions, as well as of a lung lesion, showed a similar microscopic appearance still believed to be a sweat gland carcinoma with metastases to the lung.

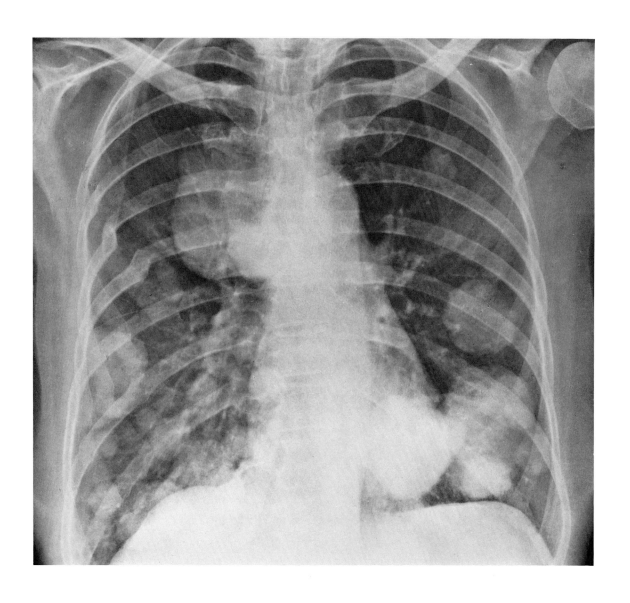

Figure 187 · Metastatic Sweat Gland Carcinoma / 493

Figure 188.—Metastatic basal cell carcinoma from the nose.

A, posteroanterior radiograph: Revealing a multilobulated mass in the right lower lobe (**x**) with irregular pseudopod extensions into the surrounding lung.

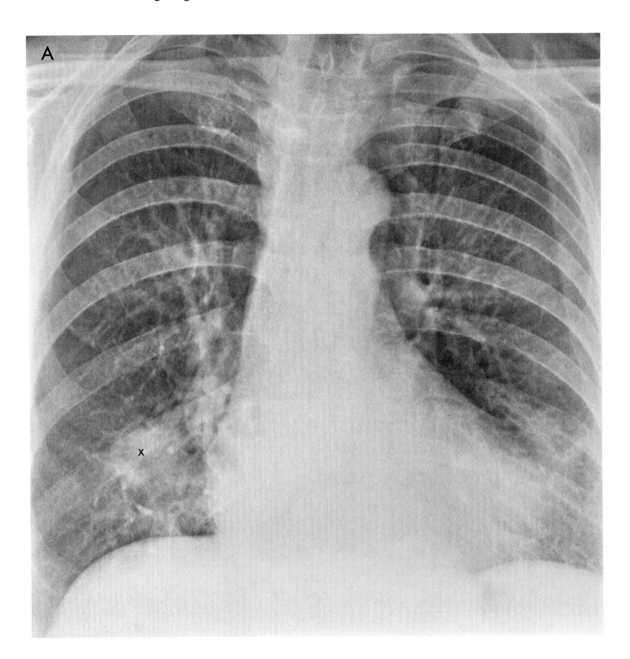

B, close-up of the lesion (**x**) in **A:** Showing displacement of several pulmonary vessels.

C, a body-section radiograph through the midportion of the mass: Demonstrating the irregular lobulated lesion (**x**). The displaced blood vessels are more clearly seen here (**arrows**).

This 70-year-old woman had a long-standing progressive basal cell carcinoma of the nose. It was totally removed with no evidence of local recurrence. Five years later, chest studies revealed the lesion shown here. Right lower lobectomy disclosed metastatic basal cell cancer similar to the ancient nasal carcinoma.

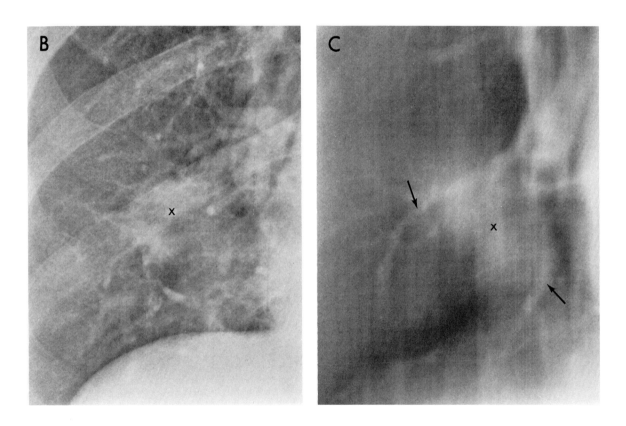

Figure 188 · Metastatic Basal Cell Carcinoma / 495

Figure 189.—Metastatic adenocystic carcinoma from the salivary gland.

Posteroanterior radiograph: Delineating diffuse ovoid, sharp-edged nodules throughout both lungs. They are of about equal size, suggesting that all must have seeded about the same time in a shower of emboli. The appearance is characteristic of blood-borne metastases.

A 68-year-old man had a lump in the right parotid gland that slowly enlarged for about a year. On removal it proved to be an adenocystic carcinoma of the parotid. The metastatic pulmonary lesions appeared about a year after excision of the parotid tumor and progressed only slowly over the next 12 months without causing clinical symptoms.

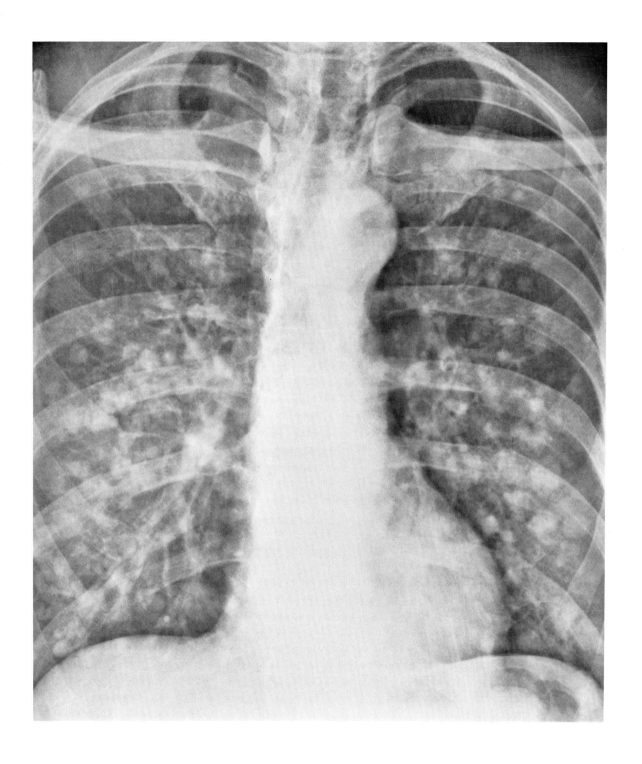

Figure 189 · Metastatic Adenocystic Carcinoma / 497

Index

A

ADENOCARCINOMA: left upper lobe, primary, 366-367
ADENOCYSTIC CARCINOMA: metastatic, salivary gland, 496
ADENOMA
  bronchial, 358-361
    general characteristics, 346-347
  parathyroid
    general considerations, 218
    mediastinal, 324-325
ADENOMATOUS GOITER, 214
ALVEOLAR CELL CARCINOMA, *see* Carcinoma, alveolar cell
AMYLOID TUMOR: of lung, 408-409
ANAPLASTIC CARCINOMA, see Carcinoma, anaplastic
ANEURYSM
  aortic, 284-288
  pulmonary artery, 312-315
  pulmonary vein, 311
  subclavian artery, 308
ANGIOCARDIOGRAPHY
  in myxoma, atrial, bilateral, 300
  in thymoma, 228
ANGIOGRAPHY
  in arteriovenous malformations, multiple, 370, 372
  chest, 14
  intravenous, in respiratory duplication, 260
  in pulmonary artery aneurysm, 314
  subclavian, bilateral, 76
ANGIOMYOMATOUS HYPERPLASIA, 404-405
  general characteristics, 351
ANGIOSARCOMA: characteristics, 412-413
ANOMALIES: arteriovenous, multiple, 370-372
AORTIC ANEURYSM, 284-288
AORTOGRAPHY
  of respiratory duplication cyst, 268
  in rhabdomyosarcoma of heart, 291
ARTERIOGRAPHY
  bronchial, 7, 92-93
  in bronchopulmonary sequestration, 376
  in hemangiopericytoma, 434
  pulmonary, 7

ARTERIOVENOUS MALFORMATIONS: multiple, 370-372
ARTERY
  pulmonary, aneurysm, 312-315
  subclavian, aneurysm, 308
ASBESTOSIS AND MESOTHELIOMA, 418-421
  with pleural effusion, 420-421
ATRIAL MYXOMA: bilateral, 296-302
AZYGOS VEIN: prominent, 317

B

BARIUM BRONCHOGRAPHY: in carcinoma, 112, 114, 118
BASAL CELL CARCINOMA: metastatic, from nose, 494-495
BIOPSY: scalene node, 22
BLEB: emphysematous, carcinoma in, 46-48
BOCHDALEK FORAMEN: hernia of, 254
BREAST, METASTATIC CARCINOMA from, 456-466
  to sternum, 454
BRONCHI
  adenoma, 358-361
    general characteristics, 346-347
  carcinoma
    anaplastic, 78-80
    left lower lobe with mediastinal invasion, 72-74
    left main stem, 54-55
BRONCHIECTATIC CAVITY: in right lower lobe, 369
BRONCHOGENIC CARCINOMA, 9-149
  anaplastic, 60
  bronchography, 12
BRONCHOGENIC CYST
  arising from trachea, 274
  mediastinal, 270-272
BRONCHOGRAPHY, 6
  barium, in carcinoma, 112, 114, 118
  in carcinoma, bronchogenic, 12
BRONCHOPULMONARY SEQUESTRATION, 374-376
  general characteristics, 348
BRONCHOSCOPY IN CARCINOMA
  bronchus, left main stem, 55
  with fissure, 52

BRONCHOSCOPY IN CARCINOMA (*cont.*)
  with granuloma, 144
  with Klebsiella pneumonia, 50
BURKITT'S LYMPHOMA, 206-208
  general considerations, 154
  kymography in, 207

C

CANCER: of lung, etiology, 13
CARCINOMA
  adenocystic, metastatic, from salivary
      gland, 496
  alveolar cell
      diffuse, 362-365
      general characteristics, 347-348
  anaplastic
      bronchi, 78-80
      bronchogenic, 60
      mediastinal invasion in, 68-70
  basal cell, metastatic, from nose, 494-
      495
  breast, metastases from, 456-466
      to sternum, 454
  bronchogenic, *see* Bronchogenic carci-
      noma
  colon, lymphangitic spread from, 482
  lung, *see* Lung, carcinoma
  prostate, metastatic, 490-491
  squamous cell
      in bleb, emphysematous, 46-48
      bronchus, left lower lobe, with medi-
          astinal invasion, 72-74
      bronchus, left main stem, 54-55
      cavitary, 34-37
      cavitating, 40
      chest wall invasion in, 95
      developing, 42-43, 122-123, 126-129
      developing adjacent to old granu-
          loma, 130-132
      excavating metastatic lesions, 486-
          487
      fissure and, interlobar, 52
      hamartoma and, 148-149
      hilus, left, and granuloma, 142-144
      left apex, 20
      local extension, 56-59
      lower lobe, left, 30-31, 96, 114, 138-
          139
      lower lobe, right, 110-113, 117-119
      lower lobe, right, and granuloma, 141
      mediastinal invasion, 82-84
      metastatic, from penis, 484-485
      middle lobe, right, 32-33
      nodal metastases in, 92-93
      nodal metastases in, hilar and para-
          tracheal, 26

  pneumonia and, Klebsiella, 50
  rib destruction in, 28
  right apex, 18-19
  silicosis and, 146
  small cavity in, 44
  trachea, primary carcinoma, 124
  tracheal invasion in, 76
  tuberculosis and, 123
  upper lobe, left, 64-65, 90, 100-102,
      104-106
  upper lobe, right, 16, 22, 62, 98, 108,
      120-121
  upper lobe, right
      —early carcinoma, 134-137
      —with mediastinal invasion, 66, 86-
          88
      —with metastases, 24
      —with multiple cavities, 38
  vena caval invasion in, 76
  stomach, lymphangitic spread, 480-481
  sweat gland, metastatic, from hand,
      492
  thyroid, metastatic
      follicular, 470-471
      medullary, 472-473
CHEMODECTOMA: of right lung, 403
CHEST
  angiography, 14
  intrathoracic splenosis, general consid-
      erations, 220
  intrathoracic thyroid gland, 242-247
  lymphomas in, *see* Lymphoma
  shadows of, 4
  wall
      fibrosarcoma of, 423-425
      hemangiosarcoma of, 431
      invasion in carcinoma, 95
      lipoma of, 428-429
      tumors of, 411-441
CHORIOCARCINOMA TESTIS: metastatic,
      452
COBALT MINERS: and lung cancer,
      13
COBALT-60 THERAPY UNIT, 4-5
  used in Hodgkin's disease, 164
COLON
  carcinoma, lymphangitic spread from,
      482
  solitary metastatic pulmonary nodule
      from, 475
CYST(S)
  bronchogenic
      arising from trachea, 274
      mediastinal, 270-272
  duplication
      enteric, 276-277
      general considerations, 215-216

respiratory, 265-269
    hydatid, 394-395
        of left lower lobe, 392-393
        of right upper lobe, 397
    neurenteric, 336-338
        general considerations, 219-220
    pericardial, 278-283
        general considerations, 216-217
    thymic, 232
CYSTIC LYMPHANGIOMA, 236

D

DUPLICATION CYSTS, *see* Cyst(s), duplication

E

EMPHYSEMATOUS BLEB: carcinoma in, 46-48
ENTERIC DUPLICATION CYST, 276-277
ESOPHAGUS: leiomyoma of, 256-259

F

FIBROMA
    general characteristics, 351
    pulmonary, 406-407
FIBROMYXOSARCOMA: of pulmonary valve, 304-306
FIBROSARCOMA
    characteristics, 412
    of chest wall, 423-425
    metastatic low-grade, 488-489
FIBROUS MESOTHELIOMA, 414-415
FILM DISTANCE-RADIATION SOURCE, 3-4
FISSURE: interlobar, in carcinoma, 52
FLUID
    extrapleural fluid collection, 438-439
    loculated in bed of resected granuloma, 440-441
FLUORODENSITOMETRY, 144
FLUOROSCOPY, 5
    of substernal extension of thyroid, 241
FORAMEN
    of Bochdalek, hernia, 254
    of Morgagni, hernia, 252-253

G

GANGLIONEUROMA, 326-327
GOITER, 214
    adenomatous, 214
    colloid, 214
    exophthalmic, 214
    nodular, 214
    simple, 214

GRANULOMA
    carcinoma of left hilus and, 142-144
    carcinoma of right lower lobe and, 141
    old, carcinoma developing adjacent to, 130-132
    resected, loculated fluid in bed of, 440-441

H

HAMARTOMA, 355-357
    carcinoma and, squamous cell, 148-149
    general characteristics, 346
    of left lower lobe, 353
HAND: metastatic sweat gland carcinoma from, 492
HEART
    osteosarcoma, 292-294
    rhabdomyosarcoma of, 291
    size variations, 4
    tumors
        metastatic, general considerations, 218
        primary, general considerations, 217-218
HEMANGIOPERICYTOMA, 432-434
HEMANGIOSARCOMA: of chest wall, 431
HEMOPOIESIS, EXTRAMEDULLARY, 340-343
    general considerations, 220
HERNIA
    of foramen of Bochdalek, 254
    of foramen of Morgagni, 252-253
HIBERNOMA, 391
HILAR METASTASES, 26
HODGKIN'S DISEASE, 156-188
    cobalt-60 therapy unit used, 164
    general considerations, 152-153
    lung involvement in, 167-168, 172-174, 186-188
    lymphoma resembling, diffuse pulmonary, 194-196
    mediastinum involved in, 167-171
        parenchymal extension in, 170-171
    pulmonary interstitial, 186-188
HYDATID CYST, *see* Cyst(s), hydatid
HYPERNEPHROMA: metastatic, 478-479
HYPERPLASIA
    angiomyomatous, 404-405
        general characteristics, 351
    of lymph node, 398-399
    lymphoid, 318-319

I

INTERCOSTAL NERVE: neurofibroma of, 427

IODINE-131 UPTAKE STUDY: of intrathoracic thyroid gland, 243, 247
IONIZATION CHAMBERS, 3
ISCHEMIC NECROSIS: in silicosis, 382-383

J

JACKSON-HUBER CLASSIFICATION, 7

K

KLEBSIELLA PNEUMONIA: and carcinoma, 50
KYMOGRAPHY: in Burkitt's lymphoma, 207

L

LEIOMYOMA
    of esophagus, 256-259
    general considerations, 215
LEIOMYOSARCOMA: general considerations, 215
LEUKEMIA
    lymphatic, 198-199
        general considerations, 153-154
    myeloid, 200-201
LIPOID PNEUMONIA, 378-379
    general characteristics, 349
LIPOMA
    of chest wall, 428-429
    general characteristics, 350
    intrapulmonary, 388-389
    of left upper lobe, 321
LIPOSARCOMA, 384-385
    general characteristics, 350-351
    of lung, 387
LUNG
    bronchopulmonary sequestration, 374-376
        general characteristics, 348
    cancer, etiology, 13
    carcinoma
        incidence, 11
        terminology, discussion, 11
    chemodectoma, 403
    fibroma, 406-407
    involvement in Hodgkin's disease, 167-168, 172-174, 186-188
    lipoma, 388-389
    liposarcoma, 387
    lymphosarcoma, primary, 204
    metastatic pulmonary nodule, solitary, from colon, 475
    plasmacytoma, 400-401
    pseudolymphoma, 204
    pulmonary interstitial Hodgkin's disease, 186-188

sarcoma, reticulum cell, 202
tumor, amyloid, 408-409
LYMPH NODE: hyperplastic, 398-399
LYMPHANGIOMA, 235, 238-239
    cystic, 236
    general considerations, 214
LYMPHANGITIC SPREAD OF CARCINOMA
    of colon, 482
    of stomach, 480-481
LYMPHOID HYPERPLASIA, 318-319
LYMPHOMA, 151-208
    Burkitt's, see Burkitt's lymphoma
    diffuse pulmonary, resembling Hodgkin's disease, 194-196
    general considerations, 152-154
    Hodgkin's disease, see Hodgkin's disease
    lymphosarcoma, see Lymphosarcoma
    pseudolymphoma, see Pseudolymphoma
    sarcoma, reticulum cell, of lung, 202
LYMPHORETICULAR TUMOR, see Burkitt's lymphoma
LYMPHOSARCOMA, 190-193
    general considerations, 153
    lung, primary, 204
    venography in, right subclavian, 193

M

MEDIASTINAL BRONCHOGENIC CYST, 270-272
MEDIASTINAL INVASION IN CARCINOMA
    anaplastic, 68-70
    bronchi, 72-74
    right upper lobe, 66, 86-88
    squamous cell, 82-84
MEDIASTINAL INVOLVEMENT IN HODGKIN'S DISEASE, 167-171
    parenchymal extension in, 170-171
MEDIASTINAL PARATHYROID ADENOMA, 324-325
MEDIASTINUM
    anatomy of, 212
    tumors, 211-343
        general considerations, 212-220
MELANOMA: metastatic, 476
MESOTHELIOMA, 416
    asbestosis and, 418-421
        with pleural effusion, 420-421
    characteristics, 412
    fibrous, 414-415
METASTASES, 443-496
    in adenocystic carcinoma from salivary gland, 496
    in basal cell carcinoma from nose, 494-495
    from breast carcinoma, 456-466

to sternum, 454
characteristics, 445-447
in choriocarcinoma testis, 452
in fibrosarcoma, low-grade, 488-489
of heart tumors, general considerations, 218
hilar, 26
in hypernephroma, 478-479
in melanoma, 476
nodal
    extensive, 92-93
    paratracheal, 26
in osteosarcoma, 469
to pleural surfaces, characteristics, 413
in prostatic carcinoma, 490-491
in seminoma, 448-450
solitary pulmonary nodule from colon, 475
sources, 445-447
in squamous cell carcinoma, 24
    excavating lesions, 486-487
    from penis, 484-485
in sweat gland carcinoma from hand, 492
in thyroid carcinoma
    follicular, 470-471
    medullary, 472-473
MORGAGNI FORAMEN: hernia of, 252-253
MYELOGRAPHY: in hemangiopericytoma, 432
MYXOMA, 217
atrial, bilateral, 296-302

N

NECROSIS: ischemic, in silicosis, 382-383
NERVE: intercostal, neurofibroma of, 427
NEURENTERIC CYST, 336-338
general considerations, 219-220
NEURILEMMOMA, 328
NEUROFIBROMA, 333-335
of intercostal nerve, 427
NEUROGENIC TUMORS: general considerations, 219-220
NOSE: metastatic basal cell carcinoma from, 494-495

O

OSTEOSARCOMA
cardiac, 292-294
metastatic, 469

P

PARAGANGLIOMA, 330-331
PARAGANGLIONIC CELL TUMORS: general considerations, 219

PARATHYROID ADENOMA, see Adenoma, parathyroid
PARATRACHEAL NODAL METASTASES, 26
PARENCHYMAL INVOLVEMENT: in Hodgkin's disease, 170-171
PARENCHYMAL TUMORS, 345-409
PENIS: metastatic squamous cell carcinoma from, 484-485
PERICARDIAL CYST, 278-283
general considerations, 216-217
PHANTOM TUMOR, 436-437
PHOTOTIMERS, 3
PLASMA CELL TUMORS: general characteristics, 350
PLASMACYTOMA: pulmonary, 400-401
PLEURA
effusion in asbestosis and mesothelioma, 420-421
extrapleural fluid collection, 438-439
metastases to pleural surfaces, characteristics, 413
tumors of, 411-441
PNEUMONIA
Klebsiella, and carcinoma, 50
lipoid, 378-379
    general characteristics, 349
PROSTATIC CARCINOMA: metastatic, 490-491
PSEUDOLYMPHOMA
general considerations, 154
lung, 204
PULMONARY ARTERY: aneurysm, 312-315
PULMONARY VALVE: fibromyxosarcoma, 304-306
PULMONARY VEIN: aneurysm, 311

R

RADIATION SOURCE-FILM DISTANCE, 3-4
RADIOGRAPHIC CONSIDERATIONS: general, 3-8
RADIOGRAPHY
body-section, 6
250 kv, 1-2 million volt, 4-5
RESPIRATORY DUPLICATION, 260-263
cyst, 265-269
RHABDOMYOMA, 217
RHABDOMYOSARCOMA
of heart, 291
malignant, 217
RIB DESTRUCTION: in squamous cell carcinoma, 28

S

SALIVARY GLAND: metastatic adenocystic carcinoma from, 496

SARCOID, 323
SARCOMA: reticulum cell, of lung, 202
SCALENE NODE BIOPSY, 22
SEMINOMA: metastatic, 448-450
SHADOWS: of chest, 4
SILICOSIS
 carcinoma and, squamous cell, 146
 conglomerate mass of, 380-381
  general characteristics, 349
  ischemic necrosis in, 382-383
SPLENOSIS: intrathoracic, general consid-
  erations, 220
SQUAMOUS CELL CARCINOMA, see Carci-
  noma, squamous cell
STERNUM: breast carcinoma metastatic to,
  454
STOMACH: carcinoma, lymphangitic
  spread, 480-481
SUBCLAVIAN ARTERY: aneurysm, 308
SWEAT GLAND CARCINOMA: metastatic,
  from hand, 492
SYMPATHETIC GANGLIONS: tumors, general considerations, 219

T

TERATOMA
 general considerations, 218-219
 vascular, 249-251
THORAX, see Chest
THYMIC CYST, 232
THYMOMA, 222-231
 general considerations, 212-213
THYROID
 carcinoma, metastatic
  follicular, 470-471
  medullary, 472-473
 extension, substernal, 240-241
 intrathoracic thyroid gland, 242-247
 tumors, general considerations, 214-215
TOMOGRAPHY, 6
TRACHEA
 bronchogenic cyst arising from, 274
 carcinoma

 primary, 124
 squamous cell, 76
TUBERCULOSIS: and carcinoma, 123
TUMORS
 chest wall, 411-441
 heart, see Heart, tumors
 lung, amyloid, 408-409
 lymphoreticular, see Burkitt's lymphoma
 mediastinum, 211-343
  general considerations, 212-220
 metastatic, see Metastases
 neurogenic, general considerations,
  219-220
 paraganglionic cell, general considerations, 219
 parenchymal, 345-409
 phantom, 436-437
 plasma cell, general characteristics, 350
 pleura, 411-441
 sympathetic ganglions, general considerations, 219
 thyroid, general considerations, 214-
  215

V

VEINS
 azygos, prominent, 317
 multiple arteriovenous malformations,
  370-372
 pulmonary, aneurysm, 311
VENA CAVA: squamous cell carcinoma of,
  76
VENACAVOGRAPHY, 76
VENOGRAPHY
 of prominent azygos vein, 317
 pulmonary, 7
 subclavian
  left, 20
  right, 22
  right, in lymphosarcoma, 193
VESSELS: malformations, general characteristics, 348